# Manual of 3D Echocardiography

Eduardo Casas Rojo
Covadonga Fernandez-Golfin
José Luis Zamorano

**Editors**

# Manual of 3D Echocardiography

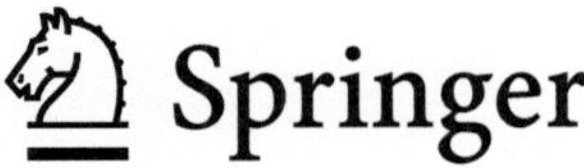 Springer

*Editors*
Eduardo Casas Rojo
Hospital Ramon y Cajal
Madrid
Spain

José Luis Zamorano
Hospital Ramon y Cajal
Madrid
Spain

Covadonga Fernandez-Golfin
Hospital Ramon y Cajal
Madrid
Spain

ISBN 978-3-319-50333-2          ISBN 978-3-319-50335-6   (eBook)
DOI 10.1007/978-3-319-50335-6

Library of Congress Control Number: 2017935459



Printed on acid-free paper

This Springer imprint is published by Springer Nature
The registered company is Springer International Publishing AG
The registered company address is: Gewerbestrasse 11, 6330 Cham, Switzerland

# Prologue

No doubt that echocardiography is the cornerstone in the non invasive diagnosis of cardiovascular diseases. It provides and accurate, fast and easy to access way of assessing morphology and function of the heart. The continuous evolution of echocardiography has lead to the *appearance* of different tools that assess heart morphology and function in abetter way. One of the most revolutionary evolutions since the beginning has been 3D echocardiography. Simply because the heart is a 3D structure and works as a 3D pump is a potent reason why cardiologist wants to see the heart in 3D.

In this book Dr. Eduardo Casas and colleagues tried to make 3D echo very practical. Indeed is a manual that aims to simplify the understanding and application of 3D echocardiography. The book comprises ten different sections. Starting with the basics, the minimum knowledge that we need to know before doing a 3D echo is explained. This section is really practical, avoiding complex terms of physics that sometimes produces confusions instead of help. We can learn the basic physics, so as the general rules for transthoracic so as transesophageal 3D echocardiography. After these basic and general aspects, the book starts with a clear clinical approach and tips and tricks for evaluating valve diseases, LV function and mechanics and the increasing use of 3D echo inside the cath lab for structural interventions. All those chapters have a clear emphasis in practical tutorials. After the routine use of 3D echo the new developments and cutting edge research information is given in the last chapters. Fusion imaging has emerged in cardiology and 3D echo is not apart from this. Finally a real expert in the field covers the use of 3D in congenital heart disease.

Dr. Eduardo Casas did an incredible job as main editor of the book. He managed to harmonise the text in an easy way of reading and producing a real practical book. He handled top authors with a lot of clinical experience in 3D echo and managed to create a Manual that for sure will help doctors both in training and in clinical application of this technique. I personally know Dr. Casas since the days he was a Cardiology Fellow. He is extremely intelligent and a doer. Once he commits to a project, he will make it possible independently of the difficulties he encounters on his way. This book is a good example of this.

Madrid, Spain                                                                                José Luis Zamorano

# Contents

# Chapter 1
# Physical and Technical Aspects and Overview of 3D- Echocardiography

Denisa Muraru and Luigi P. Badano

## Introduction

The advent of three-dimensional echocardiography (3DE) represented a real breakthrough in cardiovascular ultrasound. Major advancements in computer and transducer technology allow to acquire 3D data sets with adequate spatial and temporal resolution for assessing the functional anatomy of cardiac structures in most of cardiac pathologies. Compared to conventional two-dimensional echocardiographic (2DE) imaging, 3DE allows the operator to visualize the cardiac structures from virtually any perspective, providing a more anatomically sound and intuitive display, as well as an accurate quantitative evaluation of anatomy and function of heart valves [1]. In addition, 3DE overcomes geometric assumptions and enables an accurate quantitative and reproducible evaluation of cardiac chambers [2–4], thus offering solid elements for patient management. Furthermore, 3DE is the only imaging technique based on volumetric scanning able to show moving structures in the beating heart, in contrast to cardiac magnetic resonance (CMR) or cardiac computed tomography (CT), which are based on post-acquisition 3D reconstruction from multiple tomographic images and displaying only 3D rendered snapshots.

Data regarding clinical applications of 3DE are burgeoning and gradually capturing an established place in the noninvasive clinical assessment of anatomy and function of cardiac structures. Recently, joint European Association of Echocardiography and American Society of Echocardiography recommendations have been published, aiming to provide clinicians with a systematic approach to 3D image acquisition and analysis [5] Finally, the recent update of the recommendations for the chamber quantification using echocardiography recommended 3DE for the assessment of the left (LV) and right ventricular (RV) size and function [6].

D. Muraru • L.P. Badano (✉)
Department of Cardiac, Thoracic and Vascular Sciences, University of Padua, Padua, Italy
e-mail: lpbadano@gmail.com

© Springer International Publishing AG 2017
E. Casas Rojo et al. (eds.), *Manual of 3D Echocardiography*,
DOI 10.1007/978-3-319-50335-6_1

# Physics of 2D and 3D Ultrasound

The backbone of current 3DE technology is the transducer. A conventional 2D phased array transducer is composed by 128 piezoelectric elements, electrically isolated from each other, arranged in a single row (Fig. 1.1, Left). Each ultrasound wave front is generated by firing individual elements in a specific sequence with a delay in phase with respect to the transmit initiation time. Each element adds and subtracts pulses in order to generate a single ultrasound wave with a specific direction that constitutes a radially propagating scan line. Since the piezoelectric elements area arranged in a single row, the ultrasound beam can be steered in two dimensions – vertical (axial) and lateral (azimuthal) – while resolution in the z axis (elevation) is fixed by the thickness of the tomographic slice, which, in turn, is related to the vertical dimension of piezoelectric elements.

Modern 3DE matrix-array transducers are composed of about 3000 individually connected and simultaneously active (fully sampled) piezoelectric elements with operating frequencies ranging from 2 to 4 MHz and 5 to 7 MHz for transthoracic and transoesophageal transducers, respectively. To steer the ultrasound beam in 3D, a 3D array of piezoelectric elements needs to be used in the probe, therefore piezoelectric elements are arranged in rows and columns to form of a rectangular grid (matrix configuration) within the transducer (Fig. 1.1, right upper panel). The electronically controlled phasic firing of the elements in that matrix generates a scan

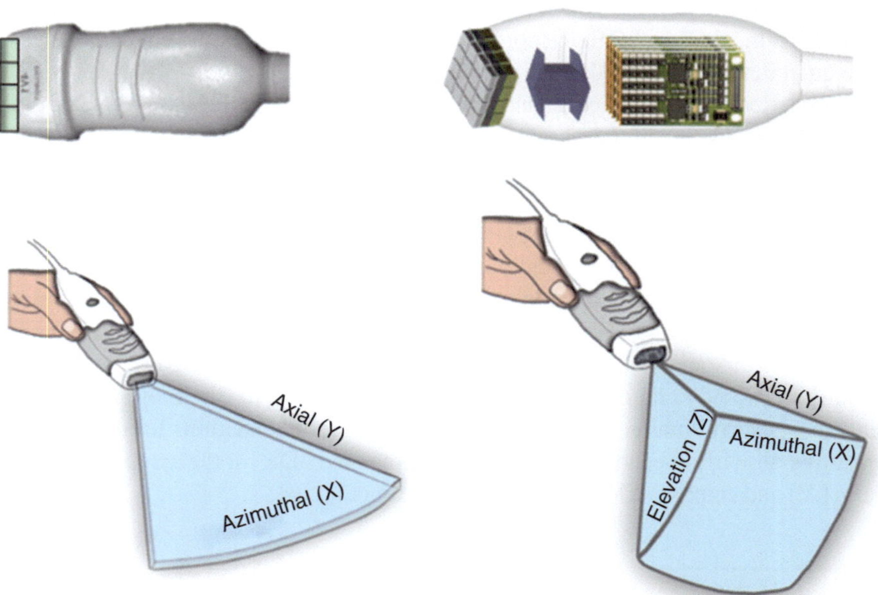


**Fig. 1.1** Two- and three-dimensional transducers. Schematic drawing showing the main characteristics of two- (*left panel*) and three-dimensional (*right panel*) transducers

line that propagates radially (y or axial direction) and can be steered both laterally (x or azimuthal direction) and in elevation (z direction) in order to acquire a volumetric pyramidal data set (Fig. 1.1, right lower panel). Matrix array probes can also provide real-time multiple simultaneous 2D views, at high frame rate, oriented in predefined or user-selected plane orientations by activacting multiple lines of piezoelectric elements within the matrix (Fig. 1.2).

The main technological breakthrough which allowed manufacturers to develop fully sampled matrix transducers has been the miniaturization of electronics that allowed the development of individual electrical interconnections for every piezoelectric element which could be independently controlled, both in transmission and in reception.

Beamforming (or spatial filtering) is a signal processing technique used to produce directionally or spatially selected signals sent or received from arrays of sensors. In 2DE, all the electronic components for the beamforming (high-voltage transmitters, low-noise receivers, analog-to-digital converter, digital controllers, digital delay lines) are inside the system and consume a lot of power (around 100 W and 1500 cm$^2$ of personal computer electronics board area). If the same beamforming approach would have been used for matrix array transducers used in

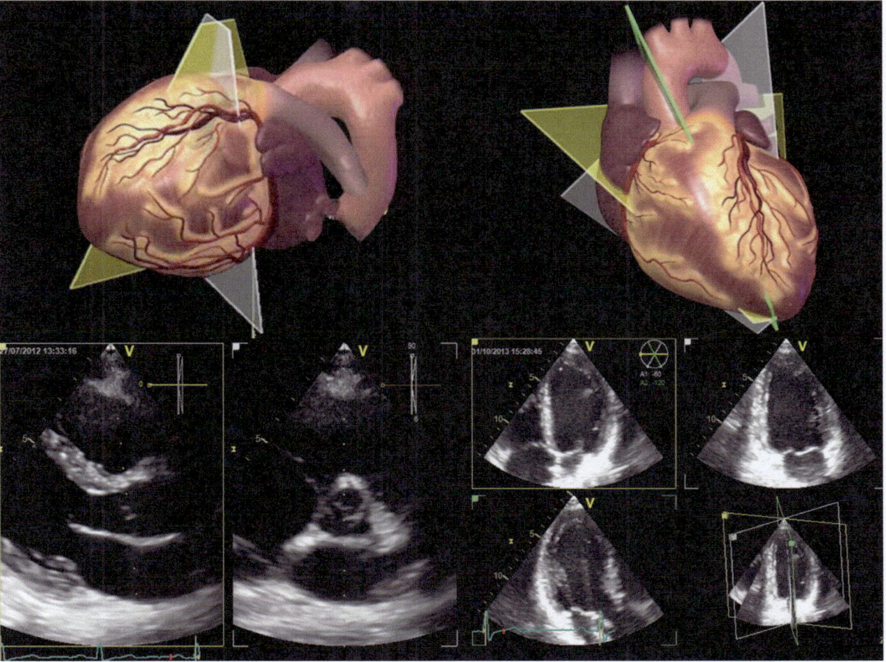

**Fig. 1.2** Multiplane acquisition using the matrix array transducer. From the left parasternal approach, the probe can be used to obtain simultaneous long- and short axis views of the left ventricle during the same cardiac cycle (*right panels*). From the apical approach, the probe can be used to obtain 2 or 3 simultaneous views (*left panels*). The orientation of the scan planes (shown in the *upper diagrams*) can be modified by the operator during acquisition to obtain the desired view

3DE, it would have required around 4 kW power consumption and a huge PC board area to accommodate all the needed electronics to control 3000 piezoeletric elements. To reduce both power consumption and the size of the connecting cable, several miniaturized circuit boards are incorporated into the transducer, allowing partial beamforming to be performed in the probe (Fig. 1.3). This unique circuit design results in an active probe which allows microbeamforming of the signal with low power consumption (<1 W) and avoids to connect every piezoelectric element to the ultrasound machine. The 3000 channel circuit boards within the transducer controls the fine steering by delaying and summing signals within subsections of the matrix, known as patches (microbeamforming, Fig. 1.3). A typical patch for a cardiac matrix probe contains approximately 25 piezoelextric elements configured in 5 × 5 matrix. Only patches are connected to the mainframe beamformer within the system. This microbeamforming works like a very small electronic beamformer by pointing its 25 elements (on both transmit and receiving) toward the desired scan line and allows to reduce the number of the digital channels to be put into the cable that connects the probe to the ultrasound system from 3000

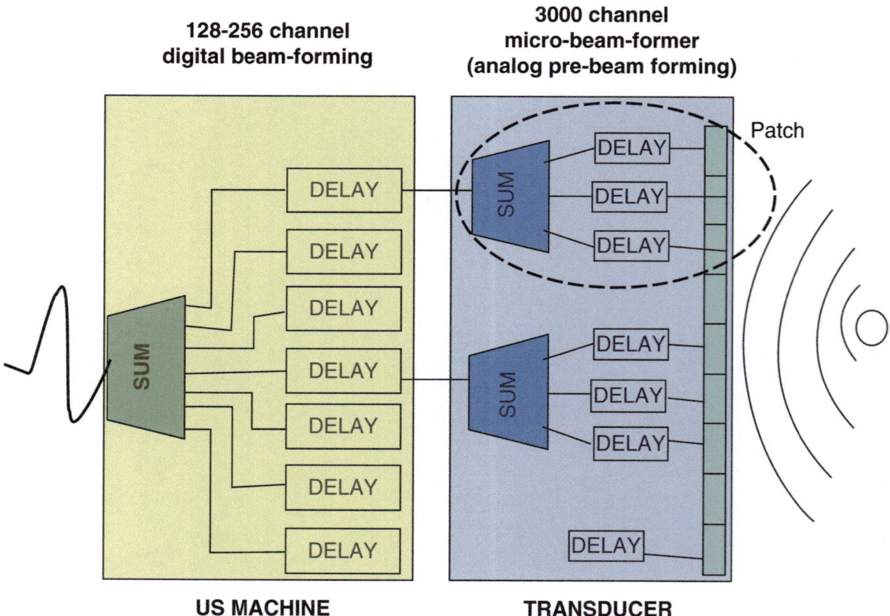


**Fig. 1.3** Three-dimensional beamforming. Beamforming with 3D matrix array transducers has been splitted in the transducer and the ultrasound machine levels. At the transducer level, interconnection technology and integrated analog circuits (DELAY) control transmit and receive signals using different subsection of the matrix (patches) to perform analog pre-beamforming and fine steering. Signals from each patch are summed to reduce the number of digital lines in the coaxial cable that connects the transducer to the ultrasound system from 3000 to the conventional 128–256 channels. At the ultrasound machine level, analog-to-digital (A/D) convertors amplify, filter and digitize the elements signals which are then focused (coarse steering) using digital delay (DELAY) circuitry and summed together ($\Xi$) to form the received signal from the desired object

(which would make the cabling too heavy for practical use) to the conventional 128–256 allowing the same size of the 2D cable to be used with 3D probes. Each micro-beamformer has its own output, which is wired back to the ultrasound systemtrough the transducer cable. Coarse steering is controlled by the ultrasound system where the patches are time-aligned to produce the parallel receive beams for each transmit beam (Fig. 1.3).

However, the electronics inside the probe produce heat whose amount is directly proportional to mechanical index used during imaging, therefore the engineering of active 3DE transducer should include thermal management.

Finally, new and advanced crystal manufacturing processes allows production of single crystal materials with homogeneous solid state technology and unique piezoelectric properties. These new transducers result in reduced heating production by increasing the efficiency of the transduction process to improve the conversion of transmit power into ultrasound energy and of received ultrasound energy into electrical power. Increased efficiency of the transduction process together with a wider bandwidth result in increased ultrasound penetration and resolution which improve image quality with the additional benefits of reducing artifacts, lowering power consumption and increase Doppler sensitivity.

Further developments in transducer technology have resulted in a reduced transducer footprint, improved side-lobe suppression, increased sensitivity and penetration, and the implementation of harmonic capabilities that can be used for both gray-scale and contrast imaging. The last generation of matrix transducers are significantly smaller than the previous ones and the quality of 2D and 3D imaging has improved significantly, allowing a single transducer to acquire both 2D and 3DE studies, as well as of acquiring the whole LV cavity in a single beat.

## 3D echocardiography physics

3DE is an ultrasound technique and the physical limitation of the constant speed of ultrasounds in human body tissues (approximately 1540 m/s in myocardial tissue and blood) cannot be overcome. The speed of sound in human tissues divided by the distance a single pulse has to travel forth and back (determined by the image depth) results in the maximum number of pulses that can be fired each second without producing interferences. Based on the acquired pyramidal angular width and the desired beam spacing in each dimension (spatial resolution), this number is related to the volumes per second that can be imaged (temporal resolution). Therefore, similar to 2DE imaging, in 3DE imaging there is an inverse relationship between volume rate (temporal resolution), acquisition volume size and the number of scan lines (spatial resolution). Any increase in one of these factors will cause a decrease in the other two.

The relation between volume rate, number of parallel receive beams, sector width, depth, and line density can be described by the following equation:

$$\text{Volume rate} = \frac{1540 \times \text{No. of parallel received beams}}{2 \times \left(\text{volume width / lateral resolution}\right)^2 \times \text{Volume depth}}$$

therefore the volume rate can be adjusted to the specific needs by either changing the volume width or depth. The 3D system allows the user to control the lateral resolution by changing the density of the scan lines in the pyramidal sector too. However, a decrease in spatial resolution also affects the contrast of the image. Volume rate can also be increased by increasing the number of parallel receive beams, but in this way the signal-to-noise ratio and the image quality will be affected.

To put all this in perspective let us assume that we would like to image up to 16 cm depth in the body and acquire a $60° \times 60°$ pyramidal volume. Since the speed of sound is approximately 1540 m/s and each pulse has to propagate 16 cm $\times$ 2 (to go forth and come back to the transducer), $1540/0.32 = 4812$ pulses can be fired per second without getting interference between the pulses. Assuming that $1°$ beam spacing in both X and Z dimension is a sufficient spatial resolution we would need 3600 beams ($60 \times 60$) to spatially resolve the $60° \times 60°$ pyramidal volume. As a result, we will get a temporal resolution (volume rate) of $4812/3600 = 1.3$ Hz, which is practically useless in clinical echocardiography.

The example above shows that the fixed speed of sound in body tissues has been a major challenge to the development of 3DE imaging. Manufacturers have developed several techniques such as parallel receive beamforming, multibeat imaging and real-time zoom acquisition to cope with this challenge but, in practice, this is usually achieved by selecting the appropriate acquisition modality for different imaging purposes (see Image acquisition and display paragraph).

Parallel receive beamforming or multiline acquisition is a technique where the system transmits one wide beam and receives multiple narrow beams formed within the bounds of the trasmit beam. In this way the volume rate (temporal resolution) is increased by a factor equal to the number of the received beams. Each beamformer focuses along a slightly different direction that was insonated by the broad transmit pulse. As an example, to obtain a $90° \times 90°$, 16-cm depth pyramidal volume at 25 vps, the system needs to receive 200,000 lines/s. Since the emission rate is around 5000 pulsed/s, the system should receive 42 beams in parallel for each emitted pulse. However, increasing the number of parallel beams to increase temporal resolution leads to an increase in size, costs and power consumption of the beamforming electronics, and deterioration in the signal-to-noise ratio and contrast resolution. With this technique of processing the received data, multiple scan lines can be sampled in the amount of time a conventional scanner would take for a single line, at the expense of reduced signal strength and resolution, as the receive beam are steered farther and farther away from the center of the transmit beam (Fig. 1.4).

Another technique to increase the size of the pyramidal volume and maintain the volume rate (or the reverse, e.g. maintain volume rate and increase the pyramidal volume) is the multibeat acquisition. With this technique, a number of small, ECG-gated subvolumes acquired from consecutive cardiac cycles are stitched together to build up the final, large pyramidal volume (Fig. 1.5). Multibeat acquisition will be effective only if the subvolumes to stitch together will be constant in position and size, therefore any transducer movement, cardiac translation motion due to respiration, change in cardiac cycle length will create subvolume malalignment and stitching artifacts (Fig. 1.6).

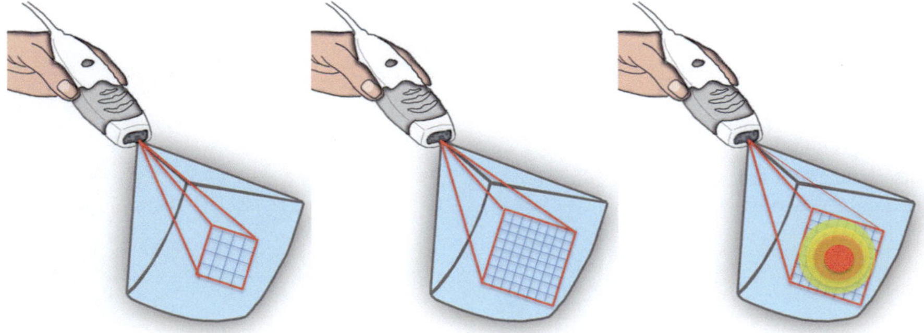

**Fig. 1.4** Parallel receive beamforming. Schematic representation of the parallel receive or multi-line beamforming technique receiving 16 (*left panel*) or 64 (*central panel*) beams (*blue squares*) for each broad transmit beam (*red pyramid*). The *right panel* shows the degradation of the power and resolution of the signal (from red maximal to bright yellow minimal) from the parallel receiving beams steered farther away from the center of the transmit beam

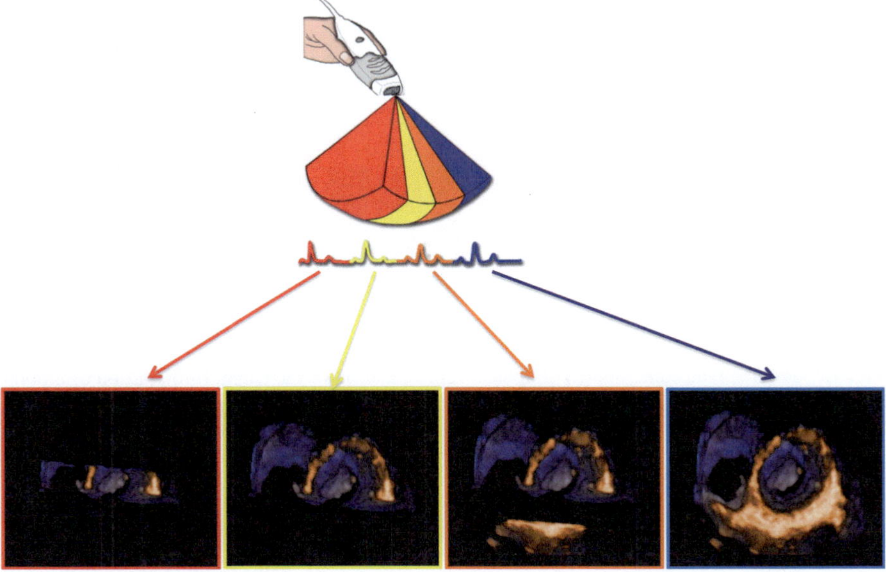

**Fig. 1.5** Multibeat acquisition. Schematic drawing of a 4-beat full-volume acquisition. The 4 pyramidal subvolumes (the colors show the relationships between the pyramidal subvolumes, the ECG beats and the way the 3D data set has been built up in the *lower part of the figure*) are obtained from consecutive heart beats and are stitched together to build up the final full volume (*blue square in the right lower part of the figure*)

Finally, the quality of the images of the cardiac structures which can be obtained by a 3DE system will be affected by the point spread function of the system. The point spread function describes the imaging system response to a point input. A point input, represented as a single pixel in the "ideal" image, will be reproduced as

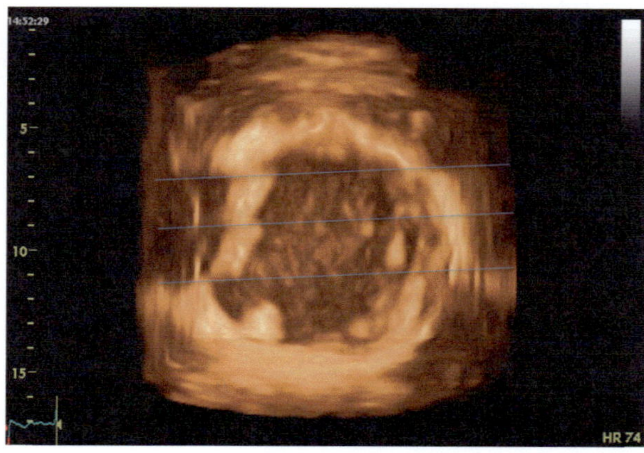

**Fig. 1.6** Stitching artifacts. Volume-rendered image of the left ventricle displayed with respiratory gating artifacts. The *blue lines* highlight the misalignment of the pyramidal subvolumes

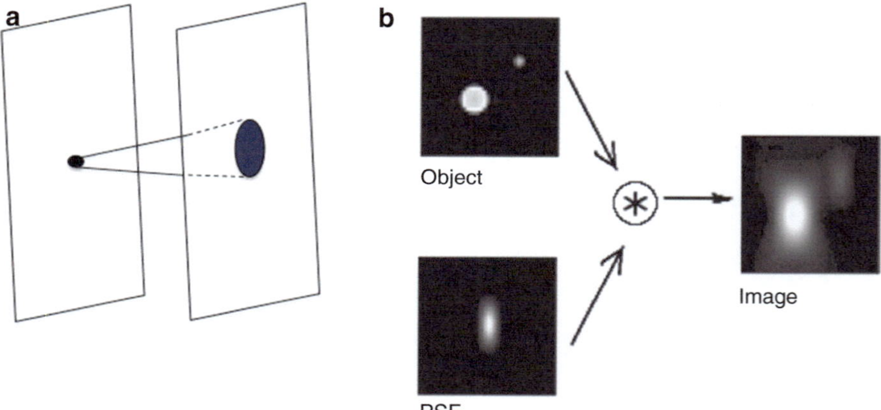



**Fig. 1.7** Point spread function. (**a**) Graphical representation of the extent of distortion of a point passing through a optical system. (**b**) Effect of the point spread function on the final image of a circular object

something other than a single pixel in the "real" image (Fig. 1.7). The degree of spreading (blurring) of any point object varies according to the dimension employed. In current 3DE systems it will be around 0.5 mm in the axial (y) dimension, around 2.5 mm in the lateral (x) dimension, and around 3 mm in the elevation (z) dimension. As a result we will obtain the best images (less degree of blurring, i.e. distortion) when using the axial dimension and the worst (greatest degree of spreading) when we use the elevation dimension.

These concepts have an immediate practical application in the choice of the best approach to image a cardiac structure. According to the point spread function of 3DE the best results is expected to be obtained by using the parasternal approach because structures are mostly imaged by the axial and lateral dimensions. Conversely, the worst result is expected to be obtained by the apical approach which mostly uses the lateral and elevation dimensions.

# History of 3D Echocardiography

Since the early days of cardiovascular imaging, the concept of 3D imaging was indisputably perceived as a need based on the recognition that depicting the complex shape of the cardiovascular system in less than three dimensions severely limited the diagnostic value of the information obtained from medical imaging (Fig. 1.8). During the last half of the twentieth century, we have witnessed an impressive technological progress driven by strong demand from the cardiology community that moved from fuzzy single-projection X-ray films to multi-slices high spatial resolution tomographic images depicting anatomical details previously seen only in anatomy atlases. The possibility to visualize these details in living patients changed completely the way cardiologists understand disease processes and resulted in new standards in the diagnosis of diseases and patients' management. Currently, both the diagnosis and treatment of most cardiovascular disease states heavily relies on information obtained by noninvasive imaging.

However, 3D imaging of the beating heart remained a challenge because of the constant motion of this organ. While 3D imaging of stationary organs was conceptually easy to solve by collecting information from different parts or from different

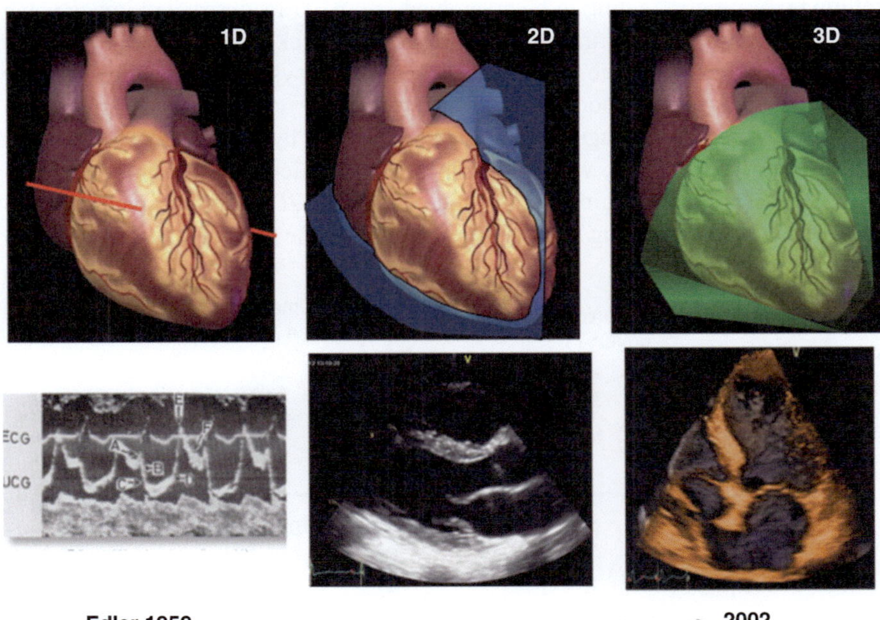


**Fig. 1.8** Progress in ultrasound technology. From the early M-mode (*1D*), when one single ultrasound beam produced a time-depth display of cardiac structures, through two-dimensional echocardiography (*2D*), when a real-time tomographic display of the beating heart was made available, to current three-dimensional technology (*3D*), with which a real-time pyramidal acquisition of data is available

angles consecutively, imaging of the beating heart required data collection to occur virtually in real time. This was a real challenge for engineers and physicists. In fact, it can be read in textbooks from the early 1970s explanations why real-time two-dimensional (2D) imaging of the beating heart is an enormous technological advancement that was believed to be unsurpasssable because of the limitations imposed by the constant speed at which ultrasound waves travel inside the human body.

Neverteless, despite the fact that the speed of sound has not changed since then, the combination of the exponential rise of computational power of computers with ingenious engineering solutions that increased the efficiency of the process of image formation from ultrasound reflections has meant that, during the last decade, 3DE has completed its transition from a predominant research tool to an imaging technique employed in everyday clinical practice [1].

This transition began in 2002 with the release of a reasonable user-friendly version of a matrix array transducer capable of real-time 3D imaging together with software which allows rapid slicing and quantification of 3DE data sets.

Before these technological achievements, attempts to develop 3DE imaging had relied in using a 2DE transducer (either tracking it in space or moving it in a pre-specified pattern) to acquire multiple 2D views. This required spatial information about the ultrasound probe itself with the aid of cardiac and, in some technological solutions, respiratory gating to be assembled into a 3D reconstructed image using dedicated software. The ultrasound probe has been tracked via a variety of means either extrinsic and intrinsic to the probe. More recent systems obviate the need for these spatial tracking methods (Fig. 1.9).

The first attempt in imaging the human heart in 3D by ultrasound was made by Dekker et al. [7] in 1974, who used a mechanical articulated arm that measured probe displacement during the acquisition of multiple 2DE views to perform free-hand transthoracic scanning (Fig. 1.10). This marked the birth of static surface ren-

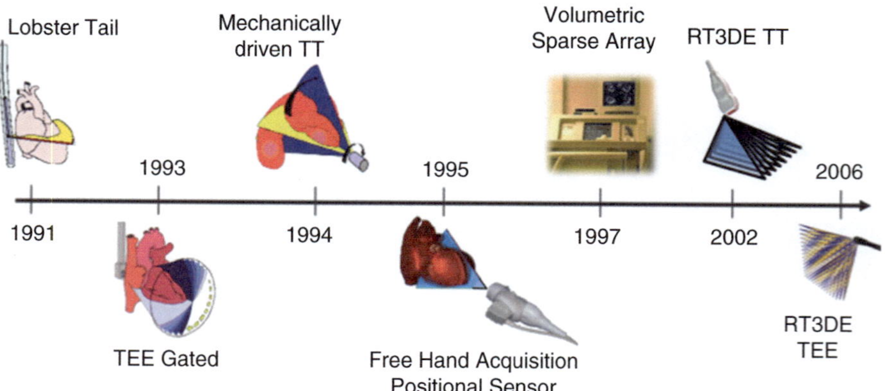


**Fig. 1.9** Temporal evolution of three-dimensional echocardiography technology (see text for details). Abbreviations: *RT3DE* real-time three-dimensional echocardiography, *TEE* transesophageal, *TT* transthoracic

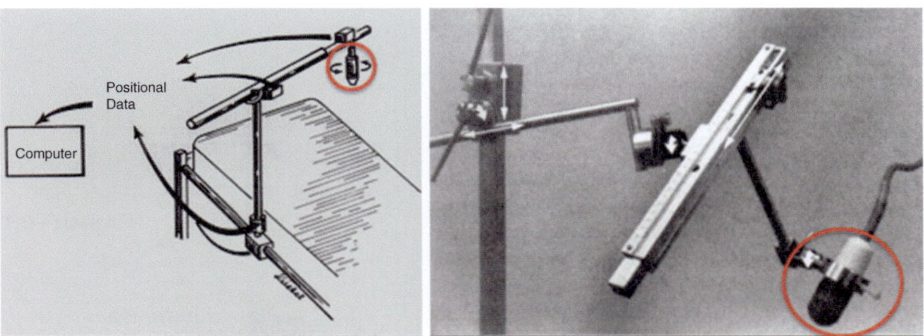



**Fig. 1.10** The mechanical arm. Schematic drawing of the scanning bed and the device (*left panel*) and actual picture of the arm with the probe (*right panel*). A large external beam device gives spatial data regarding an ultrasound probe to enable three-dimensional reconstruction. The ultrasound probe is highlighted by a *red circle*

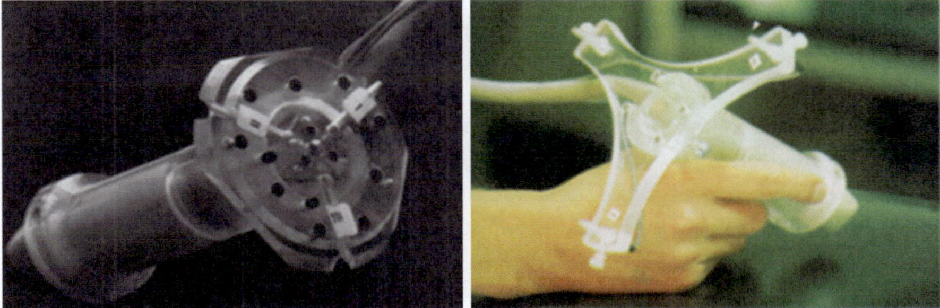

**Fig. 1.11** Acoustic locator or "spar-gaps". The ultrasound probe position is tracked by a means similar to radar technology

dering, the earliest 3D echocardiographic technique. This work demonstrated the possibility of producing a 3D data set, but the technology was impractical for clinical use.

Trying to improve the tracking method, Moritz and Shreve [8] developed an acoustic locator (the so called "spark-gap) whereby an acoustic element was attached to the ultrasoud probe and sent regular audio pulses that were detected by a fixed antenna to be included in a Cartesian locator grid (Fig. 1.11).

In 1977, Raab et al. [9] reported about an electromagnetic sensor which could be attached to the ultrasound probe allowing continuous monitoring of its position in space. Although this technique was quite advanced for 1977, it was not used systematically until the mid 1990s (Fig. 1.12). Several other Authors published early attempts to produce 3DE data sets during this time period [10–12]. Further development of these techniques led to what has been termed "free-hand scanning". With this modality, a highly developed magnetic-field system orients sequentially acquired 2DE imaging planes by tracking the movement of the ultrasound probe as it is manipulated by the operator.

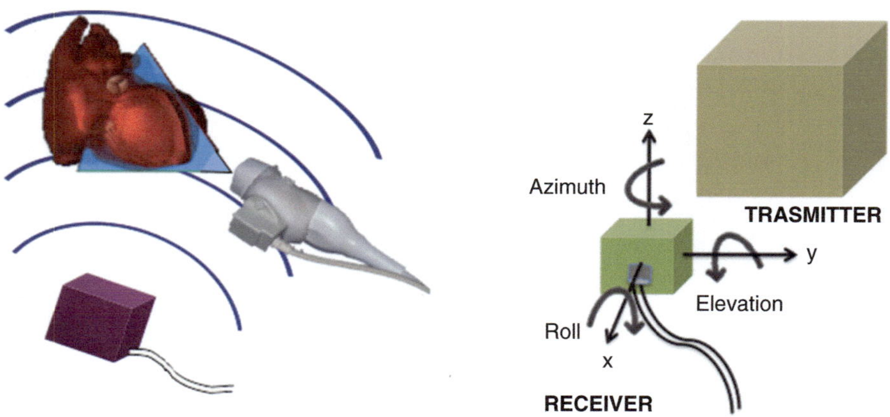


**Fig. 1.12** Freehand scanning. A modified ultrasound probe is tracked in 3D space using an electromagnetic locator system (*left panel*). Schematic drawing of the receiver and transmitting device and the Cartesian coordinate system for tracking the location of the transducer (*right panel*). Images then may be reconstructed off-line to create 3D data sets

One crucial developmental aspect for the success of 3D reconstruction from multiplane acquisition was the registration of the different planes, so that they could be combined together to create a 3D image of the heart. This was achieved by sequential gated acquisition, wherein different cut planes were acquired one-by-one with gating designed to minimize artifacts. To minimize spatial misalignment of slices because of respiration, respiratory gating was used, such that only cardiac cycles coinciding with a certain phase of the respiratory cycle were captured. Similarly, to minimize temporal misalignment because of heart rate variability, ECG gating was used, such that only cardiac cycles within preset limits of R-R interval were included. This methodology became standard in both transthoracic and transesophageal multiplane imaging aimed at 3D reconstruction and was widely used until real-time 3D imaging became possible.

To achieve effective multiplane acquisition, new techniques were developed that operated under the assumption that both the patient and the housing of the ultrasound probe remained in a relatively fixed position. The ultrasound probe was held by a device that moved the probe in a specified, preprogrammed fashion within the housing of a mechanical device. Examples were linear, fan-like and rotational acquisition methods (Fig. 1.13).

In the early 1990s, the use of linear step-by-step motion acquisition, wherein the transducer was mechanically advanced between acquisitions using a motorized driving device become commercially available [13].

However, this simple solution was not applicable for transthoracic echocardiography, because of the need to find intercostal acoustic windows for each acquisition step. This approach was implemented in a pull-back transesophageal echocardiography transducer, known as "lobster tail" probe (Fig. 1.14, Right panel). In the handle of the transducer there was a motorized unit that incrementally pulled crystals in a parallel fashion at 1 mm increments gated to electrocardiogram (ECG) and

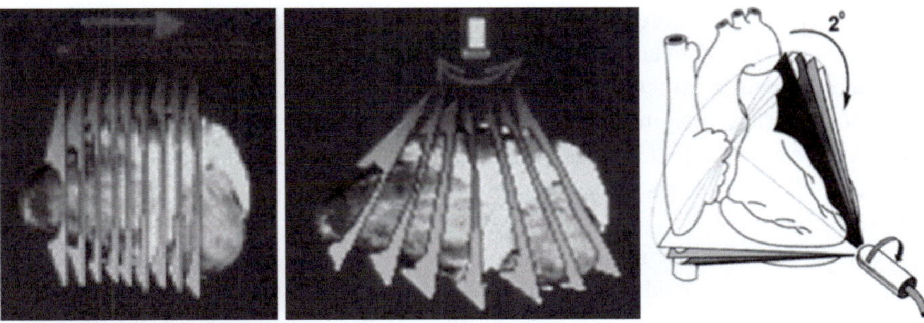

**Fig. 1.13** Gated sequential imaging. Transducer motion modalities to generate 3DE images using gated sequential imaging. Linear (*left panel*): multiple parallel equi-distantly spaced 2D images can be obtained by progressive computer-controlled linear motion of the transducer in prespecified depths. Fan-like (*central panel*): multiple two-dimensional images are obtained in a fan-like array by tilting the transducer in specified arc angles to create a pyramidal data set. Rotational (*right panel*): multiple two-dimensional images are obtained by rotating the transducer 180° and obtaining images at pedetermined intervals (e.g. every 3° or 6°) to create a conical data set

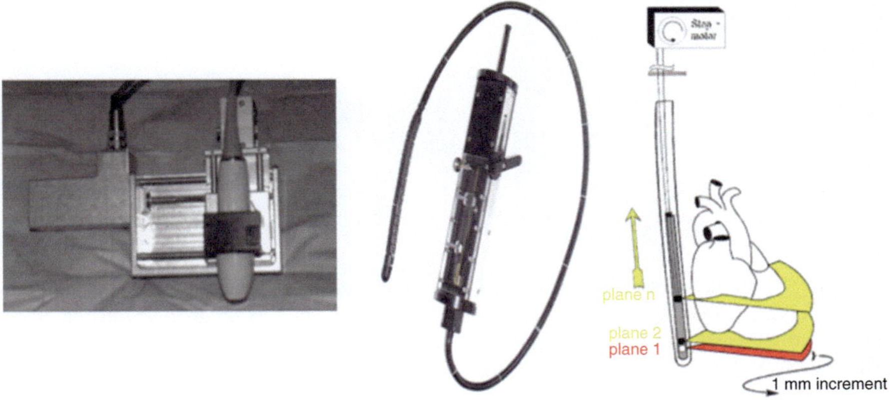


**Fig. 1.14** Motorized linear-motion device used to acquire parallel cut planes for reconstructing 3D images using linear step-by-step transducer motion (*left panel*). Pull back transoesophageal probe that employed the same approach of linear motion (*right panel*)

respiration. The first transesophageal 3DE study was performed in the early 90s using this device [14].

An alternative approach to linear scanning was to keep the transducer in a fixed position corresponding to an optimal acoustic window, and rotate the imaging plane by internally steering the imaging element in different directions (Fig. 1.15). This concept of rotational scanning in combination with gated sequential scanning was implemented into transoesophageal technology and resulted in a probe that has subsequently become the main source of multiplane images used for 3D reconstruction, both for research and clinical practice [15, 16].

This approach provided 3D reconstructions of reasonably good quality due to the high quality of the original 2D images and the fact that the transoesophageal probe is relatively well "anchored" in its position throughout image acquisition, especially in sedated patients. Nevertheless, cardiac structures, such as valve leaflets appeared jagged as a result of stitch artifacts (Fig. 1.15, right panel), reflecting the contributions of individual imaging planes that could not be perfectly aligned during reconstruction, despite the ECG and respiratory gating. Multiple studies demonstrated the clinical usefulness of this approach mostly in the context of the evaluation of valvular heart disease.

An early transthoracic implementation of rotational approach consisted of a motorized device that contained a conventional transducer (Fig. 1.16), which was mechanically rotated several degrees at a time, resulting in first transthoracic gated sequential multiplane acquisitions suitable for 3D reconstruction of the heart [17–19].

Despite the previously unseen transthoracic 3DE images that excited so many, it quickly became clear that this methodology was destined to remain limited to the research arena because image acquisition was too time-consuming and tedious for clinical use. In addition, the quality of the reconstructed images was limited.

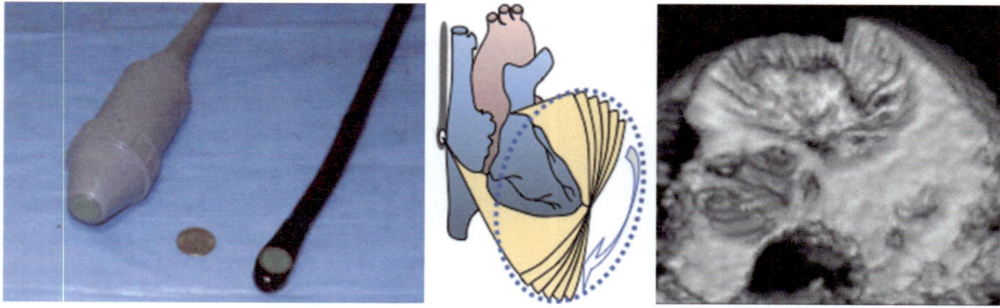

**Fig. 1.15** Rotational approach implemented into a transoesophageal multiplane transducer (*left panel*). Schematic drawing of sequential ultrasound images obtained by progressive rotation of the transducer in a prespecified fashion (*central panel*). Example of a 3D image of the mitral valve with anterior leaflet prolapse from multiplane images acquired using this transducer (*right panel*)

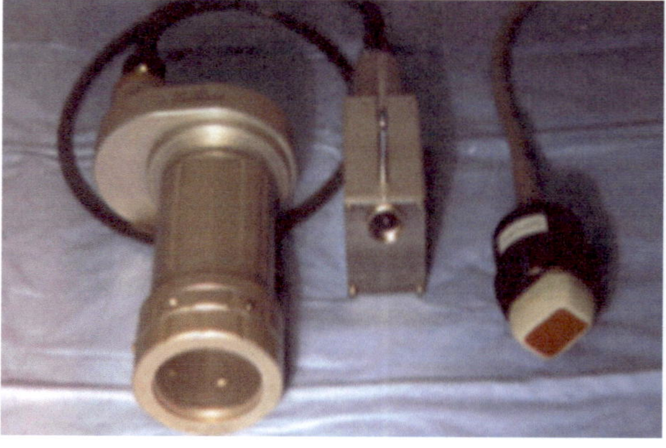

**Fig. 1.16** Motorized device that housed an external stepper motor that mechanically rotated a built-in transthoracic transducer.

With each of these methods, once the numerous 2D "planes" have been obtained according to prescribed transducer movements, the images had to be realigned and digitally reformatted into rectangular pixels that were then stacked. Gaps between adjacent images were filled by interpolation. A cubic volume of "voxels" was then derived from the stacked images that could then be volume rendered or "sliced" in any plane of interest (Fig. 1.17).

A profound limitation to each of these techniques was that they fundamentally relied on the acquisition of multiple 2D images. Image quality was therefore highly dependent on concordance between adjacent images. The inherent need to interpolate data became problematic if the adjacent images were themselves discordant due to voluntary or involuntary patient movement. Problems inherent to irregular heart rate and lung artifact were minimized by using cardiac and respiratory gating to prespecified heart rates and phases of the respiratory cycle. Images were therefore acquired over a varying period of time, often up to 2–3 min, and even longer in the presence of atrial fibrillation. This was because, from a practical standpoint, the image mismatch was too profound if the R-R gating was set to vary by more than roughly 150 ms. If a patient with atrial fibrillation was gated at 150-ms variation, the acquisition could take up to 10 min. In this setting, it was unlikely that either the patient or the physician obtaining the data could remain stationary for this length of time. Actually, to obtain a satisfactory 3D reconstruction with this technology, it was required a very skilled operator, a very cooperative patient, an operator skilled with 3D reconstruction and a bit of luck. If succesful, although image quality was suboptimal for small discrete structure like valve morphology analysis, even at this time, data sets were useful for ventricular volume assessment.

However, the presence of the locator device, which, limited significantly the portability of the ultrasound system, the need of avoiding any metallic close to the

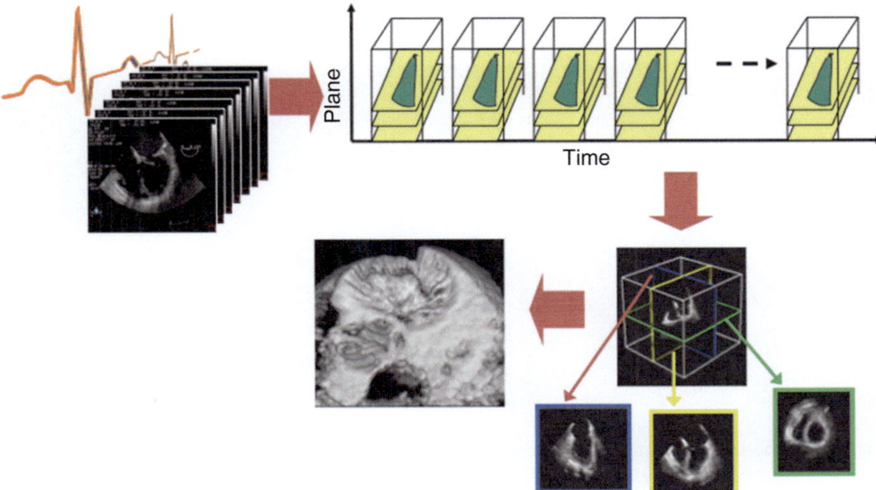


**Fig. 1.17** Reconstruction of a 3D data set from multiple 2D images. The collection of images (typically 15 to 60 cardiac cycles, with 10 to 15 frames/heart beat) were re-sampled in a cubical data set and ultimately rendered into a 3D image or sliced according to planes of interest

system and the patient, the long reconstrunction times and the unpredictability of the final results have further hindered more widespread use of this technique in clinical practice.

The collective experience and the limitations of the gated sequential acquisition and offline 3D reconstruction gradually led developers to the understanding that scanning volumes rather than isolated cut planes would intrinsically address many of the previous issues. This revolutionary idea led von Ramm et al. [20, 21] to develop the first real-time 3DE system at Duke university. This system was equipped with a phased-array transducer, in which piezoelectric elements were arranged in multiple rows, rather than one row, allowing fast sequential scanning of multiple planes. The phased array technology, that has been an integral part of the 2D transducers for decades, was modified to electronically change the direction of the beam not only within a single plane to create a fan-shaped scan, but also in the lateral direction to generate a series of such scans. Importantly this was achieved without any mechanical motion, allowing the speeds necessary for volumetric real-time imaging.

The first generation of real-time 3D transducers was bulky due to unprecedented number of electrical connections to the individual crystals, despite the relatively small number of elements in each row. This sparse array matrix transducer consisted of 256 non-simultaneously firing elements and had large footprint, which did not allow good coupling with the chest wall for optimal acoustic windows, and produced 3D images that were suboptimal in any selected plane, when compared to the quality of standard at the time 2D echocardiographic images. Nevertheless, the mere fact of successful real-time 3D imaging of an entire volume of heart using one cardiac cycle was a huge technological breakthrough.

This represented a major transition from the thin slice sector imaging obtainable with 2DE. Despite volumetric acquisition was a very positive development, the images were displayed as 2D (Fig. 1.18). The 2D images were derived from the 3D data set but were displayed as 2D orthogonal cut planes.

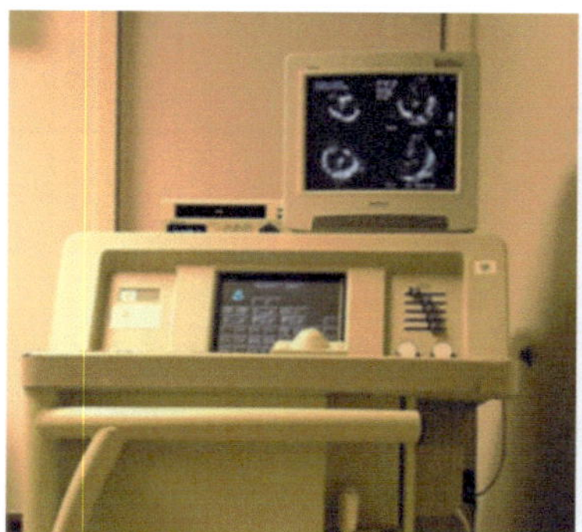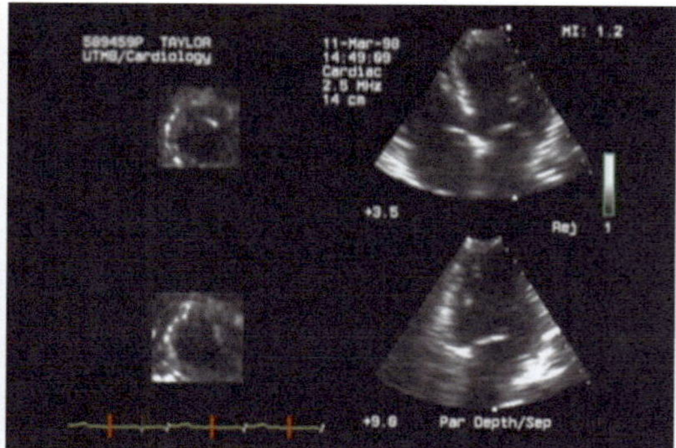


**Fig. 1.18** The first real-time 3D echocardiography system (C-scan, Volumetrics, Inc.) equipped with a sparse matrix array transducer (*left panel*). In the *right panel* the images which can be obtained with that system are shown: apical views of the heart on the right (4-chamber on *top*, and 2-chamber of the left ventricle on the *bottom*), and short axis, or C scans, of the LV derived from perpendicular cuts through the apical views on the left

However, the road was paved and in November 2002, at the time of the American Heart Association meeting, Philips released the first generation of real-time 3DE.

## Technical Features and Limitations of 3D Echocardiography

By being a tomographic technique, conventional 2DE relies heavily on the operator's experience to "mentally" reconstruct the complex shape of cardiac structures from a limited number of "slices" (Fig. 1.19). As such, 2DE is limited in its ability

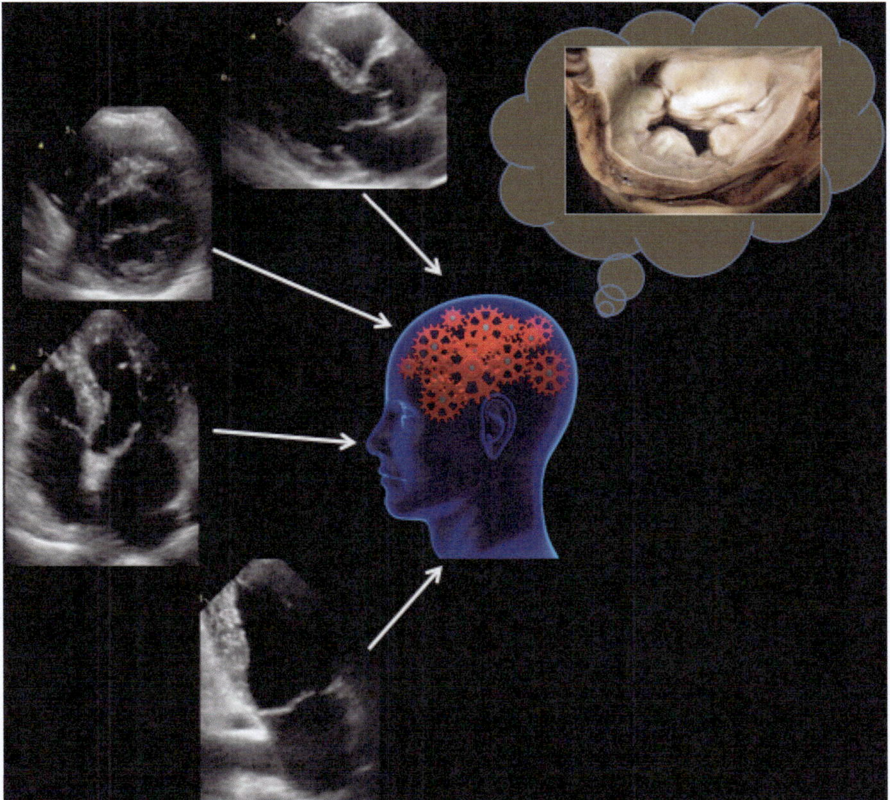

**Fig. 1.19** Mental reconstruction of complex cardiac structure from a limited number of tomographic views obtained with conventional two-dimensional echocardiography. Since no single view represents the actual 3D shape of the mitral valve, the echocardiographer acquires a number of 2DE views from different approaches and then start a mental process to integrate these views to obtain a stereoscopic representation of the actual valve. It is evident how this process (and the results) are affected by the operator experience and his/her practice of the anatomical theatre and/ or operating room

to illustrate complex cardiac strucural relationships and relies on assumptions about image plane position and cardiac structure geometry when quantitation is performed.

3DE is a volumetric technique which allows an "electronic" cutting of the data set (similar to what is done in the anatomical theatre by the anatomist) to provides a virtually unlimited sections of the heart and its structures. Compared to conventional 2DE, the operator can obtain unique views of the heart (e.g. the "surgeon view"of the cardiac, like the mitral or the tricuspid valve seen from the atrium or the aorta seen from the aortic root) and perform quantitative analyses of the geometry and function of cardiac structures without making any assumption about their shape. As an example, if we want to use 2DE to calculate the volumes of the LV we can use different formulas (Fig. 1.20) which assume that the LV has a certain shape that can be assimilated to a known geometrical figure and the volume is calculated from simple actual measurements (usually areas and linear dimensions). With 3DE, there is no calculation to be performed. The endocardium of the LV is mapped to create a beutel whch represent the cardiac cavity (Fig. 1.21) and the volume is measured by simply counting the voxels within the beutel. The ability to acquire volumetric data sets which contains the whole cardiac cavity and to measure volumes without the need of geometrical assumptions have prompted the possibility of measuring the volumes of geometrically complex structures like the right ventricle which are impossible to calculate with 2DE [22].

Accordingly, the clinical usefulness of 3DE has been shown in several areas, including: (i) measurement of cardiac chamber volumes without the need of geometric modeling and without the detrimental effect of foreshortened views [3, 22–25]; (ii) unique, anatomically sound and realistic views of cardiac valves and congenital abnormalities [26–28]. This has been proven to be extremely useful to understand the pathophysiology and quantitate the severity of the diseases and to guide and assess effectiveness of surgical and/or percutaneous transcatheter interventions [29]; (iii) Visualization of regional wall motion [30]; (iv) Localization and visualization regurgitant or shunting jets with 3D color Doppler. In some instances, the scientific evidence seems strong enough to endorse the use of 3DE as a new standard in the clinical assessment of the heart [31].

However, despite 3DE clearly offers new possibilities to acquire, display and quantify cardiac structures, current 3DE systems are not yet able to fully replace conventional high-end 2DE systems. The main shortcomings in currently available 3D echo technology are: (i) 3DE systems are technically demanding to be properly used for both data set acquisition and post-processing; (ii) both temporal and spatial resolution are suboptimal (particularly in single beat acquisition mode); (iii) Software tools for quantitative analysis of 3D echo data sets are limited (currently there is no software package to quantitate the atria and the tricuspid valve) and most of those which are available works only with vendor specific data sets; and iv. lack of a DICOM standard to quantify and crop the 3D echo data sets.

For effective application of the 3DE technique, echocardiographers need specific education and training. They have to learn how to acquire volumetric data sets without artifacts, and navigate within the data set to obtain the desired cut plane or

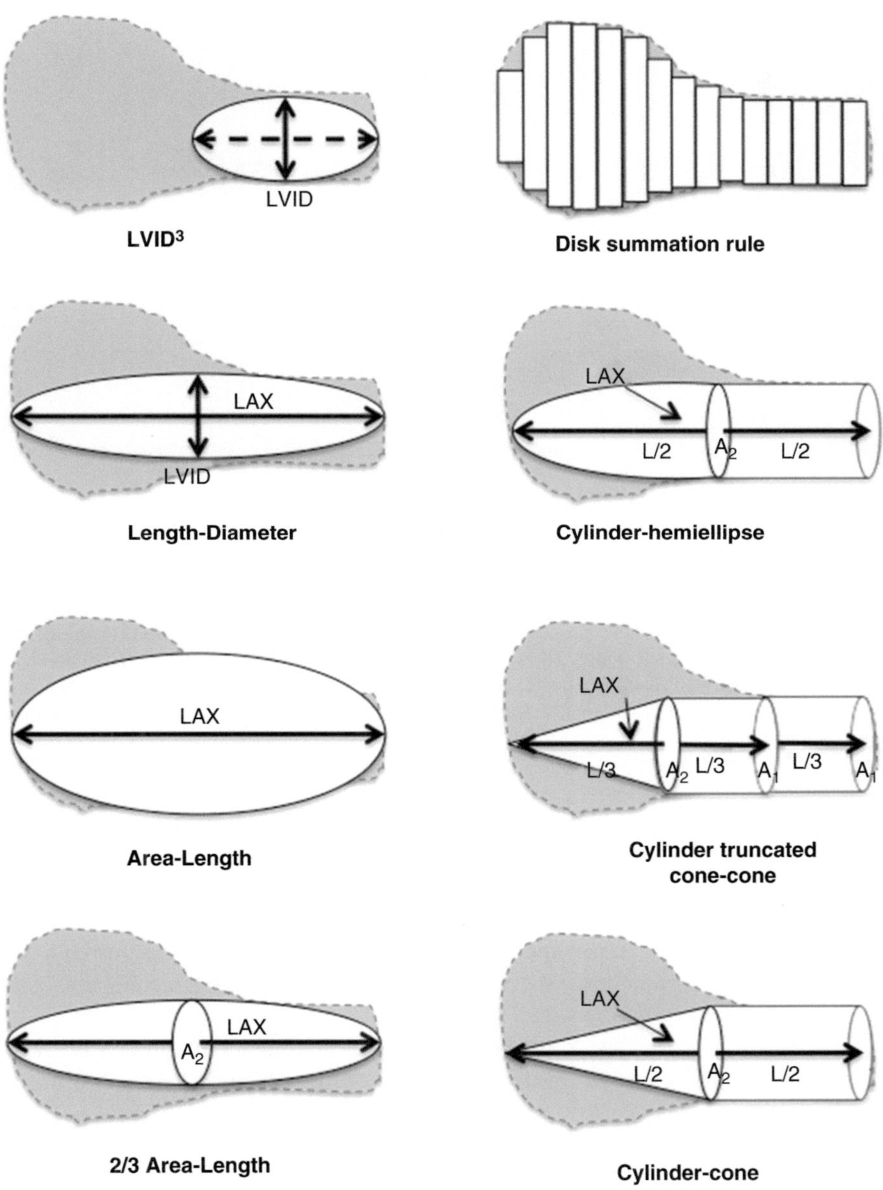


**Fig. 1.20** Schematic representation of the main geometric assumptions used to calculate left ventricular (LV) volumes by M-mode and two-dimensional echocardiography, and their correspondence to actual shape of distorted ventricle (apical aneurysm). *A1, LV* short-axis area at mitral valve level, *A2, LV* short-axis area at papillary muscle level, *L* length, *LAX* LV long axis, *LVID* LV internal diameter

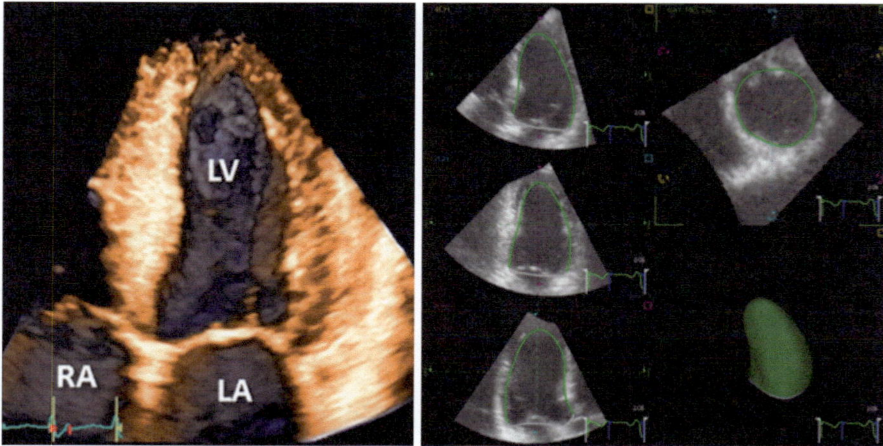


**Fig. 1.21** Three-dimensional measurement of left ventricular volume. Volume rendering of a three-dimensional multibeat acquisition focused on the left ventricle (*left panel*). The data set is segmented in 3 longitudinal (apical 4- and 2-chamber and long-axis) views and 1 transversal view (SAX) (*Right panel*). The three longitudinal views share the same apex (as it can be seen on the SAX) and their position can be adjusted by rotating the *yellow* (4CH), *purple* (3CH) and *green* (2CH) lines in order to achieve proper view orientation. Semi- or fully-automated tracing of the endocardial border in these views allows a mapping of the entire endocardial surface which is rendered in the surface rendering beutel (*right lower angle of the right panel*). The count of the voxels in the beutel at different moments of the cardiac cycle will provide the measurement of the LV volumes

extract the needed views. New tools like cropping, slicing and thresholding are available to manipulate the data sets in order to visualize the cardiac structure of interest. Various ways to display the information are available (see next paragraph). Compared with the reassuring simplicity of obtaining 2DE imaging which is virtually the same on every echocardiographic machine, the workflow for both 3D data sets acquisition and post-processing, which is specific for each company, definitely needs to be standardized and simplified.

Theoretically, spatial and temporal resolution of 3DE data sets can be similar or even higher than the one of 2DE images. This can be obtained by using a much larger number of piezoelectric crystals in the probe. All of them should be controlled independently during both the transmitting and receiving process, more efficient beam forming techniques need to be implemented, and the data should be transferred in real-time to the system to build up the final data sets. However, this implies problems of miniaturization, probe heating management, huge data streams and complex calculations that cannot be implemented in the current generation of echocardiographic systems. Several research groups have the equipment to obtain high resolution 3DE data sets, but it requires long acquisition times, off line processing and the reconstruction of a data set from a single heart beat may require hours or days. However, new materials are continuously created to improve the efficience of crystals, and the computational power of computers is growing exponential, therefore it can be expected that future echocardiographic systems will be able to handle this data and provide high frame rate 3DE imaging.

Acquiring 3DE data sets of the different cardiac structures is feasible however, availability of tools able to allow advanced 3D quantitation, display and printing of cardiac structures is relatively limited. In particular, there is a definite need of developing new software packages to assess tricuspid valve, atria, RV shape and strain and also improve the robustness and accuracy of automated measurement software packages in order to increase feasibility and reproducibility of measurements.

## Modalities of Displaying 3D Imaging

Currently, 3D data set acquisition can be easily implemented into standard echocardiographic examination by either switching among 2D and 3D probes or, with newest all-in-one-probes, by switching between 2D and 3D modalities available in the same probe. The latter probes are also capable to provide single-beat full-volume acquisition, as well as real-time 3D color Doppler imaging.

At present three different methods for 3D data set acquisition are available [5]:

- multiplane imaging
- "real-time" (or "live") 3D imaging
- multi-beat ECG-gated imaging

In the multiplane mode, multiple, simultaneous 2D views can be acquired at high frame rate using predefined or user-selected plane orientations and displayed using the split screen option (Fig. 1.2). The first view on the left is usually the reference plane that is orientated by adjusting the probe position while the other views represents views obtained from the reference view by simply tilting and/or rotating the imaging planes. Multiplane imaging is a real time acquisition and secondary imaging planes can only be selected during acquisition. Doppler colour flow can be superimposed on 2D images and in some systems both tissue Doppler and speckle tracking analysis can be performed. Although strictly not a 3D acquisition, this imaging mode is useful in situations where assessment of multiple views from the same cardiac cycle is desirable (e.g. atrial fibrillation or other irregular arrhythmias, stress echo, evaluation of interventricular dyssynchrony, analysis of regurgitant jet extension and shape, etc.)

In the real-time mode, a pyramidal 3D volumetric data set is obtained from each cardiac cycle and visualized live, beat after beat as during 2D scanning. As the data set is updated in real-time, data set orientation and cut plane can be changed by simply rotating or tilting the probe. Visualization of cardiac structures is obtained with limited post-processing and the data set can be rotated (independent of the transducer position) to view the cardiac structure of interest from different orientations. Heart dynamics is shown in a realistic way, with instantaneous on-line volume rendered reconstruction. Real-time modality allows fast acquisition of dynamic pyramidal data structures from a single acoustic view that may encompass the entire heart without the need of reference system, electrocardiographic (ECG) and respiratory gating. Real-time imaging is time-saving both for data acquisition and analysis. Although this acquisition mode overcomes rhythm disturbances or respiratory motion limitations, it still suffers of relatively low temporal and spatial resolution. Real-time imaging can be acquired in the following modes:

(a) Live 3D. Once the desired cardiac structure has been imaged in 2DE it can be converted to a volumetric image by pressing a specific button in the control panel. The 3D system automatically switch to a narrow sector acquisition (approximately $30° \times 60°$ pyramidal volume) to preserve spatial and temporal resolution. The size of the pyramidal volume can be increased to visualize larger structures, but both scan line density (spatial resolution) and volume rate (temporal resolution) will drop down. 3D live imaging mode is used to: (i) guide full-volume acquisition; (ii) Visualize small structures using the zoom mode (aortic valve, masses etc); (iii) Recording short-lived events (i.e. bubble passage); (iv) in patients with irregular rhythm/dyspnea unable to cooperate for a full-volume acquisition; (v) guiding/monitoring interventional procedures.
(b) Live 3D colour. Colour flow can be superimposed on a live 3D data set to visualize blood flow in real time. With this modality, temporal resolution is usually very low
(c) 3D zoom. This imaging mode is an extension of live 3D and allows a focussed real time view of a structure of interest. A crop box is placed on a 2D single- or multiplane image to allow the operator to adjust lateral and elevation width to include the structure of interest in the final data set, then the system automatically crops the adjacent structures to provide a real time display of the structure of interest with high spatial and temporal resolution. The draw-back of the 3D zoom mode is that the operator loses the relationships of the cardiac structure of interest with surrounding structures. This acquisition modality is mainly used during transoesophageal studies for detailed anatomical analysis of the structure of interest
(d) Full-volume. The full-volume provides has the largest acquisition volume possible (usually $90° \times 90°$ degrees). Real-time (or "single-beat") full-volume acquisition is affected by low spatial and temporal resolution and it is used for quantification of cardiac chambers when multibeat ECG gated acquisition is not possible (e.g. irregular cardiac rhythm, patient unable to cooperate for breath-holding)

In contrast to real-time/live 3D imaging, multi-beat acquisition is realized through sequential acquisitions of narrow smaller volumes obtained from several ECG-gated consecutive heart cycles (from 2 to 6) that are subsequently stitched together to create a single volumetric data set (Fig. 1.5). Once acquired, the data set cannot be changed by manipulating the probe like in live 3D imaging and analysis requires off-line slicing, rotation and cropping of the acquired data set. It provides large data sets with high temporal and spatial resolution that can be used for quantitating cardiac chamber size and function or to assess spatial relationships among cardiac structures. However, this 3D imaging mode has the disadvantage of the

ECG-gating, as the images are acquired over several cardiac cycles and the final data set is available to be visualized by the operator only after the last cardiac cycle has been acquired, it is a *"near real-time"* imaging, and it is prone to artifacts due to patient or respiratory motion or irregular cardiac rhythms. Multibeat imaging can be acquired with or without color flow mapping and usually more cardiac cycles are required for 3D color data sets.

3D data sets can be sectioned in several planes and rotated in order to visualize the cardiac structure of interest from any desired perspective, irrespective of its orientation and position within the heart. Accordingly, the operator can easily obtain unique visualizations, that may be difficult or impossible to achieve using conventional 2DE (e.g. en-face views of the tricuspid valve or cardiac defects). Three main actions are undertaken by the operator to obtain the desired view from a 3D volumetric data set: cropping, slicing and rotating. Similarly to what the anatomists or the surgeons do to expose an anatomic structure within a 3DE data set, the operator should remove the surrounding chamber walls. This process of virtually removing the irrelevant neighbouring tissue is called cropping (Fig. 1.22), and can be performed either during or after acquisition. In contrast with 2D images, displaying a cropped image requires also data set rotation (Fig. 1.22) and the definition of the viewing perspective (i.e. since the same 3D structure can be visualized *en face*

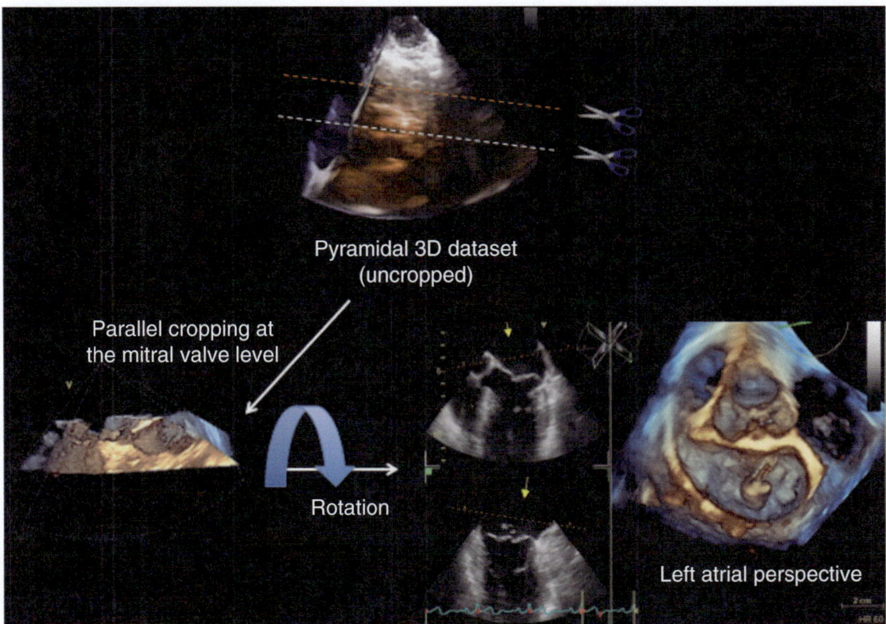


**Fig. 1.22** Data set cropping and rotation. To display the mitral valve from the left atrial perspective (surgical view) a full-volume pyramidal data set has been cropped to remove part of the left ventricle from above and part of the left atrium from below. Then, remaining data set has been rotated to the desired perspective to display the cardiac structures in an anatomical sound position

either from above or below, as well as from any desired view angle) [1]. Slicing refers to a virtual "cutting" of the 3D data set into one or more (up to 12) 2D (tomographic) grey-scale images (Fig. 1.23). Finally, irrespective of its acquisition window, a cropped or a sliced image should be displayed according to the anatomical orientation of the heart within the human body and this is usually obtained by rotating the selected images.

Acquisition of volumetric images generates the technical problem of rendering the depth perception on a flat, 2D monitor. 3D images can be visualized using three display modalities (Fig. 1.24):

- volume rendering,
- surface rendering (wireframe and solid surface rendering)
- tomographic slices

In the volume rendering modality, various color maps are applied to convey the depth perception to the observer. Generally, lighter shades (e.g. bronze, Fig. 1.24) are used for structures closer to the observer, while darker shades (e.g. blue, Fig. 1.24) are used for deeper structures. Surface rendering modality displays the 3D surface of cardiac structures, identified either by manual tracing or by using

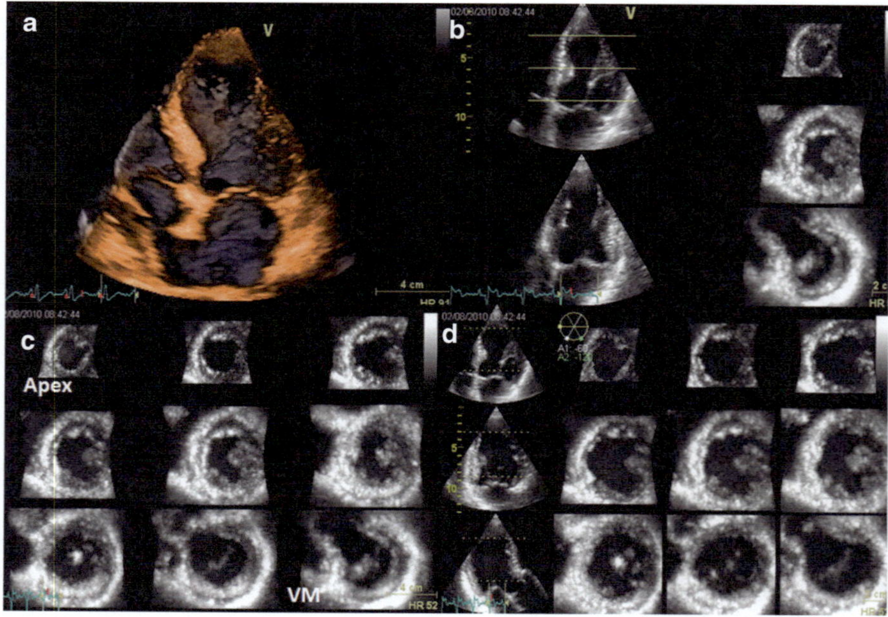

**Fig. 1.23** Data set slicing. A full-volume data set (Panel **a**) can be sliced in several ways. Two longitudinal (4-chamber and the orthogonal view) plus 3 transversal slices at different levels of the left ventricle (*yellow lines*) (Panel **b**). Nine transversal slices of the left ventricle from the mitral valve (*MV*) to the apical (*Apex*) level (Panel **c**). Three longitudinal slices (4- and 2-chamber plus the long-axis apical views) and nine transversal views (Panel **d**). The position of the lowest and the highest transversal planes are adjustable by the operator and the slices in between are automatically repositioned to be equidistant. The position of longitudinal planes are also adjustable both during acquisition and post processing

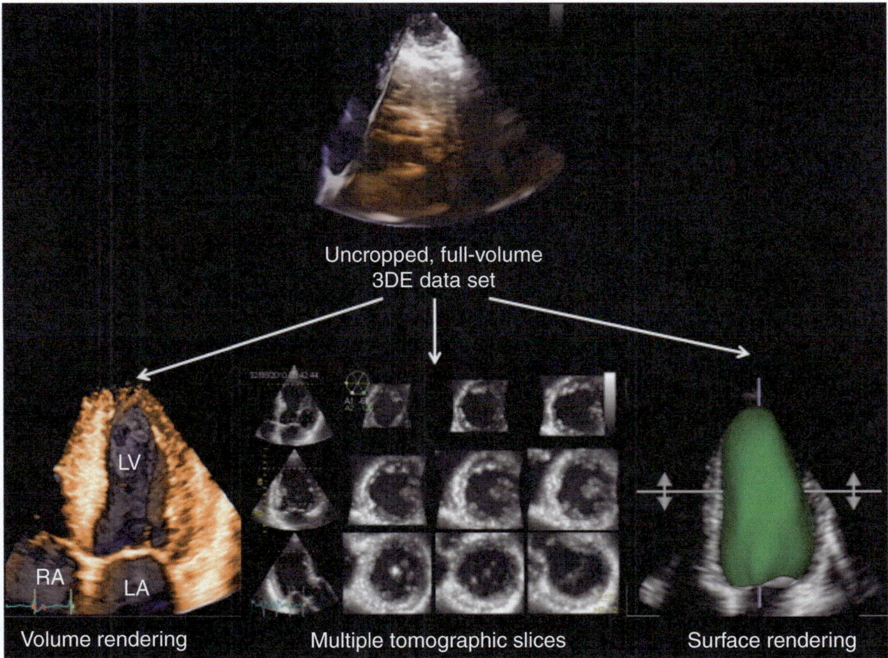



**Fig. 1.24** Techniques used to display a 3D data set of the left ventricle. Volume rendering to assess anatomy (*left panel*), multislice to evaluate regional wall motion and distribution of myocardium(*central panel*) and surface rendering to assess function (*right panel*) (see text for details)

automated border detection algorithms on multiple 2D cross-sectional images of the structure/cavity of interest. This stereoscopic approach is useful for the assessment of the shape of the cardiac chambers, great vessels and valves, and for a better appreciation of their geometry and dynamic function during the cardiac cycle.

Wireframe rendering (Fig. 1.25, left panel) is the simplest of the available surface rendering techniques. It identifies equidistant points on the surface of a 3D object obtained from manual tracing, or using semi- or fully- automated border detection algorithms, to trace the endocardial contour in cross-sectional images and then connect this points using lines (wires) to create a mesh of little polygonal tiles. Smoothing algorithms are used to smooth angles and give a realistic appearance to the structure of interest. This rendering technique processes a relatively low amount of data and it is used for relatively flat endocardial boundaries such as the cardiac chamber walls. This stereoscopic approach is particularly useful, in combination with a solid surface display of the volume change during the cardiac cycle, to visualize regional and global chamber function.

Finally, the pyramidal data set can be automatically sliced in several tomographic views simultaneously displayed (Fig. 1.23). Cut planes can be orthogonal, parallel or free (any given plane orientation), selected as desired by the echocardiographer for obtaining optimized cross-sections of the heart in order to answer specific clinical questions and to perform accurate and reproducible linear and/or area measurements.

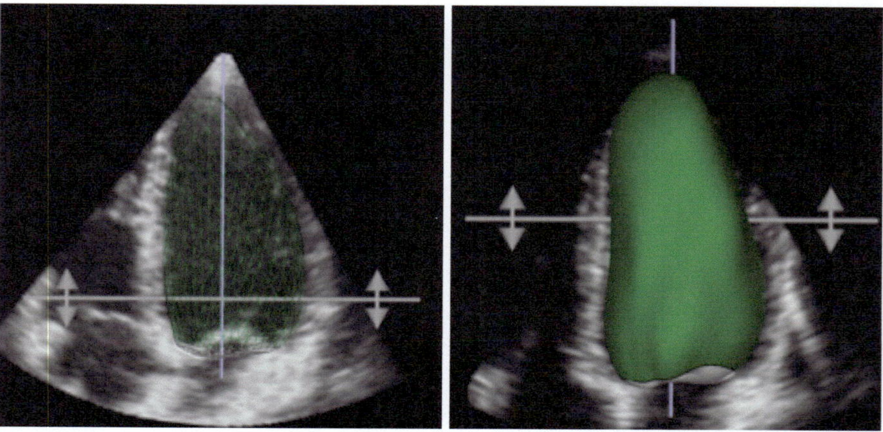

**Fig. 1.25** Surface rendering of the left ventricle. Both wireframe (*left panel*) and solid (*right panel*) surface rendering display are shown for the same 3DE data set of the left ventricle

As any other imaging technique, 3DE images may be affected by artifacts. The main artifacts that may affect the interpretation of 3DE images are stitching artifacts, dropout artifacts, blurring and blooming artifacts, and artifacts related to wrong gain settings.

As previously described, the most effective way to improve both temporal and spatial resolution of 3DE data sets is to acquire a number of narrow data sets and stitch them together (Fig. 1.5). However, since the single narrow data sets are obtained from consecutive cardiac cycles, they are not simultaneous. If the position of the cardiac structures changes from beat to beat due to heart translation within the chest during respiration, probe movements during acquisition, or different cardiac cycle length (e.g. irregular atrial fibrillation, ectopic beats, etc), the cross sections of neighbouring data sets do not match when they are stitched together. Stitching artifacts appears as lines separating adjacent subvolumes. Despite the fact that minor stitching artifacts with limited impact on image quality can be tolerated, important stitching artifacts (Fig. 1.6) not only impact on image quality and interpretation but also hinder quantitative analysis of data sets. There are some ways to prevent the occurrence of stitching artifacts: ask the patient to stop breating during acquisition, maintain a stable probe position on the chest, reduce the number of subvolumes to acquire in patients with irregular heart rhythm. Last generation 3DE systems offer single beat full volume acquisition to be used to obtain 3DE data sets in uncooperative patients and in patients with irregular arrhythmias.

Dropout artifacts appear as false holes in volume rendered 3D surfaces where no real holes are present. The cause of dopout artifacts are structures (typically normal interatrial septum, aortic valve cusps, tricuspid valve leaflets) that are too thin to reflect enough echo signal intensity and appear as a loss in the 3D surface. Visual assessment of whether a signal loss on a surface is a true defect or a dropout artifact is not always that easy. The use of 2DE and 3DE color flow is very useful since it will not show any flow through false defects.

Blurring or blooming artifacts are usually caused by inaccurate voxel interpolation among distant image lines that creates an unsharp volume rendering of structures. These artifacts are inversely proportional to line density (i.e. spatial resolution). Blurring refers to the unsharp display of thin structures (e.g. mitral leaflets, chordae tendinee etc) that appear thicker than they actually are. Blooming refers to the unsharp and excessive representation of highly echoreflective structures (e.g. pace—maker wires, mechanical valve prostheses etc.). However, in most of the cases both blurring and blooming artifacts coexist.

Gain artifacts are related to over- or under-gain setting during acquisition. Over-gain might cause the occurrence of an effect of dust or smoke within the cardiac chamber which may obscure the structures of interest. Under-gain might create dropout artifacts. To avoid these artifacts, it is recommended that acquisition should be performed with the gain set a little higher than with conventional 2DE to avoid under-gain issues. Then, 3DE data sets stored as raw data can always be postprocessed and gain settings can be adjusted at the desired level.

## Overview of Clinical Applications

3DE is currently considered one of the most versatile and promising techniques for the diagnosis, risk stratification and management of patients with cardiovascular diseases. Its introduction has revolutionized the traditional echocardiographic imaging and enabled the acquisition of all cardiac structures of interest in a single pyramidal data set which could be sliced in multiple tomographic views or/and analyzed by dedicated software packages in order to obtain reliable diagnostic information on cardiac anatomy and (patho-) physiology without using geometrical assumptions.

In 2012, the European Association of Echocardiography and American Society of Echocardiography published recommendations to provide clinicians with a systematic approach to 3D data set acquisition, display and analysis [5]. In 2015, a joint update of the recommendations for cardiac chamber quantitation using echocardiography identified 3DE as the most accurate and reproducible echocardiographic technique for accurate quantification of both LV and RV size and function [6]. Additionally, due to the development of high quality real-time 3D transesophageal echocardiography (TEE) the method has now been integrated into clinical tools for guiding complex interventional catheter procedures [29] and represents a valuable source of information for 3D printing of cardiac structures [32].

### *Left Ventricular Morphology and Function*

Accurate and reproducible assessment of LV volumes and function are pivotal for diagnosis, treatment, and risk stratification of many cardiovascular disorders. In this context, LV quantification can be considered the most important contribution of

3DE to the routine clinical practice. Modern software packages enable user-friendly and fast semi- or fully-automated volumetric analysis of LV, which unlike M-mode or Simpson's method does not rely on geometric assumptions regarding the LV shape (Fig. 1.21). Since the analysis of 3DE data only requires minimum manipulation by an operator, reproducibility of the technique is greatly improved.

3DE volumetric analysis of LV has been extensively validated against CMR and other imaging modalities (computed tomography (CT), nuclear imaging) [33]. It was demonstrated to be less labour-intensive, more reproducible and accurate compared to conventional 2DE for LV volumes and ejection fraction measurement. Re-alignment of planes and adjustment of the LV chamber size to its maximum longitudinal axis length and avoidance of any assumption about cardiac chamber shape are important advantages offered by 3DE over conventional 2DE.

Foreshortening of LV longitudinal axis is a major cause of volume underestimation by 2DE, which accounts for the larger bias observed in comparison with 3DE [6]. Results of recent meta-analyses conducted on 95 studies demonstrated that 3DE also generally underestimates LV volumes compared to CMR, while the accuracy of EF measurement is excellent [33–35]. According to another meta-analysis, underestimation of LV volume is not as significant as that observed with 2DE; there was also less variability than 2DE when compared to a reference standard [36]. Race-, age and gender-specific reference ranges of LV volumes and EF established on large cohorts of healthy individuals were published to facilitate the standardization of the technique and encourage its routine implementation in the echocardiographic laboratories [23, 37, 38]. On the basis of weighted average values derived from these studies gender-specific upper limits of the normal range for LV volumes have been established and included in the recent chamber quantification recommendations (Table 1.1) [6].

Through displaying the entire myocardial volume in a multi-slice panel (Fig. 1.29), 3DE allows for a comprehensive assessment of the whole LV circumference to be performed and improves the accuracy of visual regional wall motion assessment not limited to several predefined regions of the LV available in standard 2DE views. A more accurate evaluation of regional wall motion achieved using 3DE improves the diagnostic accuracy of pharmacological stress echocardiography in ischemic heart disease [30].

Despite this added clinical value compared with conventional 2DE and Doppler echocardiography [4], 3DE analysis of the LV is not free from specific limitations. As a rule, good image quality is a prerequisite for an accurate identification of endocardial borders. 3D image acquisition should also focus on including the entire LV within the pyramidal data set. To ensure an accurate identification of end-systole, the temporal resolution of 3D imaging should be set to a maximum without compromising spatial resolution. It also requires regular heart rate and patients' cooperation for breath holding. Nevertheless, specific advantages of 3DE over other imaging modalities including its portability, absence of ionizing radiation, and the ability to examine patients with pacemakers and defibrillators overweight aforementioned limitations in almost all clinical settings.

**Table 1.1** Two- and three-dimensional abnormality thresholds for cardiac chamber volumes

| Chamber | Parameter | 2DE Abnormality threshold | 3DE Abnormality threshold |
| --- | --- | --- | --- |
| Left ventricle [6] | EDVi (ml/m$^2$) | | |
| | Men | >74 | >79 |
| | Women | >61 | >71 |
| | ESVi (ml/m$^2$) | | |
| | Men | >31 | >32 |
| | Women | >24 | >28 |
| | EF (%) | | |
| | Men | ≤52 | <52 |
| | Women | ≤54 | <54 |
| Right ventricle [24] | EDVi (ml/m$^2$) | | |
| | Men | – | >87 |
| | Women | – | >74 |
| | ESVi (ml/m$^2$) | | |
| | Men | – | >44 |
| | Women | – | >36 |
| | EF (%) | – | <45 |
| Left atrium [3] | Vmax (ml/m$^2$) | >34 | <47 |
| | VpreA (ml/m$^2$) | >22 | <31 |
| | Vmin (ml/m$^2$) | >14 | >19 |
| Right atrium [25] | Vmax (ml/m$^2$) | >39 | >44 |
| | VpreA (ml/m$^2$) | >28 | >28 |
| | Vmin (ml/m$^2$) | >20 | >20 |

*Abbreviations*: *3DE* three-dimensional echocardiography, *EDVi* index of end-diastolic volume, *EF* ejection fraction, *ESVi* index of end-systolic volume, *Vmax* maximal volume, *Vmin* minimal volume, *VpreA* volume pre A wave on the ECG

## *Right Ventricular Morphology and Function*

Quantitative assessment of the right ventricle (RV) by conventional echocardiography is a challenging task due to its complex asymmetric geometry (complicating visualisation of both inflow and outflow tracts in the same view), highly trabeculated endocardial borders, lack of precise anatomic landmarks, and unfavourable position of the RV in the chest. Furthermore, 2DE diameters of the RV vary significantly with minor rotation or tilting the transducer and may be inaccurate leading to an under- or overestimation of RV size [2].

3DE opened a new era in echocardiographic evaluation of the RV. It allows to obtain all three parts of the RV in the same dataset with adequate temporal and spatial resolution (Fig. 1.24). This dataset can be further analysed using dedicated software packages to obtain the mapping of the RV endocardial surface and measure the RV volumes and function without using geometrical assumptions or approximations (Fig. 1.26).

RV 3DE measurements closely correlate (but slightly underestimate) with RV volumes measured by CMR [22, 39–42]. In the most recent meta-analysis aimed to explore the accuracy of different imaging modalities (2DE, 3DE, radionuclide ventriculography, CT, gated single-photon emission CT, and invasive cardiac cineventriculography) for RV ejection fraction using CMR as reference method, 3DE has proven to be the most reliable technique, overestimating the RV ejection fraction only by 1.16% (range −0.59 to 2.92%) [43]. Normative data for 3DE RV volumes and ejection fraction including age-, body size-, and sex-specific reference values based on

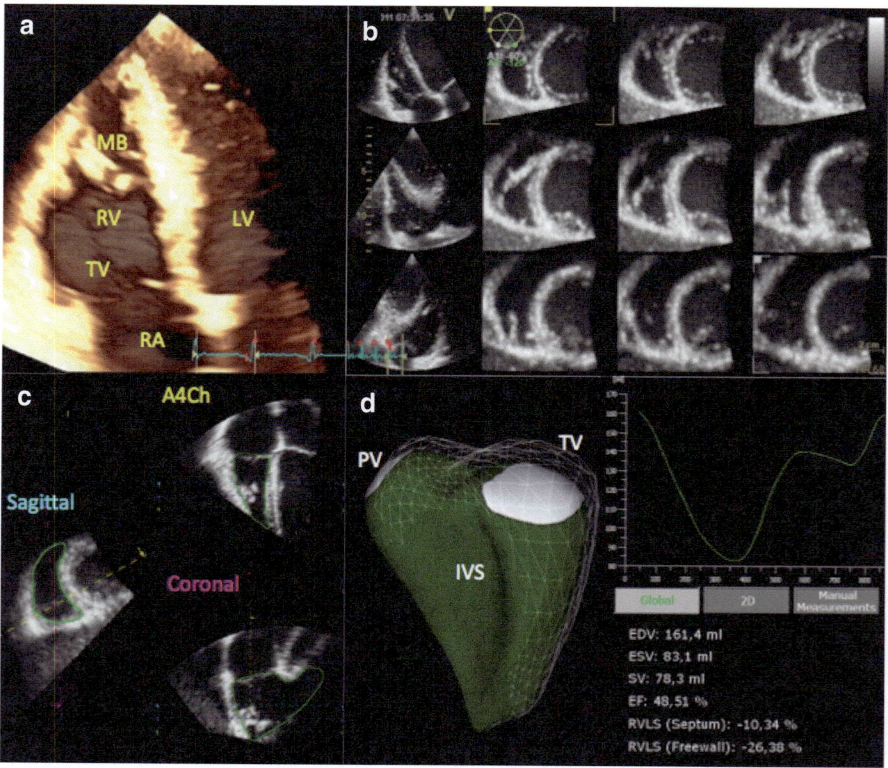


**Fig. 1.26** Display modes of a 3D data set of the right ventricular obtained from the RV-focused apical 4-chamber view using full-volume multi-beat acquisition (four to six consecutive beats) with adjusted depth and volume width to encompass the entire RV. (**a**) Volume rendering demonstrating the RV anatomy; (**b**) Multi (12)- slice mode including 3 longitudinal (0°, 60° and 120°), and 9 transversal equidistant tomographic views between the apex and the base of the RV mainly used for regional wall motion and RV shape analysis; (**c**) Semiautomatic identification of the RV endocardial surface in the right ventricular short-axis, four-chamber, and coronal views; (**d**) Surface rendered three-dimensional model of the right ventricle (*green model*) combining the wire-frame (*white cage*) display of the end-diastolic volume. Surface rendered dynamic model changes its size and shape throughout the cardiac cycle enabling the visual assessment of the RV dynamics and quantitation of RV volumes and ejection fraction. *EDV* end-diastolic volume, *EF* ejection fraction, *ESV* end-systolic volume, *IVS* interventricular septum, *LV* left ventricle, *MB* moderator band, *PV* pulmonic valve, *RA* right atrum, *RV* right ventricle, *SV* stroke volume, *TV* tricuspid valve

large cohort studies of healthy volunteers is also available (Table 1.1) [24]. Inclusion of recommendations for 3D analysis of the RV volumes and EF in laboratories with appropriate 3D platforms and experience in the most recent edition of chamber quantification guidelines highlights the importance of 3DE in the assessment of RV [6].

Limitations of 3D volumetric analysis of the RV include dependency on image quality and the position of the RV in the anterior mediastinum, immediately below the sternum. This may cause possible dropout of the RV anterior wall and incomplete inclusion of the whole RV (the RV outflow tract is often incompletely acquire) in the pyramidal data set in case of severe dilation.

## *Mitral Valve Evaluation*

3DE contributed a lot into our understanding of the mitral valve (MV) structure [44]. The unique ability of 3DE to display the MV *en-face* from either the atrial or the ventricular perspective enabling precise anatomical and functional analysis of the valve and the surrounding cardiac structures makes 3DE, especially 3D TEE, the most useful imaging modality for the diagnosis of MV diseases and to guide their management (Fig. 1.27).

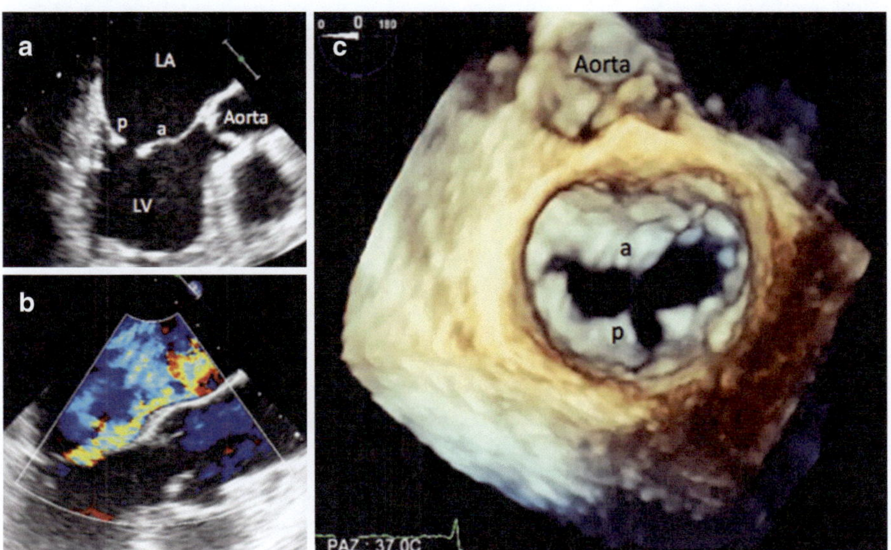


**Fig. 1.27** The added value of transesophageal 3DE in diagnosis of cleft of posterior leaflet of the mitral valve. (Panels **a, b**) Mid-esophageal long axis 2DE views showing no significant morphological abnormalities of the mitral valve leaflets, but severe mitral regurgitation with highly eccentric regurgitant jet in color Doppler. (**c**) En-face view of the mitral valve obtained by transesophageal 3DE clearly demonstrating cleft of posterior mitral valve leaflet, which was not visible from standard 2DE views. Abbreviations: *a* anterior leaflet of MV, *LA* left atrium, *LV* left ventricle, *p* posterior leaflet of MV

3DE is ideally suited to identify the mechanism and assess the severity of mitral regurgitation (MR) (Fig. 1.28) by allowing precise evaluation of the geometry of mitral annulus, leaflet tenting volume, coaptation distance, leaflets surface, and the relationship between the valve leaflets and papillary muscles. Moreover, the introduction of 3DE color mode capable of the acquisition of the whole regurgitant jet to visualize its 3D volume, origin and extension in relation to adjacent structures, has led to a change of a paradigm by understanding the vena contracta (VC) as being strongly asymmetric in the majority of patients and etiologies (Fig. 1.28d) [45]. The effective regurgitant orifice area can be directly measured from a 3D color data set

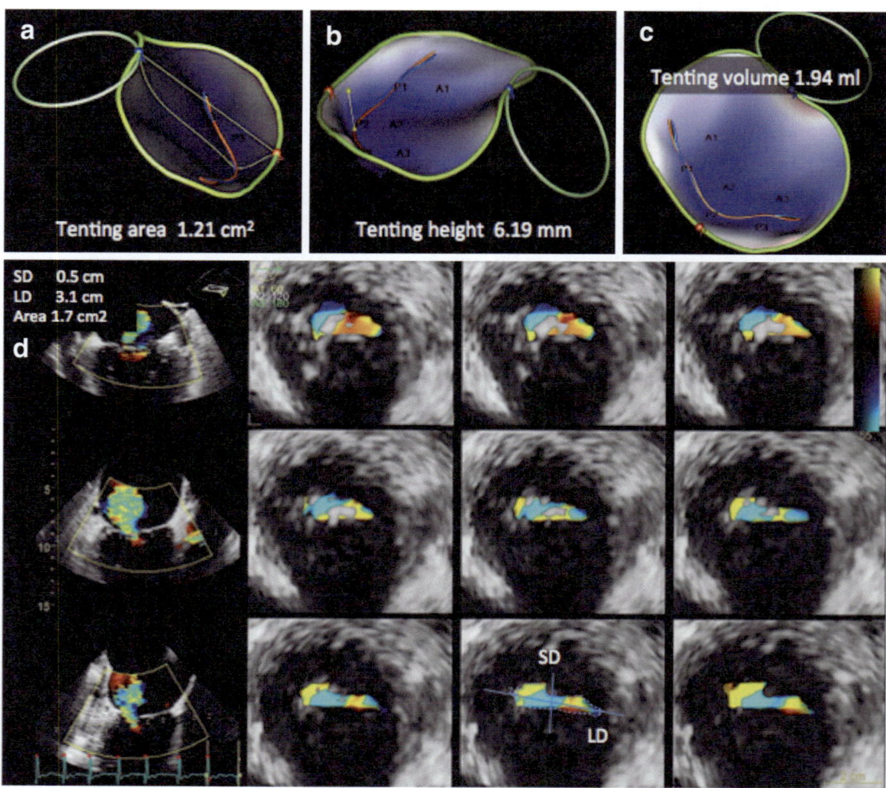


**Fig. 1.28** The role of 3DE in assessment of the mechanisms and severity of functional mitral regurgitation. (Panels **a–c**) Semi-automated quantitative analysis of mitral valve morphology and annulus geometry in a patient with functional mitral regurgitation enabling accurate measurement of several parameters (such as tenting height, tenting area and tenting volume). (Panel **d**) Multi-slice display of the 3DE color data set, demonstrating the non-circular shape of the vena contracta. Alignment of the cut-planes perpendicular to the regurgitant jet allows correct identification of the regurgitant orifice area and its quantitative analysis including largest and sortest diameters and real anatomic regurgitant orifice area, avoiding geometrical assumptions about its shape, flow convergence limitations and distorsions. Correct visualization of regurgitant flow, particularly eccentric ones, improves accuracy in effective regurgitant orifice area quantification. Abbreviations: *A* area, *LD* largest diameter, *SD* shortest diameter

without geometrical assumption about its shape or the morphology of the proximal isovelocity surface area (PISA) [46]. Application of color Doppler real-time 3DE for the assessment of MR severity based on VC area and 3D PISA has been validated in the recent studies [47–50]. To expedite its routine clinical use longitudinal observational studies evaluating the clinical and prognostic value of 3DE derived measurements of MV geometry are vitally needed.

The actual added value of 3DE is the possibility to visualize the MV in the beating heart from the same perspective as in the operating room, for a precise identification and sizing of the prolapsing scallops, assessment of disease severity and surgical planning [44, 51]. Several studies consistently reported that 3DE was superior to 2DE providing more accurate, easy and fast identification of prolapsing segment(s) [52, 53].

Finally, 3DE has significant incremental value in assessment of mitral stenosis (Fig. 1.29). It allows for a direct planimetry of MV area to be performed avoiding the numerous limitations of conventionally used Doppler (angle dependence, load dependence, influence of cardiac rhythm and hemodynamics) or 2DE techniques (overestimation of valve orifice area due to fixed orientation of the 2D plane, which is frequently not orthogonal to the direction of the mitral funnel and do not cross its narrowest area). Cropping the 3D data set helps to identify the correct orientation

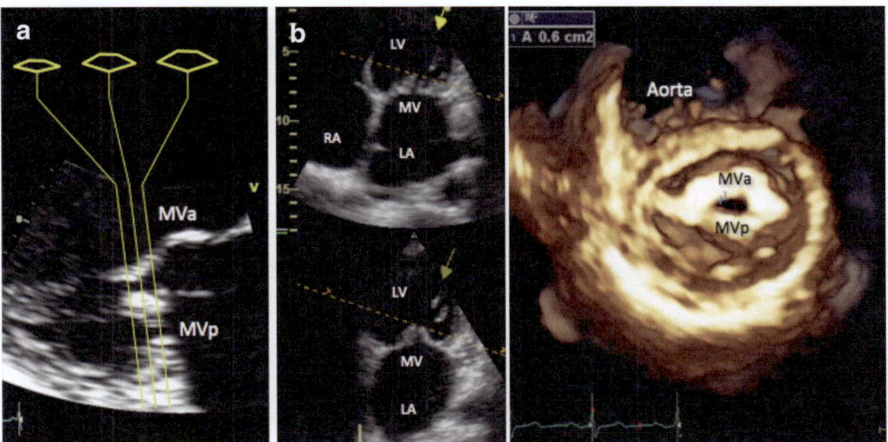


**Fig. 1.29** The added diagnostic value of 3DE in assessment of mitral stenosis. (Panel **a**) Parasternal long axis view focused on the mitral valve demonstrating the influence of correct positioning of the cut plane on the size of the residual MV orifice area (*yellow exagons*). If the cut plane does not cross the narrowest area and/or is not perpendicular to the direction of the mitral funnel, it may lead to significant underestimation of the severity of mitral stenosis. (Panel **b**) Volume rendering display of the mitral valve from the left ventricular perspective in a patient with rheumatic mitral stenosis. The limited opening of the mitral valve, thickened leaflets and fused commissures are well visualized. The cut planes (*dashed, thin yellow lines*) shown in 2DE slices are optimized to be perpendicular to the opening direction of the residual mitral orifice to obtain an accurate orifice area planimetry. Abbreviations: *A* residual MV orifice area, *LA* left atrium, *LV* left ventricle, *MV* mitral valve, *MVa* anterior leaflet of mitral valve, *MVp* posterior leaflet of mitral valve, *RA* right atrium

and position of the cut plane for obtaining the real smallest area of the stenotic valve. 3DE has shown the best agreement with cardiac catheterization for residual MV orifice area quantification and better reproducibility than 2DE [31, 54]. Recently a new 3DE scoring system for mitral stenosis has been proposed [55]. It has proven to be feasible and highly reproducible for the assessment of MV morphology and overcame the main limitations of existing 2DE systems including the ability to distinguish leaflets calcification and subvalvular apparatus involvement – the critical aspects in predicting of success of an intervention [55, 56].

## *Tricuspid Valve Evaluation*

Accurate assessment of morphology and function of the tricuspid valve (TV) is important for clinical management of cardiac patients. 3DE gained increased attention over the past decade as conventional 2DE does not allow a simultaneous visualization of the three leaflets in most of the patients [57, 58] and its accuracy in measuring the tricuspid annulus size is suboptimal [59, 60].

3DE is the single echocardiographic technique capable of providing an en-face visualization of the whole TV from both the atrial and ventricular perspective during the cardiac cycle to allow the accurate assessment of leaflet morphology, coaptation, separation of the commissures, and measurement of tricuspid annular area (Fig. 1.30) [61]. Although obtaining high quality en-face view of TV by 3DE tends to be more challenging than of MV, it was shown to be feasible in up to 90% of patients [58, 62] demonstrating an incremental benefit for definitive leaflet identification and localization of tricuspid leaflet pathology

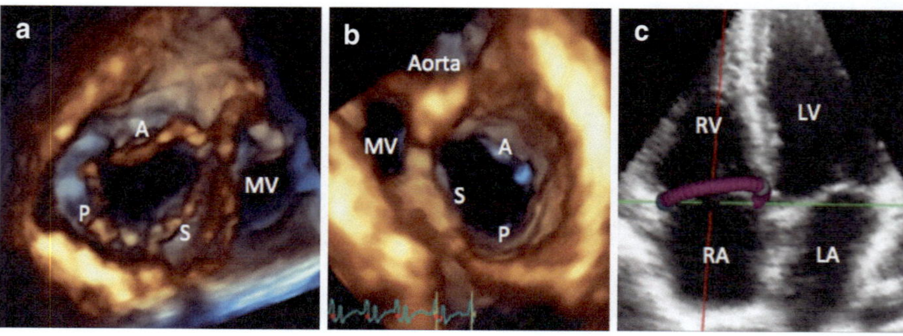


**Fig. 1.30** Comprehensive assessment of the tricuspid valve morphology and function by transthoracic 3DE. (Panel **a**) En face view of the tricuspid valve from the right ventricular perspective demonstrating the complex anatomy of tricuspid valve annulus and leaflets. (Panel **b**) En face view of the tricuspid valve from the right atrial perspective ("surgical view"). (Panel **c**) Semi-automated reconstruction of tricuspid annulus demonstrating its nonplanar shape, with the postero-septal portion being the lowest and the antero-septal portion the highest. Abbreviations: *A* anterior tricuspid valve leaflet, *LA* left atrium, *LV* left ventricle, *MV* mitral valve, *P* posterior tricuspid valve leaflet, *RA* right atrium, *RV* right ventricle, *S* septal tricuspid valve leaflet

[57, 58]. Furthermore, 3DE is the unique method enabling a reliable assessment of actual tricuspid annulus size and morphology (Fig. 1.30c) [59, 60], which is pivotal in determining the need for tricuspid annuloplasty in patients undergoing left-sided valve surgery [61] and for planning of percutaneous TV interventions [63]. Using 3DE, TV annulus under normal conditions was found to have an elliptical nonplanar shape, more flattened and oval than the saddle-shaped mitral annulus. It was shown to be highly dynamic during cardiac cycle with 25% fractional shortening and 30–40% of area decrease during atrial systole with various factors, including age, gender, and loading conditions affecting its sizing accuracy [59, 63].

The transthoracic 3DE plays an important role in visualization of device-lead position in right heart chambers. Using this technique it was demonstrated that the leads positioned against tricuspid leaflets impinge upon or restrict leaflet motion, resulting in a greater severity of TR, compared with leads positioned within the commissure or at the centre of TV (Fig. 1.31), encouraging the routine clinical use of this imaging modality for post- and intra-procedural monitoring [62, 64].

Although less clinically relevant than for MV, 3DE has been shown to have an added value in the assessment of the TV orifice area in patients with TV rheumatic stenosis [65] or carcinoid disease [66], and systematic evaluation of leaflet prolapse, flail segments and chordae rupture [27] (Fig. 1.32).

The use of color Doppler 3DE holds the great promise to provide an integrated quantitative assessment of tricuspid regurgitant volume regardless of the shape of the regurgitant orifice. Quantitative evaluation of TR severity by 3DE planimetry of VC area is feasible in most patients, even those with atrial fibrillation [67]. The reported cut-offs of VC area by color 3DE suggestive of severe TR were >0.57 cm$^2$ in functional TR and >0.36 cm$^2$ regardless of TR mechanism [67, 68]. Another approach for a more accurate quantification of TR severity is 3D PISA method (Fig. 1.33). It was demonstrated to be useful for clinical use and more accurate than 2D PISA, even though the comparison was done against non-universally recognized reference methods (3D color planimetry and quantitative 2D Doppler echocardiography based on tricuspid and pulmonary stroke volumes) [69]. The lack of validation studies and established cut-off values as well as variations introduced by technical factors (inadequate breath holding, gain changes, color baseline adjustments, low temporal/spatial resolution by transthoracic approach) and arrhythmias limit the current clinical implementation of these methods.

## *Guiding Interventional Procedures*

Regardless of the type of the intervention, 3DE plays a critical role in the (i) diagnosis of the defect, (ii) device sizing, (iii) intra-procedural guidance, and (iv) post-procedural evaluation of device function and potential complications [5, 70]. During percutaneous closure of atrial septal defects 3DE can be used to assess the location

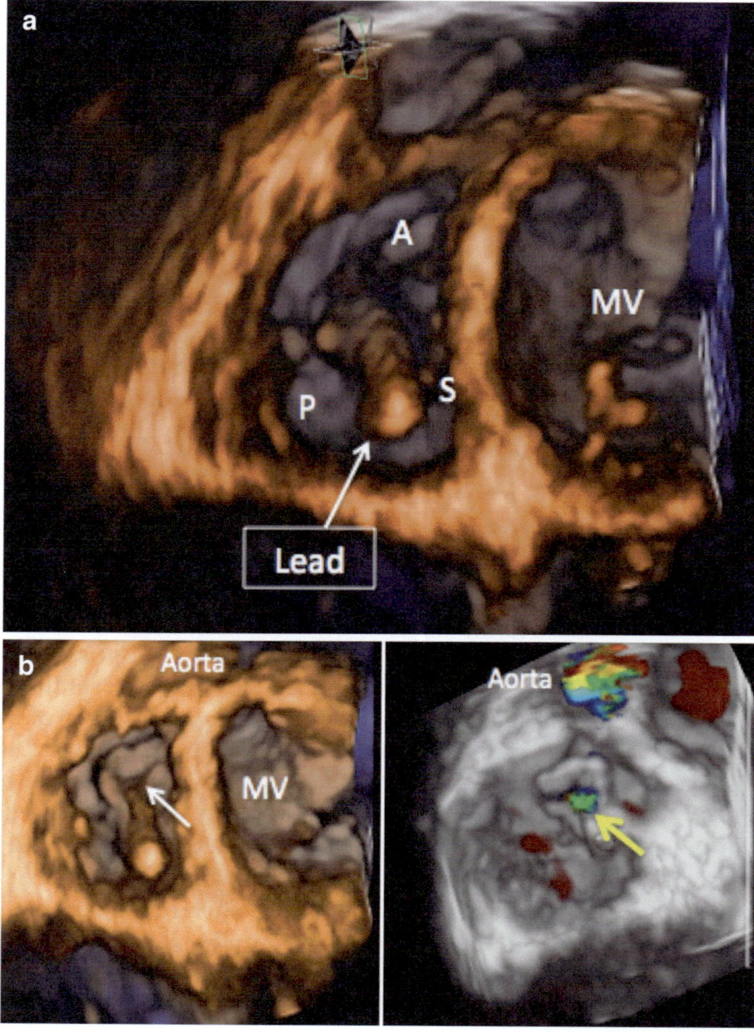



**Fig. 1.31** The role of transthoracic 3DE in visualization of the device-lead position within the tricuspid annulus and its relationships with tricuspid valve leaflets. (Panel **a**) En-face view of the tricuspid valve in diastole from the ventricular perspective showing a pacemaker lead positioned in the centre of opened tricuspid valve with non interference with leaflet motion. (Panel **b**) 3D volume rendering and 3D color of tricuspid valve during systole demonstrating minimal coaptation defect at the basis of the lead (*white arrow*) corresponding to minimal tricuspid regurgitant orifice area at 3D color during systole (*yellow arrow*). Abbreviations: *A* anterior tricuspid valve leaflet, *MV* mitral valve, *P* posterior tricuspid valve leaflet, *S* septal tricuspid valve leaflet

and size of the defect as well as its spatial relationship with the other cardiac structures. An advantage of 3D TEE over conventional TEE is its ability to obtain en-face views of the defect from both the atria, that helps to evaluate the dynamic morphology of complex atrial septal defects (such as those with elliptical shape or with

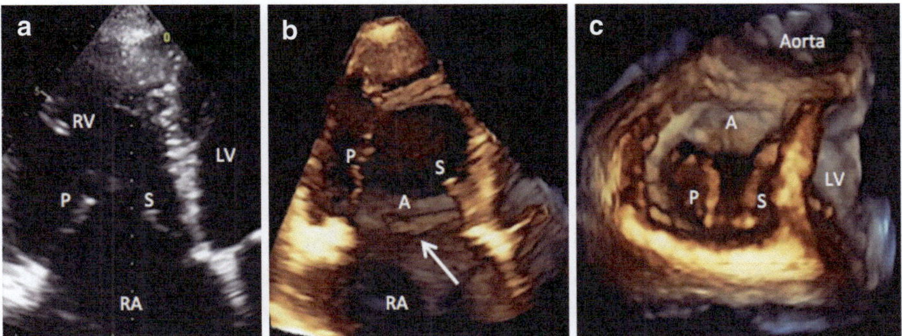

**Fig. 1.32** The added value of transthoracic 3DE in diagnosis of the flail tricuspid valve leaflet. (Panel **a**) Conventional 2DE apical view focused on the tricuspid valve demonstrating dilatation of the tricuspid annulus with no significant abnormalities of visible parts of the leaflets in a patient with severe tricuspid regurgitation. (Panel **b**) 3DE volume rendering of the tricuspid valve and right heart chambers demonstrating the flailing of the anterior tricuspid leaflets (*arrow*) located beyond the cut-plane, explaining why it was not visible by 2DE. (Panel **c**) En-face view of the tricuspid valve from ventricular perspective allowing to assess spatial relationship of tricuspid leaflets with the other cardiac structures and the correct identification of the flailing leaflet as the anterior one. Abbreviations: *A* anterior tricuspid valve leaflet, *LV* left ventricle, *P* posterior tricuspid valve leaflet, *RA* right atrium, *RV* right ventricle, *S* septal tricuspid valve leaflet

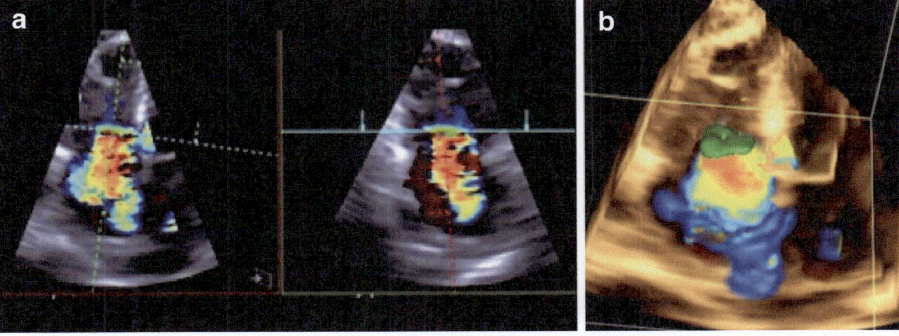

**Fig. 1.33** Quantification of tricuspid regurgitation severity by 3D proximal isovelocity surface area method (3D PISA). (**a**) Two orthogonal cut-planes demonstrating asymmetric shape of regurgitant jet. (**b**) Volume rendering of the tricuspid regurgitant color flow jet at mid-systole shows the complex non-circular and flat shape of the PISA

multiple fenestrations), and assess the device deployment position post procedure. It also helps to appreciate the location of wires and devices in real time, and to display 3D color demonstrating the presence and direction of potential leaks around the device.

3D TEE is widely used in patients scheduled for transcatheter aortic valve implantation (TAVI) for aortic annulus sizing, characterization of the periannular region (cusps, LV outflow tract, and proximal aortic root) and assessment of the position of coronary ostia relative to valve cusps [71]. Several studies demonstrated that 3D TEE measurements of annular aortic annulus are accurate and reproducible and correlate well with the reference standard CT [72, 73], however 3DE still may be hindered by severe calcification, limited image resolution and operator inexperience. During the TAVI procedure, 3D TEE helps in positioning of the catheters and prosthetic valve, whereas after the transcatheter valve deployment, it provides rapid and accurate assessment of valve location and function, coronary patency, MV and ventricular function, and allows monitoring for complications [71].

TTE is the primary screening tool in candidates for percutaneous edge-to-edge MV repair technique using MitraClip. Moreover, 3D TEE imaging provides the clear delineation of the involved segment(s), intra-procedural guidance (optimizing the position of the trans-septal puncture, correct placing the device, clip deployment), and en-face visualization and quantitation of the residual MR by 3DE planimetry of VC area after the clip has been placed [29].

3DE has also proven accurate in the assessment of prosthetic valves, as 3D 'en-face' surgical view of the valve is extremely helpful for determining its function and defining the presence, origin, and direction of regurgitant jets [74]. 3D TEE has become increasingly important in patients with paravalvular leaks as it is uniquely capable of demonstrating the irregular shape of the defects, able to identify multiple defects, and provide accurate sizing. During the interventional procedures, 3D TEE is used to continuously assist wire and device deployment, and then to assess residual regurgitation [70].

Finally, 3D TEE is pivotal to assess the suitability of the left atrial appendage anatomy for the device closure. It is used for selecting the optimal device type and size, guidance in trans-septal puncture, post-deployment device assessment, and for follow-up imaging after the device implantation [70].


## Future Directions

3DE is the most recent among the various echocardiography techniques and the one with the largest room for future improvement.

The expected improvement in both temporal and spatial resolution will allow to acquire larger data sets which will include the whole heart and to change our way of thinking. Not anymore considering LV, RV, atrial function as the various cardiac structures work in isolation, but we will assess and understand the "cardiac function", being able to appreciate the interrelationships among cardiac structures (i.e. atrio-ventricular coupling, ventricular interdependence etc) and assess their relative contribution to "cardiac function".

Highly performant fully automated software packages will allow accurate and reproducible quantitative analysis of the geometry and function of cardiac chambers [75] and valve structures [76, 77] independent on the expertise of the single echocardiographer, to provide clinicians, interventionists and cardiac surgeons reliable data to be used to address management, plan and monitoring interventions, and assess their outcome.

3DE data sets potentially allow morphometric quantitation of every cardiac structure. However, to obtain this goal we need dedicated software packages taking into account morphological the same software cannot be used to display and quantitate the aorta and the mitral valve) and functional (e.g. the atria have a three phases function and not just diastole and systole like ventricles) peculiarities of the various cardiac structures. In particular, we lack software packages to assess the right heart structures. 3DE analysis of RV shape and mechanics in various directions (i.e. longitudinal, circumferential and area strain) is a promising area in future clinical practice. In pulmonary hypertension patients significant correlation with RV ejection fraction was demonstrated for 3D global longitudinal strain [78] and for area strain with the latter being a strong independent predictor of death [79]. Finally, recently developed methodology for analysis of 3DE-derived global and regional RV shape indices based on analysis of the RV curvature demonstrated good results in patients with pulmonary arterial hypertension, showing that the curvature of the RV inflow tract is a more robust predictor of death than RV ejection fraction, volumes, or other regional curvature indices [80].

Finally, 3DE data set can be shown in more effective ways than just displayed on flat screen monitors. Availability of volumetric data allows both the 3D printing [32] and the holographic display [81, 82] of cardiac structures. Printing solid three-dimensional models of cardiac structures or displaying them in holographic modality will allow detailed morphological and quantitative analysis of their geometry and has the potential for rapid integration into clinical practice to assist with decisionmaking, surgical or interventional planning and teaching.


## Conclusions


3DE is an established imaging technique, which permits a comprehensive evaluation of cardiac anatomy and function without pre-established geometrical assumptions regarding cardiac structures' morphology. BY displaying anatomically sound images of the heart it allows for a more reproducible and objective echocardiographic assessment of cardiac structures and improve the communication with non echocardiographers. Over the last decade it has evolved into an essential clinical tool offering new diagnostic and prognostic capabilities almost free from 2DE limitations. It has changed the paradigm in assessment of the atrio-ventricular valves morphology and function; the 3DE-based volumetric analysis of the LV and RV has developed into the most accurate, reproducible and extensively validated method of evaluation of the ventricular size and function; and, finally, 3DE became a critical step in guiding intervention procedures, providing both anatomic and haemodynamic information. Further improvements in image quality, spatial and temporal resolution, acquisition process, and data analysis will make 3DE the standard echocardiographic examination procedure in the nearest future.

# References


1. Surkova E, Muraru D, Aruta P, et al. Current clinical applications of three-dimensional echocardiography: When the technique makes the difference. Curr Cardiol Rep. 2016;18:19.
2. Surkova E, Muraru D, Iliceto S, Badano LP. The use of multimodality cardiovascular imaging to assess right ventricular size and function. Int J Cardiol. 2016;214:54–69.
3. Badano LP, Miglioranza MH, Mihaila S, et al. Left Atrial Volumes and Function by Three-Dimensional Echocardiography: Reference Values, Accuracy, Reproducibility, and Comparison With Two-Dimensional Echocardiographic Measurements. Circ Cardiovasc Imaging. 2016;9:pii: e004229.
4. Badano LP. The clinical benefits of adding a third dimension to assess the left ventricle with echocardiography. Scientifica. 2014;2014:1–18.
5. Lang RM, Badano LP, Tsang W, et al. EAE/ASE recommendations for image acquisition and display using three-dimensional echocardiography. Eur Heart J Cardiovasc Imaging. 2012;13:1–46.
6. Lang RM, Badano LP, Mor-Avi V, et al. Recommendations for cardiac chamber quantification by echocardiography in adults: an update from the American Society of Echocardiography and the European Association of Cardiovascular Imaging. Eur Heart J Cardiovasc Imaging. 2015;16:233–70.
7. Dekker DL, Piziali RL, Dong Jr E. A system for ultrasonically imaging the human heart in three dimensions. Comput Biomed Res. 1974;7:544–53.
8. Moritz WE, Shreve PL. A microprocessor based spatial locating system for use with diagnostic ultrasound. IEEE Trans Biomed Eng. 1976;64:966–74.
9. Raab FH, Blood EB, Steiner TO. al. e. Magnetic position and orientation tracking system. IEEE Trans Aerospace Elec Sys. 1979;15:709–18.
10. Geiser EA, Lupkiewicz SM, Christie LG, Ariet M, Conetta DA, Conti CR. A framework for three-dimensional time-varying reconstruction of the human left ventricle: sources of error and estimation of their magnitude. Computers and biomedical research, an international journal. 1980;13:225–41.
11. Ghosh A, Nanda NC, Maurer G. Three-dimensional reconstruction of echo-cardiographic images using the rotation method. Ultrasound Med Biol. 1982;8:655–61.
12. Matsumoto M, Matsuo H, Kitabatake A, et al. Three-dimensional echocardiograms and two-dimensional echocardiographic images at desired planes by a computerized system. Ultrasound Med Biol. 1977;3:163–78.
13. Matsumoto M, Inoue M, Tamura S, Tanaka K, Abe H. Three-dimensional echocardiography for spatial visualization and volume calculation of cardiac structures. J Clin Ultrasound. 1981;9:157–65.
14. Nanda N, Pinheiro L, Sanyal R, et al. Multiplane transesophagal echocardiographic imaging and three-dimensional reconstruction. Echocardiography. 1992;9:687–94.
15. Pandian NG, Nanda NC, Schwartz SL, et al. Three-dimensional and four-dimensional transesophageal echocardiographic imaging of the heart and aorta in humans using a computed tomographic imaging probe. Echocardiography. 1992;9:677–87.
16. Flachskampf FA, Franke A, Job FP, et al. Three-dimensional reconstruction of cardiac structures from transesophageal echocardiography. Am J Card Imaging. 1995;9:141–7.
17. Vogel M, Losch S. Dynamic three-dimensional echocardiography with a computed tomography imaging probe: initial clinical experience with transthoracic application in infants and children with congenital heart defects. Br Heart J. 1994;71:462–7.
18. Ludomirsky A, Vermilion R, Nesser J, et al. Transthoracic real-time three-dimensional echocardiography using the rotational scanning approach for data acquisition. Echocardiography. 1994;11:599–606.
19. Kupferwasser I, Mohr-Kahaly S, Stahr P, et al. Transthoracic three-dimensional echocardiographic volumetry of distorted left ventricles using rotational scanning. J Am Soc Echocardiogr. 1997;10:840–52.

20. Sheikh K, Smith SW, von Ramm O, Kisslo J. Real-time, three-dimensional echocardiography: feasibility and initial use. Echocardiography. 1991;8:119–25.
21. von Ramm OT, Smith SW. Real time volumetric ultrasound imaging system. Journal of digital imaging: the official journal of the Society for Computer Applications in Radiology. 1990;3:261–6.
22. Muraru D, Spadotto V, Cecchetto A, et al. New speckle-tracking algorithm for right ventricular volume analysis from three-dimensional echocardiographic data sets: validation with cardiac magnetic resonance and comparison with the previous analysis tool. Eur Heart J Cardiovasc Imaging. 2016;17:1279–89.
23. Muraru D, Badano LP, Peluso D, et al. Comprehensive analysis of left ventricular geometry and function by three-dimensional echocardiography in healthy adults. JAmSocEchocardiogr. 2013;26:618–28.
24. Maffessanti F, Muraru D, Esposito R, et al. Age-, body size-, and sex-specific reference values for right ventricular volumes and ejection fraction by three-dimensional echocardiography: a multicenter echocardiographic study in 507 healthy volunteers. Circ Cardiovasc Imaging. 2013;6:700–10.
25. Peluso D, Badano LP, Muraru D, et al. Right atrial size and function assessed with three-dimensional and speckle-tracking echocardiography in 200 healthy volunteers. Eur Heart J Cardiovasc Imaging. 2013.
26. Muraru D, Cattarina M, Boccalini F, et al. Mitral valve anatomy and function: new insights from three-dimensional echocardiography. J Cardiovasc Med (Hagerstown). 2013;14:91–9.
27. Muraru D, Badano LP, Sarais C, Solda E, Iliceto S. Evaluation of tricuspid valve morphology and function by transthoracic three-dimensional echocardiography. Curr Cardiol Rep. 2011;13:242–9.
28. Muraru D, Badano LP, Vannan M, Iliceto S. Assessment of aortic valve complex by three-dimensional echocardiography: a framework for its effective application in clinical practice. Eur Heart J Cardiovasc Imaging. 2012;13:541–55.
29. Zamorano JL, Badano LP, Bruce C, et al. EAE/ASE recommendations for the use of echocardiography in new transcatheter interventions for valvular heart disease. Eur Heart J. 2011;32:2189–214.
30. Badano LP, Muraru D, Rigo F, et al. High volume-rate three-dimensional stress echocardiography to assess inducible myocardial ischemia: a feasibility study. J Am Soc Echocardiogr. 2010;23:628–35.
31. Zamorano J, Cordeiro P, Sugeng L, et al. Real-time three-dimensional echocardiography for rheumatic mitral valve stenosis evaluation: an accurate and novel approach. J Am Coll Cardiol. 2004;43:2091–6.
32. Farooqi KM, Sengupta PP. Echocardiography and three-dimensional printing: sound ideas to touch a heart. J Am Soc Echocardiogr. 2015;28:398–403.
33. Rigolli M, Anandabaskaran S, Christiansen JP, Whalley GA. Bias associated with left ventricular quantification by multimodality imaging: a systematic review and meta-analysis. Open Heart. 2016;3:e000388.
34. Badano LP, Boccalini F, Muraru D, et al. Current clinical applications of transthoracic three-dimensional echocardiography. J Cardiovasc Ultrasound. 2012;20:1–22.
35. Shimada YJ, Shiota T. A meta-analysis and investigation for the source of bias of left ventricular volumes and function by three-dimensional echocardiography in comparison with magnetic resonance imaging. Am J Cardiol. 2011;107:126–38.
36. Dorosz JL, Lezotte DC, Weitzenkamp DA, Allen LA, Salcedo EE. Performance of 3-dimensional echocardiography in measuring left ventricular volumes and ejection fraction: a systematic review and meta-analysis. J Am Coll Cardiol. 2012;59:1799–808.
37. Aune E, Baekkevar M, Rodevand O, Otterstad JE. Reference values for left ventricular volumes with real-time 3-dimensional echocardiography. Scand Cardiovasc J. 2010;44:24–30.
38. Chahal NS, Lim TK, Jain P, Chambers JC, Kooner JS, Senior R. Population-based reference values for 3D echocardiographic LV volumes and ejection fraction. JACC Cardiovasc Imaging. 2012;5:1191–7.

39. Leibundgut G, Rohner A, Grize L, et al. Dynamic assessment of right ventricular volumes and function by real-time three-dimensional echocardiography: a comparison study with magnetic resonance imaging in 100 adult patients. J Am Soc Echocardiogr. 2010;23:116–26.

40. Gopal AS, Chukwu EO, Iwuchukwu CJ, et al. Normal values of right ventricular size and function by real-time 3-dimensional echocardiography: comparison with cardiac magnetic resonance imaging. J Am Soc Echocardiogr. 2007;20:445–55.

41. Lu X, Nadvoretskiy V, Bu L, et al. Accuracy and reproducibility of real-time three-dimensional echocardiography for assessment of right ventricular volumes and ejection fraction in children. J Am Soc Echocardiogr. 2008;21:84–9.

42. Zhang QB, Sun JP, Gao RF, et al. Feasibility of single-beat full-volume capture real-time three-dimensional echocardiography for quantification of right ventricular volume: validation by cardiac magnetic resonance imaging. Int J Cardiol. 2013;168:3991–5.

43. Pickett CA, Cheezum MK, Kassop D, Villines TC, Hulten EA. Accuracy of cardiac CT, radionucleotide and invasive ventriculography, two- and three-dimensional echocardiography, and SPECT for left and right ventricular ejection fraction compared with cardiac MRI: a meta-analysis. Eur Heart J Cardiovasc Imaging. 2015;16:848–52.

44. Chandra S, Salgo IS, Sugeng L, et al. Characterization of degenerative mitral valve disease using morphologic analysis of real-time three-dimensional echocardiographic images: objective insight into complexity and planning of mitral valve repair. Circ Cardiovasc Imaging. 2011;4:24–32.

45. Buck T, Plicht B. Real-Time Three-Dimensional Echocardiographic Assessment of Severity of Mitral Regurgitation Using Proximal Isovelocity Surface Area and Vena Contracta Area Method. Lessons We Learned and Clinical Implications. Curr Cardiovasc Imaging Rep. 2015;8:38.

46. Chandra S, Salgo IS, Sugeng L, et al. A three-dimensional insight into the complexity of flow convergence in mitral regurgitation: adjunctive benefit of anatomic regurgitant orifice area. Am J Physiol Heart Circ Physiol. 2011;301:H1015–24.

47. Shanks M, Siebelink HM, Delgado V, et al. Quantitative assessment of mitral regurgitation: comparison between three-dimensional transesophageal echocardiography and magnetic resonance imaging. Circ Cardiovasc Imaging. 2010;3:694–700.

48. Marsan NA, Westenberg JJ, Ypenburg C, et al. Quantification of functional mitral regurgitation by real-time 3D echocardiography: comparison with 3D velocity-encoded cardiac magnetic resonance. JACC Cardiovasc Imaging. 2009;2:1245–52.

49. Thavendiranathan P, Liu S, Datta S, et al. Quantification of chronic functional mitral regurgitation by automated 3-dimensional peak and integrated proximal isovelocity surface area and stroke volume techniques using real-time 3-dimensional volume color Doppler echocardiography: in vitro and clinical validation. Circ Cardiovasc Imaging. 2013;6:125–33.

50. Zeng X, Levine RA, Hua L, et al. Diagnostic value of vena contracta area in the quantification of mitral regurgitation severity by color Doppler 3D echocardiography. Circ Cardiovasc Imaging. 2011;4:506–13.

51. Tamborini G, Muratori M, Maltagliati A, et al. Pre-operative transthoracic real-time three-dimensional echocardiography in patients undergoing mitral valve repair: accuracy in cases with simple vs. complex prolapse lesions. Eur J Echocardiogr. 2010;11:778–85.

52. de Groot-de Laat LE, Ren B, McGhie J, et al. The role of experience in echocardiographic identification of location and extent of mitral valve prolapse with 2D and 3D echocardiography. Int J Cardiovasc Imaging. 2016;32:1171–7.

53. Izumo M, Shiota M, Kar S, et al. Comparison of real-time three-dimensional transesophageal echocardiography to two-dimensional transesophageal echocardiography for quantification of mitral valve prolapse in patients with severe mitral regurgitation. Am J Cardiol. 2013;111:588–94.

54. Zamorano J, Perez de Isla L, Sugeng L, et al. Non-invasive assessment of mitral valve area during percutaneous balloon mitral valvuloplasty: role of real-time 3D echocardiography. Eur Heart J. 2004;25:2086–91.

55. Anwar AM, Attia WM, Nosir YF, et al. Validation of a new score for the assessment of mitral stenosis using real-time three-dimensional echocardiography. J Am Soc Echocardiogr. 2010;23:13–22.
56. Soliman OI, Anwar AM, Metawei AK, McGhie JS, Geleijnse ML, Ten Cate FJ. New Scores for the Assessment of Mitral Stenosis Using Real-Time Three-Dimensional Echocardiography. Curr Cardiovasc Imaging Rep. 2011;4:370–7.
57. Addetia K, Yamat M, Mediratta A, et al. Comprehensive Two-Dimensional Interrogation of the Tricuspid Valve Using Knowledge Derived from Three-Dimensional Echocardiography. J Am Soc Echocardiogr. 2016;29:74–82.
58. Stankovic I, Daraban AM, Jasaityte R, Neskovic AN, Claus P, Voigt JU. Incremental value of the en face view of the tricuspid valve by two-dimensional and three-dimensional echocardiography for accurate identification of tricuspid valve leaflets. J Am Soc Echocardiogr. 2014;27:376–84.
59. Miglioranza MH, Mihaila S, Muraru D, Cucchini U, Iliceto S, Badano LP. Dynamic changes in tricuspid annular diameter measurement in relation to the echocardiographic view and timing during the cardiac cycle. J Am Soc Echocardiogr. 2015;28:226–35.
60. Miglioranza MH, Mihaila S, Muraru D, Cucchini U, Iliceto S, Badano LP. Variability of Tricuspid Annulus Diameter Measurement in Healthy Volunteers. JACC Cardiovasc Imaging. 2015;8:864–6.
61. Badano LP, Agricola E, Perez de Isla L, Gianfagna P, Zamorano JL. Evaluation of the tricuspid valve morphology and function by transthoracic real-time three-dimensional echocardiography. Eur J Echocardiogr. 2009;10:477–84.
62. Mediratta A, Addetia K, Yamat M, et al. 3D echocardiographic location of implantable device leads and mechanism of associated tricuspid regurgitation. JACC Cardiovasc Imaging. 2014;7:337–47.
63. Fukuda S, Saracino G, Matsumura Y, et al. Three-dimensional geometry of the tricuspid annulus in healthy subjects and in patients with functional tricuspid regurgitation: a real-time, 3-dimensional echocardiographic study. Circulation. 2006;114:I492–8.
64. Nucifora G, Badano LP, Allocca G, et al. Severe tricuspid regurgitation due to entrapment of the anterior leaflet of the valve by a permanent pacemaker lead: role of real time three-dimensional echocardiography. Echocardiography. 2007;24:649–52.
65. Faletra F, La Marchesina U, Bragato R, De Chiara F. Three dimensional transthoracic echocardiography images of tricuspid stenosis. Heart. 2005;91:499.
66. Muraru D, Tuveri MF, Marra MP, Badano LP, Iliceto S. Carcinoid tricuspid valve disease: incremental value of three-dimensional echocardiography. Eur Heart J Cardiovasc Imaging. 2012;13:329.
67. Chen TE, Kwon SH, Enriquez-Sarano M, Wong BF, Mankad SV. Three-dimensional color Doppler echocardiographic quantification of tricuspid regurgitation orifice area: comparison with conventional two-dimensional measures. J Am Soc Echocardiogr. 2013;26:1143–52.
68. Song JM, Jang MK, Choi YS, et al. The vena contracta in functional tricuspid regurgitation: a real-time three-dimensional color Doppler echocardiography study. J Am Soc Echocardiogr. 2011;24:663–70.
69. de Agustin JA, Viliani D, Vieira C, et al. Proximal isovelocity surface area by single-beat three-dimensional color Doppler echocardiography applied for tricuspid regurgitation quantification. J Am Soc Echocardiogr. 2013;26:1063–72.
70. Zamorano J, Goncalves A, Lancellotti P, et al. The use of imaging in new transcatheter interventions: an EACVI review paper. Eur Heart J Cardiovasc Imaging. 2016;17:835–835af.
71. Hahn RT, Little SH, Monaghan MJ, et al. Recommendations for comprehensive intraprocedural echocardiographic imaging during TAVR. JACC Cardiovasc Imaging. 2015;8:261–87.
72. Jilaihawi H, Doctor N, Kashif M, et al. Aortic annular sizing for transcatheter aortic valve replacement using cross-sectional 3-dimensional transesophageal echocardiography. J Am Coll Cardiol. 2013;61:908–16.

73. Khalique OK, Kodali SK, Paradis JM, et al. Aortic annular sizing using a novel 3-dimensional echocardiographic method: use and comparison with cardiac computed tomography. Circ Cardiovasc Imaging. 2014;7:155–63.
74. Lancellotti P, Pibarot P, Chambers J, et al. Recommendations for the imaging assessment of prosthetic heart valves: a report from the European Association of Cardiovascular Imaging endorsed by the Chinese Society of Echocardiography, the Inter-American Society of Echocardiography, and the Brazilian Department of Cardiovascular Imaging. Eur Heart J Cardiovasc Imaging. 2016;17:589–90.
75. Tsang W, Salgo IS, Medvedofsky D, et al. Transthoracic 3D Echocardiographic Left Heart Chamber Quantification Using an Automated Adaptive Analytics Algorithm. JACC Cardiovasc Imaging. 2016;9:769–82.
76. Calleja A, Poulin F, Woo A, et al. Quantitative Modeling of the Mitral Valve by Three-Dimensional Transesophageal Echocardiography in Patients Undergoing Mitral Valve Repair: Correlation with Intraoperative Surgical Technique. J Am Soc Echocardiogr. 2015;28:1083–92.
77. Calleja A, Thavendiranathan P, Ionasec RI, et al. Automated quantitative 3-dimensional modeling of the aortic valve and root by 3-dimensional transesophageal echocardiography in normals, aortic regurgitation, and aortic stenosis: comparison to computed tomography in normals and clinical implications. Circ Cardiovasc Imaging. 2013;6:99–108.
78. Ozawa K, Funabashi N, Takaoka H, et al. Utility of three-dimensional global longitudinal strain of the right ventricle using transthoracic echocardiography for right ventricular systolic function in pulmonary hypertension. Int J Cardiol. 2014;174:426–30.
79. Smith BC, Dobson G, Dawson D, Charalampopoulos A, Grapsa J, Nihoyannopoulos P. Three-dimensional speckle tracking of the right ventricle: toward optimal quantification of right ventricular dysfunction in pulmonary hypertension. J Am Coll Cardiol. 2014;64:41–51.
80. Addetia K, Maffessanti F, Yamat M, et al. Three-dimensional echocardiography-based analysis of right ventricular shape in pulmonary arterial hypertension. Eur Heart J Cardiovasc Imaging. 2016;17:564–75.
81. Bruckheimer E, Rotschild C, Dagan T, et al. Computer-generated real-time digital holography: first time use in clinical medical imaging. Eur Heart J Cardiovasc Imaging. 2016;17:845–9.
82. Beitnes JO, Klaeboe LG, Karlsen JS, Urheim S. Mitral valve analysis using a novel 3D holographic display: a feasibility study of 3D ultrasound data converted to a holographic screen. Int J Cardiovasc Imaging. 2015;31:323–8.

# Chapter 2
# General Aspects of Transthoracic 3D-Echo

José-Julio Jiménez Nácher, Gonzalo Alonso Salinas, and Marina Pascual Izco

## Introduction: General Advices for Acquisition of a 3D TTE Study

### *Introduction*

Three-dimensional transthoracic echocardiography (3D TTE) has been one of the biggest advances in ultrasound technology. However, its advantages and limitations should be known before using it routinely.

The introduction of fully sampled-matrix transthoracic probe was crucial to establish 3D TTE as a revolutionary technology used to improve visualization of anatomical structures of the heart, provide accurate measurement of the cardiac chambers and guide interventional procedures.

Nowadays, most ultrasound companies have transthoracic probes that are able to obtain 2D, Doppler, Doppler-color and 3D images. These 3D transducers have more than 3000 elements arranged in a matrix and more efficient electronics, which enable simultaneous 2D imaging and immediate one-beat 3D volumetric imaging on-line [1].

**Electronic supplementary material** The online version of this chapter (doi:10.1007/978-3-319-50335-6_2) contains supplementary material, which is available to authorized users.

J.-J.J. Nácher (✉) • G.A. Salinas • M.P. Izco
Cardiology Department, Hospital Ramón y Cajal, Madrid, Spain
e-mail: jjjimenezn@gmail.com

© Springer International Publishing AG 2017
E. Casas Rojo et al. (eds.), *Manual of 3D Echocardiography*,
DOI 10.1007/978-3-319-50335-6_2

## *General Advices for Acquisition of a 3D TTE Study*

*Image Acquisition* The finite speed of sound in tissue (1540 m/s) is a major challenge to obtain large volumes with adequate frame rate because limits the number of ultrasound pulses that can be fired per second. As the frame rate is inversely proportional to the volume size (width and depth) and the spatial resolution, increasing the requirement of one of these, causes a drop in the other two [2]. Given these assumptions, the acquisition of 3D images is divided based on several parameters [1–4]:

(a) *Acquisition beats*

- Single-beat

Acquisition of multiple pyramidal data sets per second in a single heart-beat. This type of acquisition is also called real-time live 3D imaging. Although arrhythmias and respiratory movements are no longer a problem, it is limited by the temporal-spatial resolution.

- Multi-beat

Acquisition of images of higher temporal resolution through multiple acquisitions of narrow volumes of data over several heart beats (2–7 beats). Nonetheless, this type of acquisition may be affected by stich artifacts (see below) caused by patient breathing or irregularity of the cardiac cycles.

(b) *Acquisition mode*

- Simultaneous multiplane mode (x-plane)

A double screen where two real-time images simultaneously appear. The image on the left is the reference view and the image on the right shows a plane rotated 30–150° from the reference plane, selected by the operator. This has the advantage of being able to compare directly two individual planes side by side (Fig. 2.1).

- Narrow-angled acquisition

To decrease sector size and depth improves the spatial and temporal resolution. However, the sector size may be insufficient to display an entire anatomical structure.

- Zoom acquisition (Focused wide sector)

The volume widths and depth can be reduced to a minimum to focus mainly on an anatomical structure giving the highest achievable frame rate.

- Full volume acquisition

This mode allows a large acquisition volume that covers the complete chamber of interest. This is achieved by the acquisition of several sub volumes over 2–7

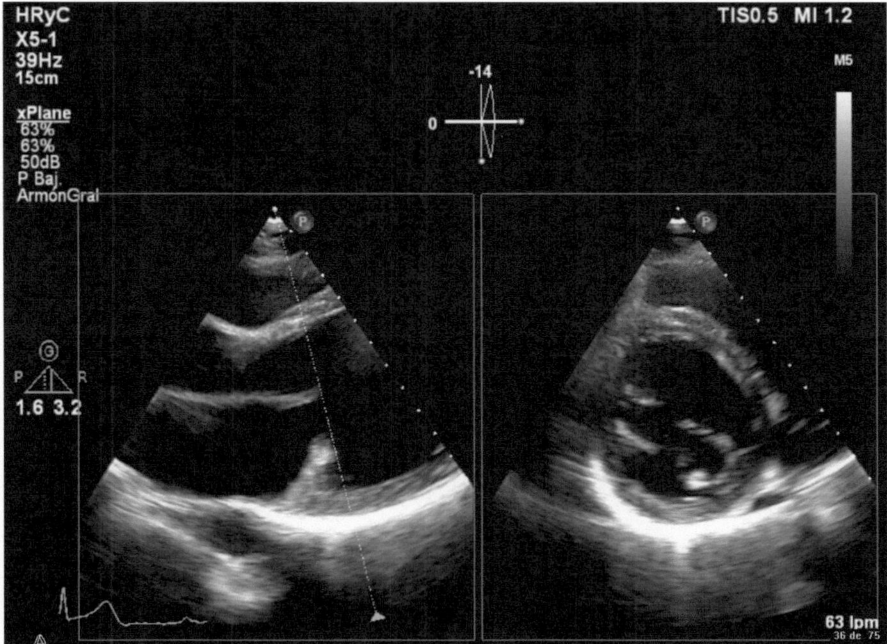


**Fig. 2.1** Simultaneous multiplane mode (X-plane): on the left, a four-chamber apical view focusing on mitral valve. On the right, a plane rotated approximately 90°

cardiac cycles ECG gated, with the same frame rate as the smaller subvolume. This type of acquisition is prone to stich artifacts (see below) (Fig. 2.2).

– 3D color Doppler

This mode combines grey scale volumetric data with Color Doppler. The acquisition can be performed using live 3D or full-volume. The first one is limited by smaller color Doppler volumes and low temporal resolution while the second one is restricted by stitching artifacts. It is primarily used for the evaluation of regurgitation lesions and shunts. To analyze 3D color Doppler regurgitation jets, it is advisable to crop (see below) to show two long-axis views of the jet, the narrowest and the broadest width of the jet with a short-axis view of the jet at the level of the vena contracta (Fig. 2.3) (Video 2.1).

(c) *Optimization mode*

To optimize the final image, follow these steps:

- A good ECG signal is necessary if you want to acquire full volume.
- Adjust gain setting: low gain results in echo drop-out (see below); excess gain produces a loss in resolution as well as a decrease in 3D perspective.
- Adjust smoothness setting: This prevents the image has minor roughness.

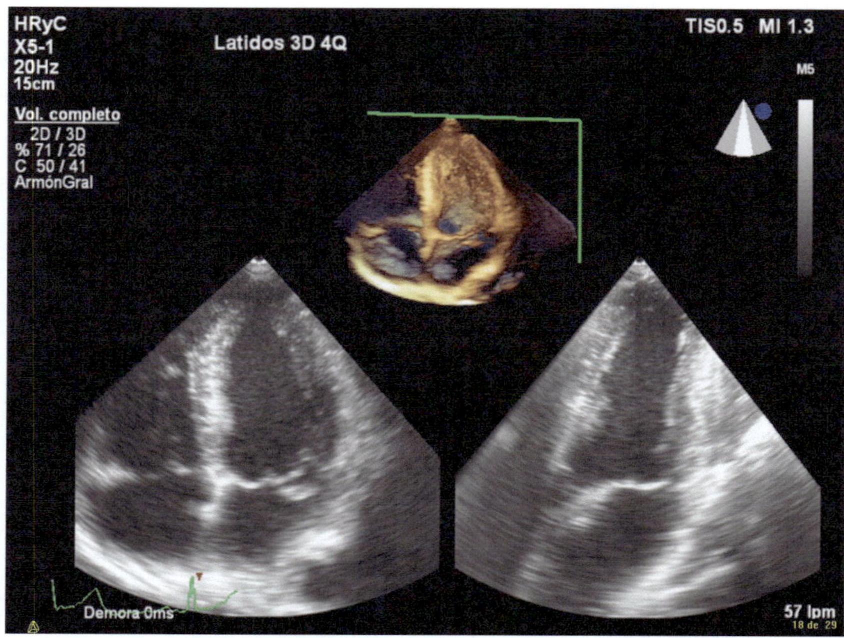

**Fig. 2.2** Full volume acquisition: This mode allows a large acquisition volume that covers the complete chamber of interest as in this case, the left ventricle

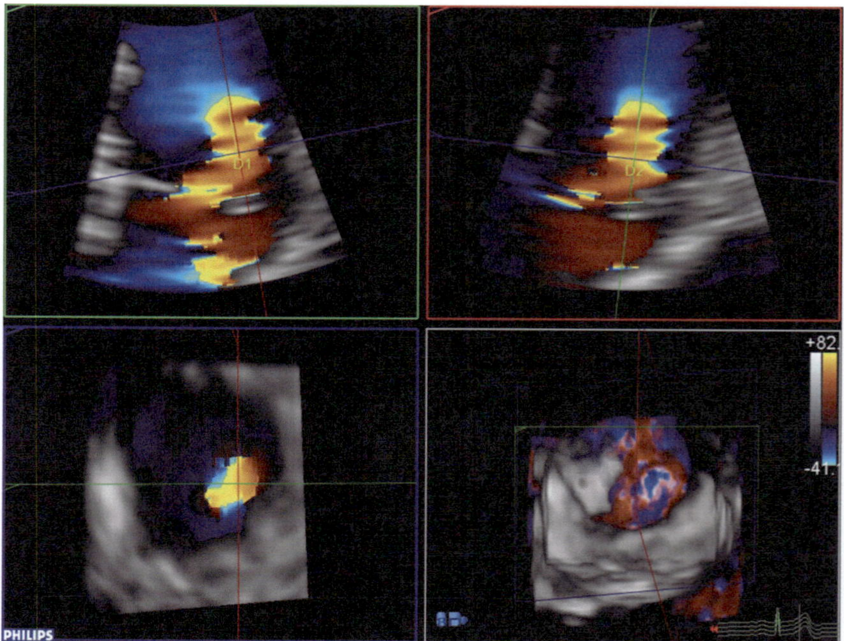

**Fig. 2.3** Doppler color 3D: To analyze 3D color Doppler regurgitation jets, it is advisable to crop (see below) to show two long-axis views of the jet, the narrowest and the broadest width of the jet with a short-axis view of the jet at the level of the vena contracta

- Adjust compression setting: This provides solid or transparent images so that the less compression, the greater transparency and vice versa.
- Adjust brightness setting: It is advisable to compensate the brightness of the image with time gain compensation rather than using the gain setting.
- Make sure the anatomical structure is within the volume sector and minimize the sector (angle and depth) to focus on the anatomical structure you want to acquire.
- Ask the patient not to breathe to avoid motion artifacts.
- Select appropriate line density. The higher densities allow better spatial resolution although at the expense of narrower angle sector.
- Magnification: The image can be enlarged to assess finer structures in more detail.

(d) *Which acquisition mode to choose?*

It is important to know what information is to be obtained from the study. For instance, if you want to assess a mitral valve prolapse, a high frame rate is necessary because the prolapse may only be appreciated in a few frames in late systole. Therefore, it is advisable to reduce the volume size to only cover the mitral valve to increase the frame rate. On the other hand, if you are evaluating a large anatomical structure such as the left ventricle, it is better to use the full volume acquisition. It is not always necessary to achieve high frame rates. Sometimes it is better to get large volumes with low frame rate as when assessing an atrial septal defect.

*3D Image Display*  There are several methods [1–4]:

Slice rendering

It is possible to obtain multiple simultaneous 2D images from a 3D acquisition that cannot be available in transthoracic 2D echocardiography (2D TTE). Virtually any plane can be achieved either as equidistant parallel slices or as slices rotated around a common axis. The current 3D systems normally show four screens where 3 simultaneous orthogonal 2D planes (coronal, sagittal and transverse or axial) plus a volumetric 3D image can be observed. These views allow accurate measurements of chamber dimensions, valve areas and regurgitant jets (Fig. 2.4).

Volume rendering

It is a method designed to produce images with 3D depth perception. It provides very useful 3D images to assess cardiac valves and complex anatomic structures.

Surface rendering

Another way of visualization of cardiac structures in a 3D scene. To obtain the images, they have to outline either manually or automatically via border detection, the anatomical structure (usually the left ventricle). This type of

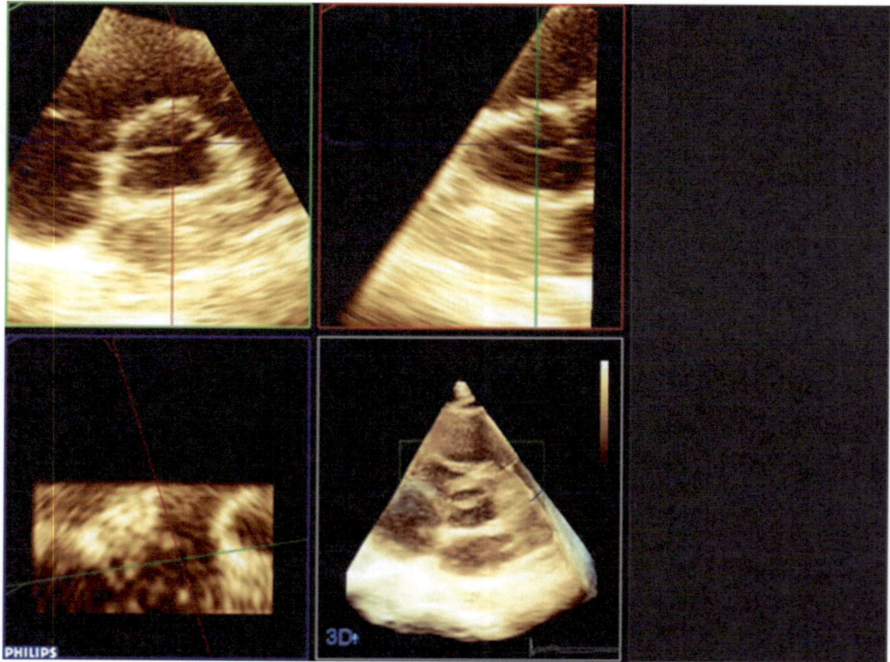

**Fig. 2.4** Slice rendering: An aortic valve is shown from the parasternal long-axis view (upper right), short-axis view (upper left), transverse-cut view (lower left) and the real-time three-dimensional echocardiography volume dataset (lower right)

reconstruction enable us to appreciate geometric shape, and superimpose information on the surface such as timing of contraction (Fig. 2.5) (Video 2.2).

Cropping method

This technique allows to remove anatomical structures from the initial data set to focus exclusively on the target anatomy. For example, cropping the left atrium to see the mitral valve from the base of the heart. 3D cropping can be done either during or after data acquisition (Fig. 2.6).

*3D Artefacts* Several types of artefacts are described [4]:

(a) *Stitch artefacts*

These occur when the mode of acquisition is 3D full volume where subvolumes are recorded and triggered by ECG. The stitch artifacts are displayed when acquired subvolumes do not perfectly merge together and instead the boundaries between the different subvolumes are clearly seen.
Stitch artifacts are caused by irregular rhythms, transductor or patient motion, including respiratory movements (Fig. 2.7).

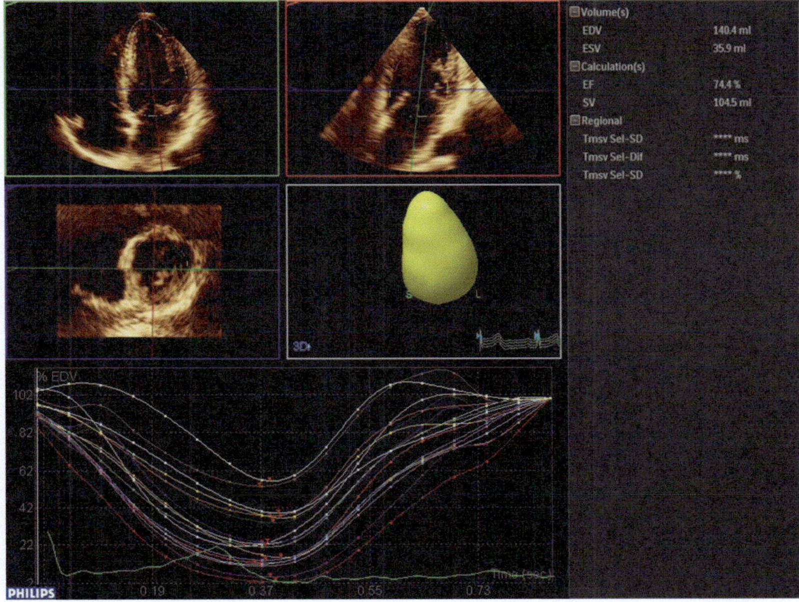

**Fig. 2.5 and Video 2.1** Surface rendering: Left ventricle (LV). LV analysis using a semiautomated border detection software allows quantification of LV volumes and ejection fraction. Once having a geometrical description of the LV, surface rendered images of the anatomy can be generated (middle right). Also, a 3D analysis of regional LV wall motion can be obtained (bottom)

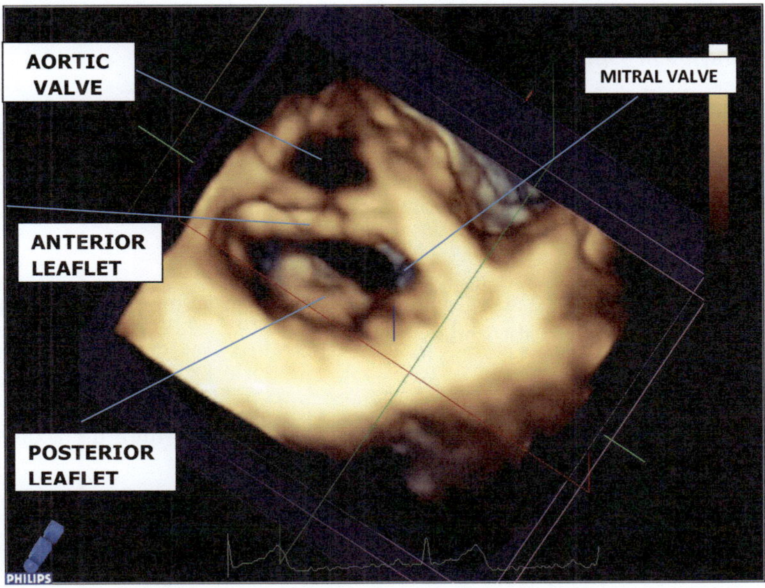


**Fig. 2.6** Cropping method: The left atrium has been removed to focus on the mitral valve, showing a flail segment (P2)

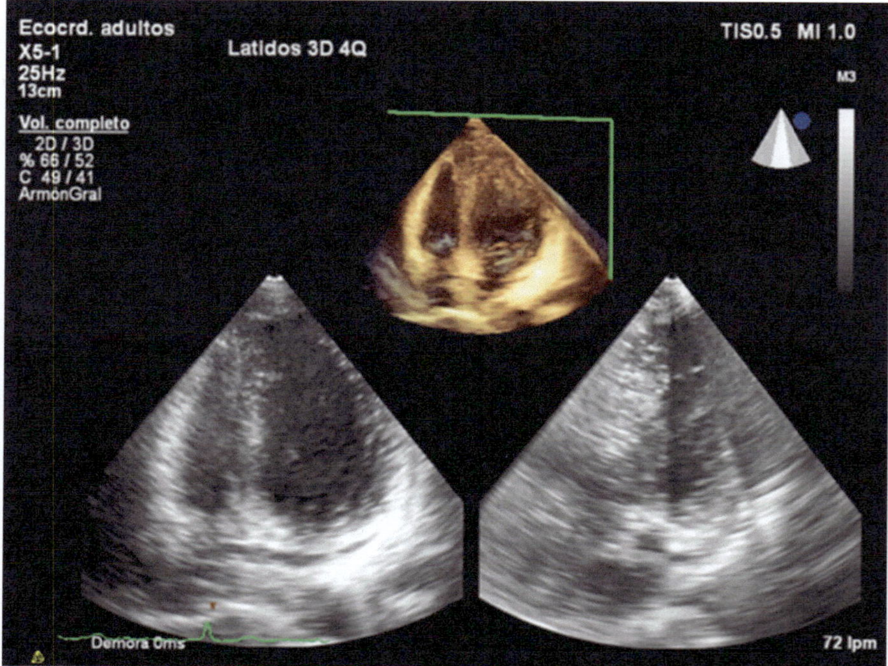


**Fig. 2.7** Stich artifact: When using ECG gated stitching of sub-volumes from multiples cardiac cycles (full volume acquisition), there is a danger of getting motion artifacts caused by respiration and heart rate variability as in this case (right image)

(b) *Shadowing or Drop-out artefacts*

These are highly echo-reflective structures such as prosthesis, providing areas of drop-out in the rendered image. It also occurs when a suboptimal gain setting is used. For example, when imaging the tricuspid valve, as the three leaflets used to be very thin, if the gain setting is low, then a drop-out may occur.

(c) *Attenuation artefacts*

Gradual deterioration of the signal intensity distal to the volume target because of reduced backscatter and absorption.

(d) *Reverberations*

Multiple reflections between structures giving false echoes within the acquisition volumes.

(e) *Aberrations*

Distortions of the ultrasound beam generating clutter noise as occur within the chamber cavities that obscures the true cardiac wall.

*3D TTE Protocol Examination* From a clinician point of view, it is more useful to perform a focused 3D TTE examination than a complete 3D TTE study. A focused

3D TTE examination is used to complete a 2D study: this depends on the target anatomical structure, so that a full volume will be acquired if you want to assess left ventricular function. In contrast, if we need to calculate a mitral stenosis area, a 3D zoom acquisition focused on mitral valve will be performed.

**Take Home Message**
- To obtain large volumes with adequate frame rate is the major challenge in 3D TTE.
- There are several methods of data acquisition in 3D TTE. Choose the best method suited to the information to be obtained: To assess left ventricular function, choose full volume acquisition. To evaluate mitral or aortic valves, choose zoom acquisition.
- Optimize 3D images by adjusting the different settings.
- There are also various methods of 3D image display: slice rendering allows accurate measurements of chamber dimensions, valve areas and regurgitant jets. Cropping is very useful to remove anatomical structures to focus exclusively on the target anatomy.
- Be aware of the artifacts in 3D TTE, especially drop-out and stich artifacts.

# Left Ventricle and Right Ventricle

## *Left Ventricle*

### Limitations of 2DE LV Assessment and 3D Advantages

Assessment of the left ventricle (LV) size and function are essential for the study of structural heart diseases. This assessment is predominantly performed using 2D echocardiography (2DE), but 2D echocardiographic data requires assumptions regarding geometric modeling of the LV. The main advantage of 3D imaging is that provides volume and ejection fraction measurements independent of geometric assumptions regarding LV shape [5], which gives more accurate and reproducible chamber quantification compared to other imaging modalities.

### Data Acquisition

- Apical four-chamber is the preferred view to 3D LV data acquisition.
- The full-volume data (data set) should be acquired during a breath hold to minimize the risk for artifacts.
- The data set acquisition should be guided by a display of orthogonal views that can be used for simultaneous imaging in two or more planes.
- Although there is no general agreement about imaging orientation and display, the apex is showed up and right-sided structures on the left-hand, normally.

**Data Analysis**

Most 3DE software provides analysis techniques that are fundamentally two-dimensional [6]. In this way, after a few anatomic landmarks in the LV (such as the mitral annulus or apex), 3DE data are usually segmented into several 2D longitudinal planes [1]. Endocardial and epicardial contours can be traced manually [7] or obtained using fully automated contouring algorithms [5]. These algorithms allow the calculation of cavity contours providing a cavity cast of the LV, from which its volume is computed without geometric assumptions [1] (Fig. 2.5) (Video 2.2).

**Clinical Application**

The application of 3D echocardiography (3DE) is particularly advantageous in these situations:

- LV mass or thrombus assessment: 3D imaging provides a 3D impression of the structure.
- LV volumes and ejection fraction (LVEF): 3DE is more accurate and reproducible than 2DE, with a high correlation with cardiovascular magnetic resonance reference values [9]. Moreover, 3D is particularly attractive in segmental wall motion assessment. As we explained in "*Data analysis*" section, 3D imaging provides a full-volume data set to create standard 2D images in which the cut planes are optimized to ensure that they are "on axis".

Several studies have published 3D echocardiographic LV volumes and LVEF reference values for healthy normotensive subjects. On the basis of weighted averages of three studies, 3D echocardiographic LV volumes were larger than 2D echocardiographic values, and corresponding upper limits of the normal range were [10]:

- End-diastolic volumes (EDVs) of 79 mL/m$^2$ for men and 71 mL/m$^2$ for women.
- End-systolic volumes (ESVs) of 32 mL/m$^2$ for men and 28 mL/m$^2$ for women.

Ultimately, a large study in a diverse population will be needed to establish normal reference ranges for 3DE for different ethnic groups.

- LV mass: Although 3DE is really attractive for LV volume and LVEF assessment, 3D echocardiography overestimates LV mass in comparison with magnetic resonance imaging measurements. The main reason is that endocardial and epicardial contours are usually traced manually [7], but this problem could be solved using automated contouring algorithms [8]. Nonetheless, because 3DE is the only echocardiographic technique that measures myocardial volume without geometric assumptions, this may be used in abnormally shaped ventricles or in patients with asymmetric or localized hypertrophy [10]. No LV mass reference values are available yet.
- LV dyssynchrony: In a left ventricle with dyssynchrony there is dispersion in the timing of regional segments, as the diseased segments achieve minimal volume

later in systole. The systolic dyssyncrhrony index is calculated from the basal and mid segments of the three standard 2D apical views, and consequently does not reflect the motion pattern of all LV segments in 3D space [11]. In contrast, 3D echocardiography evaluates all LV segments simultaneously, which represents an advantage over 2D echo.

## 3D TTE LV Assessment Limitations

The main disadvantages of 3D TTE LV assessment are the lower temporal resolution and the lack of published data on normal 3D values [10].

> **Take Home Message**
> - 3D TTE LV volumes and EF measurements are more accurate and reproducible than 2D and should be used when available and feasible.
> - Apical four-chamber is the preferred view to 3D TTE LV data acquisition.
> - A display of orthogonal views can be used to guide the 3D TTE LV data set acquisition.
> - 3D data analysis must be done by analysis software, which provides LV measures without geometric assumptions.
> - The American and European Society of Cardiac Imaging`s consensus document for Cardiac Chamber Quantification by Echocardiography (January, 2015) included normal values for LV parameters obtained with 3D TTE.

## *Right Ventricle*

### Limitations of 2DE RV Assessment and 3D Advantages

Because of its peculiar morphology and function, RV global assessment is difficult using 2D echocardiography. In contrast, 3DE enables complete assessment of RV geometry, volumes, and ejection fraction displaying the surfaces of the entire chamber including the inflow, apex, and outflow tracts. In this way, 3DE provides RV assessment without geometric assumptions.

### Data Acquisition

- RV–focused apical four-chamber is the preferred view to 3D RV data acquisition [10].
- Multibeat 3D acquisition, with minimal depth and sector angle (for a temporal resolution >20–25 volumes/sec) must be picked up [10].

## Data Analysis

In the 3DE RV data analysis it is critically important to manually define end-diastolic and end-systolic frames using maximal and minimal RV volumes; myocardial trabeculae and moderator band should be included in the cavity. After this manual initialization, the right ventricular endocardial surface is semiauto-matically identified in the right ventricular short-axis, four-chamber, and coronal views in both end-systole and end-diastole. The generated 3D surface model of the RV enables the quantitation of right ventricular ESV and ESV, stroke volume, and EF [10].

## Clinical Application

Data on RV volumes and function are of diagnostic and prognostic importance in a variety of cardiac diseases [1], including: valve disease, congenital heart disease, pulmonary hypertension, heart failure, etc.

- RV volumes: Even though 3DE tends to underestimate RV volumes compared CMR, 3DE volumes values are very similar to those described by cardiac magnetic resonance (CMR). Normal 3D echocardiographic values of RV volumes need to be established in larger groups of subjects, but current published data suggest [10]:

  - End-diastolic volumes (EDVs) of 87 mL/m$^2$ for men and 74 mL/m$^2$ for women.
  - End-systolic volumes (ESVs) of 44 mL/m$^2$ for men and 36 mL/m$^2$ for women.

- RV Ejection Fraction (RV EF): RVEF assessed by 3D TTE correlates with RV EF by CMR. Roughly, an RV EF of <45% usually reflects abnormal RV systolic function.

This is especially attractive in patients after cardiac surgery (in the absence of marked septal shift), when conventional indices of longitudinal RV function are generally reduced and no longer representative of overall RV performance [10].

## 3D TTE RV Assessment Limitations

The main limitation is that 3D TTE RV assessment depends on image quality, load, regular rhythm and patient cooperation. As same as in 3D TTE LV assessment, normal 3D echocardiographic values of RV need to be established in larger groups of subjects.

> **Take Home Message**
> - 3D TTE enables complete assessment of RV geometry including the inflow, apex and outflow tract.
> - RV-focus apical four-chamber is the preferred view to 3D TTE RV data acquisition.
> - 3D TTE RV data analyses includes manually and semiautomatically offline analyses.
> - The American and European Society of Cardiac Imaging's consensus document for Cardiac Chamber Quantification by Echocardiography (January, 2015) included normal values for RV parameters obtained with 3D TTE.

## Left and Right Atria

### *Limitations of 2DE LA Assessment and 3D Advantages*

3DE left atria (LA) assessment is, as same as LV and RV, more accurate than 2DE compared with CMR [10]. The main advantage of 3D TTE LA and right atria (RA) assessment is that not geometrical assumptions about LA shape are necessary with 3DE.

### *Data Acquisition*

- Apical view is the preferred one to 3D TTE atria assessment.
- Multibeat full-volume acquisition is needed.

### *Clinical Application*

3DE atria assessment is particularly interesting in:

- Diagnosis and management of patients with atrial fibrillation and diastolic dysfunction [10]. For example, one study showed that 3D echocardiography classified enlarged left atria more accurately than 2DE, resulting in fewer patients with undetected atrial enlargement and potentially undiagnosed diastolic dysfunction [12].

- Electrophysiologic procedures: Although fluoroscopy is routinely used to localize atrial anatomic landmarks during electrophysiologic procedures, this technique is limited by its 2D projection of complex 3D structures that may render difficult interpretation and analysis [1]. In these cases 3D TTE analyses can be useful.
- LA mass or thrombus assessment.


## *3D TTE LA and RA Assessment Limitations*

Because the atria are close to the esophagus, 3D transesophageal echocardiography provides more anatomic data than transthoracic one. Thus, we have a lack of a standardized methodology and limited normative 3D TTE data.

> **Take Home Message**
> - There is promise that 3D transthoracic echocardiography will improve the accuracy of left atrial measurements. However, no studies to date have evaluated right atrial values.
> - 3D TTE atria assessment is especially useful in electrophysiologic procedures.


# Mitral, Aortic, Tricuspid and Pulmonary Valve

## *Mitral Valve*

### Anatomy of the Mitral Apparatus and Limitations of 2D–Echocardiography Assessment

The mitral apparatus is formed from the annulus, the leaflets connected by opposing anterolateral and posteromedial commissures, the subvalvular apparatus composed of variable chordae tendineae arrangement with dual papillary muscles, and the left ventricle wall attachments. Three-dimensional echocardiographic imaging modalities are ideal for interrogating the anatomy and function of each of the individual components of the mitral apparatus. It provides additional information in patients with complex mitral valve lesion [1].

*Mitral Leaflets* The mitral valve has two leaflets that are attached at their bases to the fibromuscular ring, and by their free edges to the subvalvular apparatus. The anterior mitral valve leaflet has the larger radial surface and is attached to about one third of the annular circumference. The posterior leaflet has a quadrangular shape and is attached to approximately two-thirds of the annular circumference. The posterior leaflet usually has two indentations which divide the leaflet into three individual scallops identified as P1, P2, and P3. The P1 scallop corresponds to the anterolateral portion of the posterior leaflet, close to the anterior commissure and the left atrium (LA) appendage, the P2 scallop is medium and more developed and the P3 scallop is internal, close to the posterior commissure and the tricuspid annulus. The anterior leaflet is in continuity with the non-coronary cusp of the aortic valve, known as the intervalvular fibrosa. The free edge of the anterior leaflet is typically continuous, but it is artificially divided into three portions A1, A2, and A3, corresponding to the posterior scallops P1, P2, and P3. Leaflet segmentation is particularly useful to precisely localize prolapsing segments and anatomic lesions of the mitral valve [13].

In contrast to conventional 2D echocardiography (2DE), which displays the leaflets from the LV perspective, 3D echo enables "en face" visualization from LV and LA perspectives. The view from LA is known as the "surgical view," because it reproduces the intraoperative image of the mitral valve after the surgeon opens the LA. Furthermore, 3D echocardiography (3DE) allows any cut plane of an apical or parasternal data set for describing the display of the mitral valve leaflets. This may be necessary to precisely localize the abnormal mitral valve segment.

*Subvalvular Apparatus* The integrity of the subvalvular mitral apparatus can be appreciated from LV long-axis planes. Mitral valve "en face" view from the LV perspective allows evaluation of the chordal insertions. However, chordal rupture with flail or prolapse can be well visualized from left atrial views or by selected longitudinal cut planes.

*Mitral Annulus* Mitral annular shape exact description cannot be achieved by 2DE. Reconstruction from separate 2D views cannot provide the same information as the volume-rendered 3D reconstruction. Commercial software has been developed to precisely quantitate the size, shape, and degree of non-planarity of the mitral valve annulus. This has improved our understanding of mitral valve mechanics and has assisted surgeons in evaluating the feasibility of mitral valve repair or annuloplasty.

*Left Ventricle* Changes in LV geometry result in poor leaflet coaptation. Dynamic 3D rendering of the mitral valve can identify tethered leaflets due to regional wall motion abnormalities or global LV enlargement.

## Data Acquisition

*Multiplane Mode* This mode allows the mitral valve to be seen in two planes in real-time. The first image is usually the reference, while the second image or "lateral plane" represents a plane rotated 30–150° from the reference plane. Color flow Doppler imaging can be performed onto the 2DE images (Fig. 2.1).

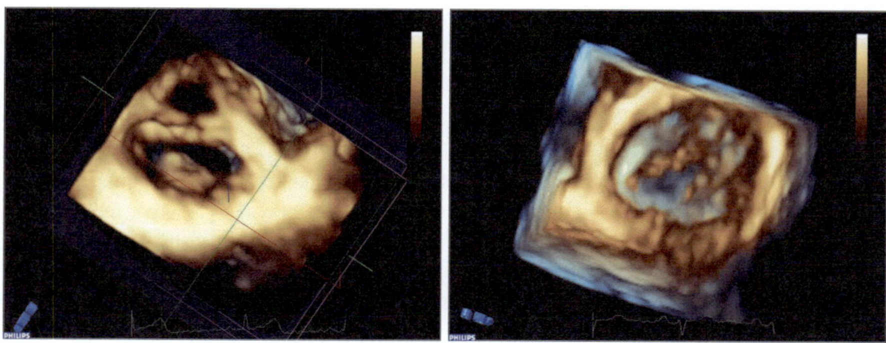

**Fig. 2.8 and 2.9**  Mitral valve: After cropping, the mitral valve is shown from the left atrium (left) and from the left ventricle (right). A flail segment of the posterior leaflet (P2) can be demonstrated

*Real-Time 3D Mode*  Live 3D permits a real-time display of a $30 \times 60°$ pyramidal volume. This is usually not enough to visualize the entire mitral apparatus, however, the superior spatial and temporal resolution permits accurate diagnoses of complex pathologies, preserving optimal temporal resolution.

*Focused Wide Sector: Zoom 3D*  The zoom mode permits a focused, wide-sector view of the mitral valve apparatus. It must be noted that excessive enlarging of the region of interest will decrease the temporal and spatial resolution (Figs. 2.6, 2.8, and 2.9) (Videos 2.3 and 2.4).

*Full Volume: Gated Acquisition*  The full-volume mode has the largest acquisition sector possible, an optimal spatial resolution and a high temporal resolution, which is desirable when diagnosing mechanisms of abnormal mitral functioning. Color flow Doppler can also be performed in this mode improving assessment of mitral regurgitation jets.

## Application

3DE may be superior to 2DE techniques diagnosing the location and extent of complex mitral valve disease. The evaluation of mitral prosthetic valve function may also be facilitated, especially in identifying the location and severity of perivalvular leaks [14]. Commercial software has been developed to provide an objective quantification of mitral valve changes. Using 3DE data sets, volumetric measurements of mitral annular height, mitral leaflet surface area, mitral annular dimensions, and papillary muscle location can be obtained. These dimensions have provided insight into the effects of various mitral valve pathologies and may be useful for directing repair techniques.

> **Take Home Message**
> - 3DE may be superior to 2DE techniques diagnosing complex mitral valve disease.
> - It enables "en face" visualization of the mitral valve from LV and LA perspectives. The view from LA with the aortic valve at the top is known as "the surgical view" because it reproduces the image after LA opening.
> - The comprehensive exam begins using the 2D multiplane modality.
> - 3D – zoom mode permit visualization from the annulus to the papillary muscles, with reduced spatial and temporal resolution.
> - Color flow Doppler should be added if needed. The size of the region of interest should be limited to the mitral apparatus and color flow Doppler jet to optimize frame rate.

## *Tricuspid Valve*

### Anatomy of the Tricuspid Valve and Limitations of 2DE Assessment

The tricuspid valve (TV) is composed of the annulus, leaflets, and chordal and papillary muscle apparatus. The annulus is a fibrous ring from which the leaflets are suspended. The normal tricuspid annulus area measures 8–12 cm$^2$ and is approximately 20% larger than the mitral annulus, it is saddle shaped with superior points, toward the right atrium (RA), along the anterior and posterior aspects of the annulus, and inferior points along the medial and lateral aspects of the annulus.

The TV has three leaflets of unequal size: the anterior leaflet is usually the largest and extends from the infundibula region anteriorly to the inferolateral wall posteriorly; the septal leaflet extends from the interventricular septum to the posterior ventricular border; the posterior leaflet attaches along the posterior margin of the annulus from the septum to the inferolateral wall.

The three main TTE views allowing the tricuspid valve visualization are the parasternal short-axis, the apical four-chamber and the subcostal views. Parasternal short-axis view, apical four-chamber (apical 4C) view and subcostal four-chamber view visualize the septal and the anterior tricuspid leaflets. Besides, parasternal long-axis view of the right ventricle (RV) reveals the anterior and the posterior tricuspid leaflets. The tricuspid apparatus has two main papillary muscles, located anteriorly and posteriorly, and frequently a third one located in the RV outflow track. Chords from each papillary muscle attach to all three tricuspid leaflets.

**Data Acquisition**

Conventional 2DE imaging of the TV requires reconstruction from multiple planes. Three-dimensional TTE approaching allows visualization of all aspects of the TV from a single full-volume data set or a focused examination using a narrower imaging acquisition mode with higher resolution, however, it is limited by a low temporal resolution compared with 2DE.

Standard 3DE data sets should be obtained from parasternal and apical windows. A subcostal 3DE data set can also be acquired but will depend on the acoustic window. The full-volume data set should englobe the TV and the RV. When displaying the TV "en face", the septal leaflet should be located in the 6 o'clock position irrespective of perspective. These "en face" views may be especially helpful in localizing leaflet disease.

*Parasternal Views*  The TV in the parasternal long-axis view of the right ventricle should be optimized for 3D full-volume data acquisition, the cropping plane should be oriented to display the anterior and posterior leaflets of the TV. This should also display the orifice of the coronary sinus and Eustachian valve. A second parasternal data set should be acquired in the short axis.

*Apical Views*  The cropping plane should obtain an apical 4C view of the TV with anterior and septal leaflets and its chordal attachments. Then, the cropping plane should be oriented along the sagittal plane to visualize the posterior and anterior leaflets. Finally, the cropping plane should be rotated over 45° clockwise to include the aortic valve (AV), this should display the septal and anterior leaflets (Figs. 2.10 and 2.11) (Videos 2.5 and 2.6).

**Application**

3DE of the TV has provided insights into normal and abnormal TV anatomy. 3DE has described the bimodal shape of the annulus and its changes due to some pathologies. In some studies it has been proved superior to 2DE in describing the pathological mechanism of TV disease [15].

> **Take Home Message**
> - Parasternal long and short axis, apical 4C and the subcostal views are the preferred to display the TV.
> - When displaying the TV "en face", the septal leaflet should be located in the 6 o'clock position irrespective of perspective.
> - In apical 4C view the plane should firstly display anterior and septal. Secondly, oriented along the sagittal plane, it visualizes the posterior and anterior leaflets. Finally, rotate over 45° clockwise (including the AV) to display septal and anterior leaflets.

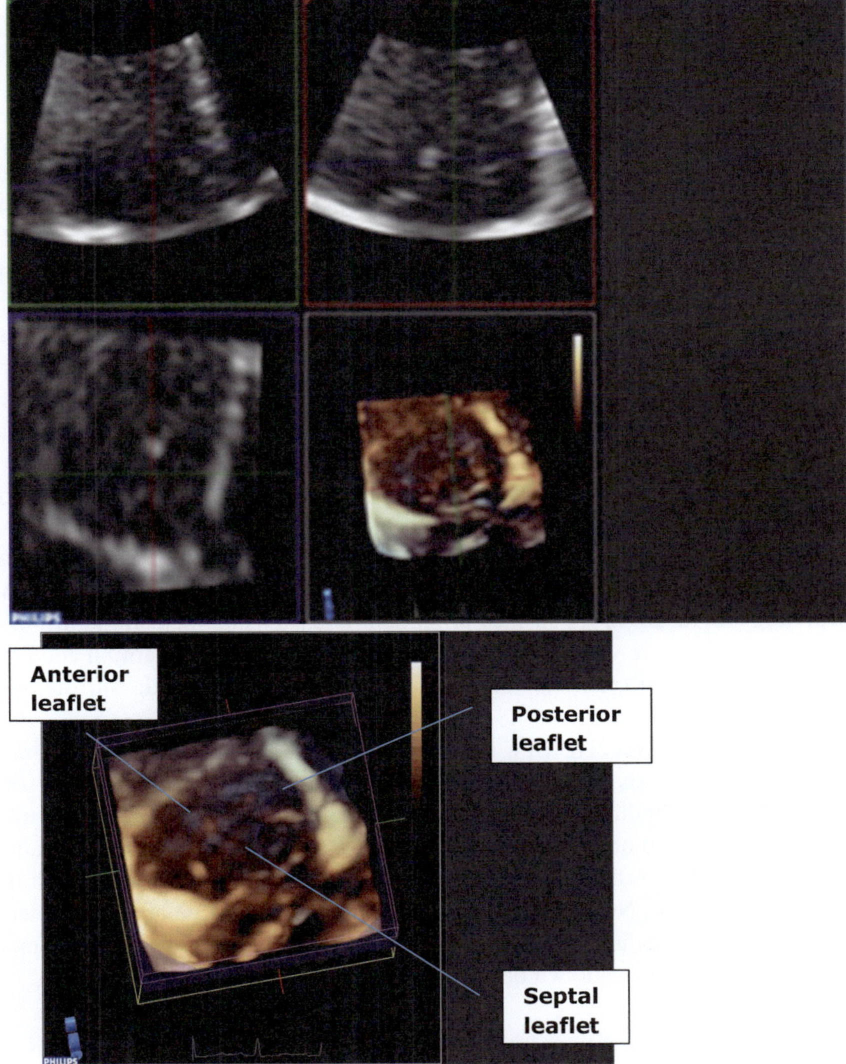


**Fig. 2.10 and 2.11** Tricuspid valve: Zoom tricuspid valve view. On the left, a normal tricuspid valve is acquired from apical views. Four-chamber view (upper left), the orthogonal view (upper right) and the short-axis of these views (lower left) with a volume-rendered image of the tricuspid valve (lower right) that is orientated with the interatrial septum posteriorly. The valve is displayed from the right atrium. On the right, the same volume-rendered image is enlarged

## *Aortic Valve*

### Anatomy of the Aortic Valve (AV) and Limitations of 2DE Assessment

The AV is composed of its three semilunar cusps and the fibrous interleaflet triangles. The aortic cusps are identified by the corresponding coronary arteries: left coronary, right coronary, and noncoronary cusps. The sinuses of Valsalva and the sinotubular junction are integral parts of the valvular mechanism, any significant dilatation of these structures will cause AV incompetence. The common approaches for imaging the aortic valve by transthoracic 3DE are from the parasternal and apical views. It can be visualized from the aortic and the ventricular perspective, as well as sliced in any desired longitudinal or oblique plane. The aortic perspective is usually suited for assessing valve morphology. The ventricular perspective identifies aortic tumors, vegetations or subvalvular obstructions.

Obtaining an exact en face alignment of the AV orifice in the 2D short-axis view is sometimes impossible, especially in hearts with dilated aortic root or a horizontal position. Moreover, the motion of the annulus throughout the cardiac cycle often hinders adequate visualization of the true AV opening orifice and morphology. With 3DE, its en face alignment is easily obtained. In addition, it allows comprehensive visualization of the entire AV complex in motion and provides additional information on the spatial relationship with surrounding structures.

Parasternal long-axis 2DE view often underestimates LV outflow tract area, as it presumes a circular shape. The true shape is demonstrated by 3DE. It can also confirm abnormal findings when structures visualized in one plane are real-time examined in a second orthogonal plane. Apical 4C allows the en face visualization of the AV by 3DE, even though the spatial resolution is lower compared with the parasternal approach. Nonetheless, adequate visualization can be at times difficult by transthoracic 3D echocardiography either in normal or in heavily calcified aortic valves, or when the acoustic window is inadequate [16].

### Data Acquisition and Examination

*Biplane Imaging* Firstly, a preliminary survey of the AV should be performed using the 2DE multiplane modality with and without color flow Doppler.

*Real-Time 3D* After the 2D image is optimized, narrow-angled acquisitions can be used to optimize the 3D image and to examine AV and root anatomy. When displayed en face, the AV should be oriented with the right coronary cusp inferiorly, regardless of the perspective (Figs. 2.4, 2.12, and 2.13) (Videos 2.7 and 2.8).

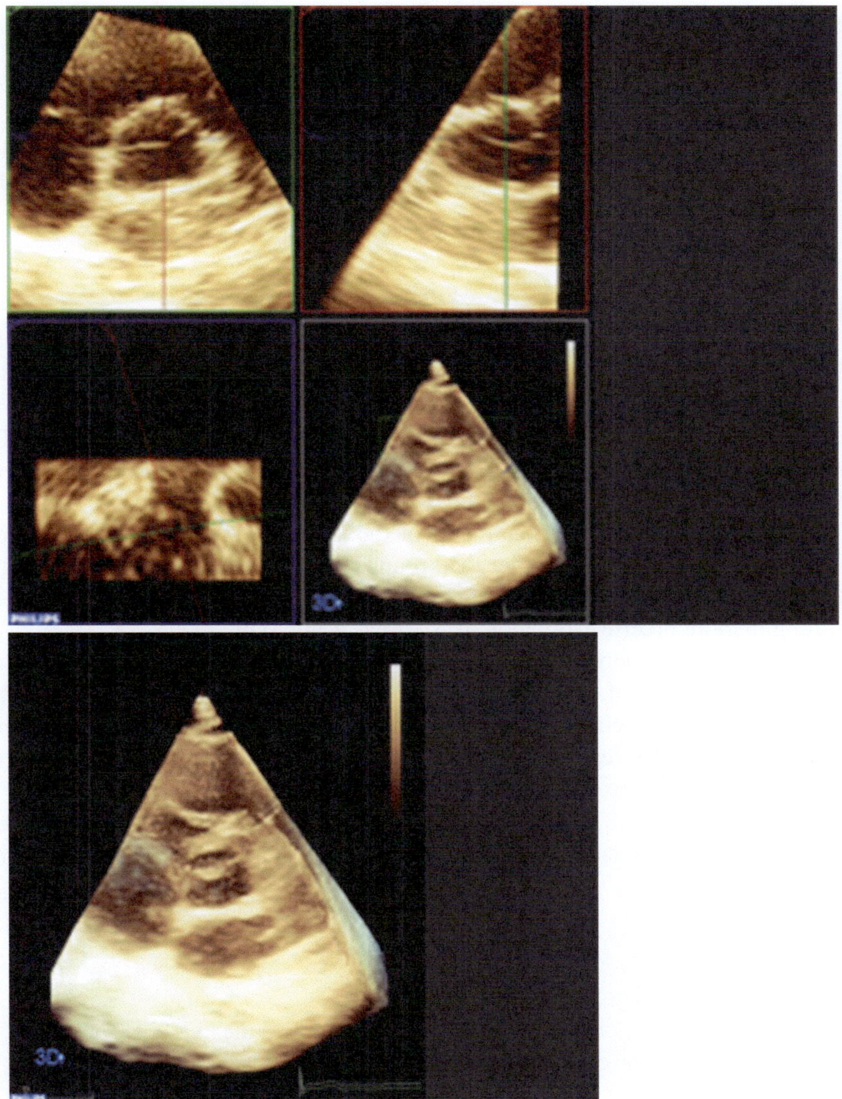

**Fig. 2.12 and 13** Aortic valve: On the left, a normal aortic valve is shown from the parasternal long-axis view (upper right), short-axis view (upper left), transverse-cut view (lower left) and the real-time three-dimensional echocardiography volume dataset (lower right). On the right, the real-time three-dimensional volume dataset is displayed

*Focused Wide-Sector Zoom and Full Volume*  The cropping plane should be aligned parallel to the aortic valve orifice, identified from the long-axis view. This results in a short-axis 3D image of the aortic valve orifice, used for planimetry. Last, the cropping planes can be placed perpendicular and parallel to the aortic annulus to assess supravalvular and subvalvular anatomy.

*Full Volume with Color Flow Doppler* Color Doppler should also be performed to detect the initial appearance of flow at the onset of systole. These color Doppler signals can also be cropped at the valve level using a parallel plane to estimate the orifice area and the vena contracta.


## Application

AV area quantification has been improved by 3DE with either planimetry or the continuity equation. 3DE TTE planimetered aortic valve area has been reported to be feasible in 92% of patients, correlating well with 2D TEE planimetry and TTE continuity values. 3DE TTE AV areas were also found to have better correlation to invasively measured AV area compared with 2D TEE values [1, 16].

3DE also allows accurate planimetry of the LV outflow tract, which has been demonstrated to be elliptical rather than round. With accurate measurement of the LV outflow tract, geometric assumptions used in the continuity equation are avoided, resulting in more precise estimation of AV areas using 3DE.

Using 3DE color Doppler, the exact perpendicular plane to the aortic regurgitation jet can be identified, from which the area of the vena contracta can be planimetered. As well, geometric assumptions of the vena contracta, which are invalid when the shape of the regurgitant orifice is nonsymmetric, are avoided with direct measurement, thus improving measurement precision.

Three-dimensional TTE assessment of the AV should be incorporated when available into the assessment of aortic stenosis and to elucidate the mechanism of aortic regurgitation.

**Take Home Message**
- 3D-TTE AV area measurement is more precise than the 2D-TEE approach.
- The comprehensive exam begins using the 2D multiplane modality.
- Parasternal long-axis 2DE assessment presumes a circular LV outflow tract. The true shape is demonstrated by 3DE.
- Exact "en face" alignment of the AV orifice in the 2D short-axis view is sometimes impossible, and using 3DE is easily obtained. 3DE short-axis view allows real AV orifice planimetry.
- 3DE color Doppler can identify the exact perpendicular plane to the aortic regurgitation jet, from which the area of the vena contracta can be planimetered avoiding geometrical assumptions.

## *Pulmonary Valve*

### Anatomy of the Pulmonary Valve and Limitations of 2DE Assessment

The pulmonary valve (PV) is composed of its three leaflets, the sinuses of Valsalva and the interleaflet triangles. The three pulmonic valve leaflets are identified by their position in relation to the septum and the aortic valve. The two septal leaflets are named left and right leaflets, and face the right and left AV leaflets. The third leaflet is called the anterior leaflet. Visualizing the PV cusps by 2DE is difficult, and usually only two cusps can be simultaneously assessed. 3DE allows simultaneous evaluation of the three cusps, as well as assessment of the RV outflow tract and main pulmonary artery (PA). This has improved quantitative assessment of pulmonary regurgitation and stenosis.

### Data Acquisition

The best possible images can be obtained from the parasternal view. After optimizing the image on 2DE, live 3DE TTE images of the valve can be obtained with greater success.

*Biplane*   Firstly, a preliminary survey of the PV should be performed using the 2DE multiplane modality with and without color flow Doppler.

*Real-Time 3D*   After the 2DE image is optimized, narrow-angled acquisitions can be used to optimize the 3DE image and to examine the PV, the RV outflow track and the main PA anatomy. When displayed in the enface view, the anterior leaflet should be located superiorly, in the 12 o'clock position, irrespective of perspective.

*Focused Wide-Sector Zoom and Full Volume*   The zoom mode allows visualization of the PV leaflets, the main PA and the RV outflow tract. Once the pyramidal volume is captured, the enface view of the valve can be displayed and the cropping plane can assess the dimensions of the main PA and the RV outflow tract. Moreover, the cropping plane also shows the RV outflow tract, PV, and main PA in a single image.

*Full Volume with Color Flow Doppler*   Color Doppler should also be performed to detect the initial appearance of flow at the onset of systole. These color Doppler signals can also be cropped at the valve level using a parallel plane to estimate the orifice area and the vena contracta.

### Application

Evaluation of the PV using 3DE can exactly define the location of pathology and the mechanism and severity of valvular dysfunction. 3DE also provides accurate RV outflow tract supravalvular, subvalvular, and valvular measurements and improved the accuracy in the assessment of pulmonary regurgitation.

There is no current evidence supporting the routine use of 3D transthoracic echocardiography or transesophageal echocardiography for the evaluation of pulmonic valve disease [1].

> **Take Home Message**
> - 3DE allows simultaneous evaluation of the three PV cusps, the RV outflow tract and main PA.
> - The best possible images can be obtained from the parasternal view.
> - When displayed in the "en face" view the anterior leaflet should be located at the 12 o'clock position, irrespective of perspective.

## *Aorta*

### Anatomy and Limitations of 2DE Assessment

Thoracic aorta should be routinely evaluated by TTE, which provides good images of the aortic root, adequate images of the ascending aorta and aortic arch in most patients, adequate images of the descending thoracic aorta in some patients, and good images of the proximal abdominal aorta.

The aortic root and proximal ascending aorta are best imaged in the left parasternal long-axis view. The left lung and sternum often limit imaging of the more distal portion of the ascending aorta. In patients with aortic dilatation, the right parasternal long-axis view can provide supplemental information. 2DE view often underestimates aortic root area, as it presumes a circular shape. The true shape is demonstrated by 3DE, which has improved the assessment of the aorta by TTE.

There is no clear echocardiographic differentiation between the sinus and tubular portion of the ascending aorta. Occasionally a fibrotic ridge, located at the sinotubular junction, is visualized. The maximum diameter of the aorta is normally in the root, at the sinus level, which is immediately distal to the aortic valve. 3DE improve this measurement, identifying the real maximum diameter and area.

Echocardiographic measurements of the aortic root will vary in an individual patient at different levels. The aortic diameter is smallest at the annulus, the tubular portion of the ascending aorta is typically about 10% smaller than the diameter at the sinus level. The aortic arch is usually easily visualized from the suprasternal view. Portions of the ascending and descending aorta can be visualized simultaneously by 2DE TTE. 3DE can visualize real diameters and improve these measurements.

The descending thoracic aorta is incompletely imaged by TTE. A cross-sectional view may be seen in the parasternal long-axis view, as it passes posteriorly to the left. The midportion of the descending thoracic aorta can also be seen in short axis in the apical four-chamber view, by rotating the transducer 90 degrees. A portion of the descending thoracic aorta can also be imaged from a suprasternal view. The normal descending thoracic aorta is smaller than both the aortic root and ascending aorta. The aorta is consistently about 2 mm smaller in female than it is in male subjects.

A substantial portion of the upper abdominal aorta can be easily imaged in sub-costal views, to the left of the inferior vena cava. This should be routinely performed as a part of a 2D echocardiographic study. When present, aneurysmal dilatation, external compression, intra-aortic thrombi, protruding atheromas, and dissection flaps can be imaged, and flow patterns in the abdominal aorta can be assessed.

**Data Acquisition**

The best possible images can be obtained from the parasternal long-axis view. After optimizing the image on 2DE, live 3DE TTE images of the valve can be obtained with greater success.

*Biplane*  Firstly, a preliminary survey of the aortic root and the aortic arch should be performed using the 2DE multiplane modality with and without color flow Doppler.

*Real-Time 3D*  After the 2DE image is optimized, narrow-angled acquisitions can be used to optimize the 3DE image and to examine the aorta, the LV outflow track and the AV. In suprasternal view arotic arch should be identified.

*Focused Wide-Sector Zoom and Full Volume*  The zoom mode allows visualization of the AV, the LV outflow track and the aortic root. Once the pyramidal volume is captured, the enface view of the aortic root can be displayed to show real shape and size.

*Full Volume with Color Flow Doppler*  Color Doppler should also be performed to detect flaps if suspected.

**Application**

TTE is particularly useful for evaluating the aortic root, and the ascending aorta and arch may also be adequately visualized in patients with good acoustic windows. 3DE can improve these measurements by identifying real maximum diameters of each part.

TTE is less helpful for evaluating the descending thoracic aorta. However, TTE is an excellent screening tool for detecting aneurysms of the upper abdominal aorta [17].

> **Take Home Message**
> - 2DE view often underestimates aortic area at any level, mostly by presuming a circular shape. 3DE demonstrate true aortic shape and improve aorta assessment by TTE.
> - The best possible 3DE TTE images of ascending aorta can be obtained from the parasternal long-axis view.
> - Suprasternal view may identify aortic arch.

## *General Aspects of Congenital Diseases from 3D TTE (See also Chap. 9)*

- Congenital heart diseases (CHD) are complex entities that often occur in the first year of life and require early treatment, most often surgery, to correct partially or completely so that nowadays CHD are frequently seen later in life, either as first presentation or as follow-up of a previously corrected CHD.
- 2D transthoracic echocardiography (TTE) has traditionally been the tool of choice for the initial approach to CHD by its non-invasive nature, high spatial and temporal resolution and immediate and easy availability. However, its main limitation compared to other techniques (MRI and CT) is the inability to represent extremely complex 3-dimensional anatomical structures such as those occurring in CHD.
- 3D TTE has emerged as a technique to overcome this limitation, although less time-space resolution of 3D echocardiography remains a problem. Nonetheless, there are, at least, three areas of potential clinical use, namely:

  (a) Improved understanding of the anatomy of CHD
  (b) Quantitation of chamber sizes, cardiac mass, volumes and ventricular function.
  (c) Planning and guiding therapeutic interventions.

(a) *Improved understanding of the anatomy of CHD.*

  - 3D TTE provides different views such as "en face" views not available with 2D TTE that provide cardiologists with better perspective of cardiac structures, a more accurate assessment of their morphologies, their size, position and their variations throughout the cardiac cycle [18].
  - 3D images allow an easier interpretation of the congenital abnormality and a greater confidence cardiologists resulting in a better management of these patients [19].
  - 3D TTE provides incremental value over 2D TTE in evaluating atrial and ventricular septal defects, atrioventricular valves anomalies such as Ebstein' disease and cleft mitral valve and also in complex left and right outflow obstructions (aortic subvalvar membrane, pulmonic subvalvar stenosis) [20].

(b) *Quantitation of chamber sizes, cardiac mass, volumes and ventricular function (see above and Chap. 5)*

- Right ventricular size and function are paramount in CHD because many therapeutic decisions are made according to their functionality. 3D TTE has shown to be a sensitive tool for detection of right ventricular dysfunction [21, 22]. It is superior to 2D TTE in assessing right ventricular volumes [18].

(c) *Planning and guiding therapeutic interventions (see also Chap. 7).*

- 3D TTE has demonstrated to be useful in guiding successfully the performance of endomyocardial right ventricle biopsy, without causing damage to the tricuspid valve or pericardial effusion [23].

> **Take Home Message**
> - 3D TTE has proved to be a useful tool in CHD in three specific areas:
>   - Improved understanding of the anatomy of the CHD.
>   - Quantification of volumes and ventricular function, especially of the right ventricle.
>   - Guiding therapeutic interventions.

# References


1. Lang RM, Badano L, Tsang W, Adams DH, et al. EAA/ASE recommendations for image acquisition and display using three dimensional echocardiography. Eur Heart J Cardiovasc Imaging. 2012;13:1–46.
2. Salgo IS. Three-dimensional echocardiography technology. Cardiol Clin. 2007;25:231–9.
3. Morbach C, Lin BA, Sugeng L. Clinical application of three-dimensional echocardiography. Prog Cardiovasc Dis. 2014;57:19–31.
4. Rabben SI. Technical principles of transthoracic three-dimensional echocardiography. In: Badano LP, Lang RM, Zamorano JL, editors. Textbook of real-time three dimensional echocardiography. London/New York: Springer; 2011. p. 9–24.
5. Monaghan MJ. Role of real time 3D echocardiograpny in evaluating the left ventrice. Heart. 2006;92:131–6.
6. Caiani EG, Corsi C, Sugeng L, et al. Improved quantification of left ventricular mass based on endocardial and epicardial surface detection with real time three dimensional echocardiography. Heart. 2006;92:213–9.
7. Mor-Avi V, Sugeng L, Weinert L, et al. Fast measurement of left ventricular mass with real-time three-dimensional echocardiography: comparison with magnetic resonance imaging. Circulation. 2004;110:1814–8.
8. Thavendiranathan P, Liu S, Verhaert D, et al. Feasibility, accuracy, and reproducibility of real-time full-volume 3D transthoracic echocardiography to measure LV volumes and systolic function: a fully automated endocardial contouring algorithm in sinus rhythm and atrial fibrillation. JACC Cardiovasc Imaging. 2012;5(3):239–51.
9. Gutiérrez-Chico JL, Zamorano JL, Pérez de Isla L, et al. Comparison of left ventricular volumes and ejection fractions measured by three-dimensional echocardiography versus by two-dimensional echocardiography and cardiac magnetic resonance in patients with various cardiomyopathies. Am J Cardiol. 2005;95(6):809–13.

10. Lang RM, Badano LP, Mor-Avi V, et al. Recommendations for cardiac chamber quantification by echocardiography in adults: an update from the American Society of Echocardiography and the European Association of Cardiovascular Imaging. J Am Soc Echocardiogr. 2015;28(1):1–39.

11. Takeuchi M, Jacobs A, Sugeng L, et al. Assessment of left ventricular dyssynchrony with real-time 3-dimensional echocardiography: comparison with Doppler tissue imaging. J Am Soc Echocardiogr. 2007;20:1321–9.

12. Mor-Avi V, Yodwut C, Jenkins C, et al. Real-time 3D echocardiographic quantification of left atrial volume: multicenter study for validation with CMR. JACC Cardiovasc Imaging. 2012;5(8):769–77.

13. Lancellotti P, Moura L, Pierard LA, et al. European Association of Echocardiography recommendations for the assessment of valvular regurgitation. Part 2: mitral and tricuspid regurgitation (native valve diseases). Eur J Echocardiogr. 2010;11:307–32.

14. Tsang W, Lang RM, Krozon I. Role of real-time three dimensional echocardiography in cardiovascular interventions. Heart. 2011;97:850–7.

15. Anwar AM, Geleijnse ML, Soliman OI, et al. Assessment of normal tricuspid valve anatomy in adults by real-time three-dimensional echocardiography. Int J Card Imaging. 2007;23(6): 717–24.

16. Gutiérrez-Chico JL, Zamorano JL, Prieto-Moriche E, et al. Real-time three-dimensional echocardiography in aortic stenosis: a novel, simple, and reliable method to improve accuracy in area calculation. Eur Heart J. 2008;29(10):1296–306.

17. Goldstein SA, Evangelista A, Abbara S, et al. Multimodality imaging of diseases of the thoracic aorta in adults: from the American Society of Echocardiography and the European Association of Cardiovascular Imaging: endorsed by the Society of Cardiovascular Computed Tomography and Society for Cardiovascular Magnetic Resonance. J Am Soc Echocardiogr. 2015;28(2):119–82.

18. Bleich S, Nanda NC, Hage FG. The incremental value of three-dimensional transthoracic echocardiography in adult congenital heart disease. Echocardiography. 2013;30:483–94.

19. Salustri A, Spitaels S, McGuie J, et al. Transthoracic three-dimensional echocardiography in adult patients with congenital heart disease. J Am Coll Cardiol. 1995;26:759–67.

20. Hage FG, Raslam S, Dean P, et al. Real time three-dimensional transthoracic echocardiography in congenital heart disease. Echocardiography. 2012;29:220–31.

21. Van der Zwaan HB, Helbing WA, Boersma E, et al. Usefulness of real-time three-dimensional echocardiography to identify right ventricular dysfunction in patients with congenital heart disease. Am J Cardiol. 2010;106:843–50.

22. Vettukattil JJ. Three-dimensional echocardiography in congenital heart disease. Heart. 2012;98:79–88.

23. Scheurer M, Bandisode V, Ruff P, et al. Early experience with real-time three-dimensional echocardiography guidance of right ventricular biopsy in children. Echocardiography. 2006;23(1):45–9.

# Chapter 3
# General Aspects of Transesophageal 3D-Echo

Ana García Martín, Teresa Segura de la Cal, and Cristina Fraile Sanz

## Abbreviations

| | |
|---|---|
| AV | Aortic valve |
| ECG | Electrocardiography |
| LA | Left atrium |
| LAA | Left atrial appendage |
| LV | Left ventricle |
| LVOT | Left ventricular out flow tract |
| ME | Mid esophageal |
| MV | Mitral valve |
| PV | Pulmonary valve |
| RA | Right atrium |
| RV | Right ventricle |
| TEE | Transesophageal echocardiography |
| TTE | Transthoracic echocardiography |
| TV | Tricuspid valve |

**Electronic supplementary material** The online version of this chapter (doi:10.1007/978-3-319-50335-6_3) contains supplementary material, which is available to authorized users.

A.G. Martín (✉) • T.S. de la Cal • C.F. Sanz
Cardiology Department, Hospital Ramon y Cajal, Madrid, Spain
e-mail: aggarciamartin@gmail.com

© Springer International Publishing AG 2017
E. Casas Rojo et al. (eds.), *Manual of 3D Echocardiography*,
DOI 10.1007/978-3-319-50335-6_3

# Introduction: General Advices for Acquisition of a TEE 3D Study

## *Introduction*

3D echocardiography has many advantages over 2D echocardiography although they are both available and complementary techniques. 3D echocardiography gives us information on the spatial relationships of different cardiac structures, offers a lot of projections and different views and we can obtain volumetric data without geometric assumptions.

3D transthoracic (TTE) and transesophageal echocardiography (TEE) have several applications in clinical practice. 3D TTE (discussed in the previous chapter) is usually more useful for evaluation of the cardiac chambers and for the ventricular volume evaluation. However, 3D TEE is a more accurate technique for the study of intracardiac masses, septal defects and specially to define the valve function and morphology. It plays a relevant role in the decision-making process and in monitoring catheter-based procedures.

Therefore, 3D echocardiography technology allows us to obtain anatomical and functional data of different cardiac structures, and a comprehensive and complementary information to that obtained by 2D echocardiography.

## *Acquisition*

3D TEE imaging acquisition is similar to TTE and it is based on the same grounds. Globally, we have two different ways for 3D data acquisition:

- Multiple-beat 3D imaging: This mode needs electrocardiography (ECG) gating and it is based on creation a single volumetric data set though the join of several narrow volumes of data along 2–6 cardiac beats.
- Live 3D (Real time): Information proceeds from a single cardiac cycle and it displays a thin pyramidal scan data without need for ECG gating. It is important to know that the spatial and temporal resolution is worse than in previous mode.

In a practical way, current transducers have four different acquisition modes [1]:

- Narrow angle live acquisition mode (Real-time 3D): In this mode, pyramidal volumes of variable dimensions are acquired. Usually the size of the sector is not sufficient to study the target structure in a single plane.
- Zoom mode (Wide sector): This mode is useful to visualize cardiac valves and other small structures. We must determine the size of the region of interest and image can be rotated to orient structure as we want and to obtain a concrete point of view (such as "en face" view in valvular pathology).
- Full Volume: This mode needs gating and obtains a wider volume of the structures, from 4 to 8 heartbeats. It can generate >90° scanning volumes and still maintain

high temporal resolution (at a frame rate of >30 Hz) with good spatial resolution. It can be used in large structures to get information about full ventricular volumes, which can be offline analyzed and processed. A regular cardiac rhythm and adequate breath-holding are needed to reduce the incidence of artefacts when the subvolumes are merged together. The final image formed is not 'live'.
– Color Doppler mode: This mode combines grey scale volumetric data with colour Doppler. It can be displayed using real-time 3D and full volume. It is useful for examination of regurgitant lesion and shunts.

In comparison with 3D TTE, TEE is the method of choice to get more accurate information about color flow abnormalities.


**Transesophageal 3DE Examination Protocol** [1, 2]

A systematic and comprehensive examination must be carried out in all patients. However, some pathologies require different, unconventional and out of protocol views [3]. Good quality 2D image of the structure of interest must be obtained to switch to live 3D mode and the gain should be adjusted to get an optimized image, trying to avoid both excess and defect of it.

A preliminary study of the structure of interest by using the 2D multiplane modality of TEE is useful. After this first approach 3D TEE study starts using real-time 3D (narrow angle). Full volume data set or Zoom mode can also be acquired, with and without color Doppler depending on the structure to study [4]:

1. *Cardiac Chambers*: It is reasonable to start with mid esophageal (ME) four chamber view, and to acquire a full volume data to study some eventual valve disease and specially to get information about global function of left ventricle (LV) and right ventricle (RV).

   – LV:

     • 0–120° ME.
     • Real time 3D and full volume acquisition (offline analyses).
     • Volume and ejection fraction information.

   – RV:

     • 0–120° ME.
     • Real time 3D and full volume acquisition (offline analyses).
     • Volume and ejection fraction information.

   – Left atrial appendage:

     • 90° ME.
     • Real time 3D and Zoom mode "en face view" (offline or online analyses).
     • Rule out thrombus inside LAA.
     • Measuring diameters (Sagittal, coronal and transverse sections).
     • Guide and monitoring catheter-based procedure.

2. *Mitral Valve (MV):* 3D TEE is an exceptional method to study the MV and all the different modes can be used to do a precise examination of this structure.

- 0–120° ME.
- Zoom mode: Zoom box must be adjusted to include the entire valve.

    - "En face" view from the left atrium: the points of reference are the LAA and aortic valve. Image can be rotated to place the aortic valve at 12 o'clock position (surgeon's view).
    - "End face" view from the LV: the point of reference is the LV outflow tract (LVOT).

- Full volume (Gated acquisition): This acquisition includes a wide sector such as the entire mitral apparatus.
- Full volume with Color Doppler (Gated acquisition): Mitral regurgitation severity by quantification of PISA, vena contracta area and direction flow.

3. *Aortic Valve (AV):*

- 60° ME – Short axis.
- 120° ME – Long axis.
- Zoom mode and Full volume with and without Color Doppler.
- Valve disease, measurements of aortic annular size, aortic valve area, LVOT area, distance between aortic annulus and coronary ostium.

4. *Interatrial Septum:*

- 60–90° ME with the probe rotated to the interatrial septum.
- Zoom mode and Full volume.
- "En face" view from left or right atrium.
- Complex atrial septal defects and transcatheter closure.

5. *Tricuspid Valve (TV):*

- 0–30° *ME*- four chamber view, with the probe rotated to get adequate view of TV.
- 40° transgastric view.
- Zoom mode and Full volume with and without Color Doppler.
- Morphologic and functional data of tricuspid valve.

6. *Pulmonary Valve (PV):*

- 90° high esophageal.
- 120° ME- three chamber view.
- Zoom mode with and without Color Doppler.
- "En face" view from RV and pulmonary artery. Image can be rotated to place the anterior leaflet at 12 o'clock position.

7. *Other structures:*

Bicaval plane.

- 90° ME.
- Position of central catheters and pacemaker leads. Presence of masses, thrombus or vegetations.

## Cardiac Chambers and Devices

### *Left Ventricle (LV)*

The LV study must include data about its size, mass and global and regional function. For this reason, 2D and 3D TTE and TEE images should be routinely obtained from all the patients.

The main advantage of 3D echocardiography is that this technique does not make geometric assumptions to get information about volume and ejection fraction of LV. Therefore, 3D echocardiography is a useful tool especially in that ventricles with complex geometries [4]. Other advantages to keep in mind are that 3D imaging is unaffected by foreshortening and it is more accurate and reproducible compared to other imaging modalities [5]; In addition, the multiplane transducer provides multiple cross-sections without changing the position of the probe.

3D image acquisition should focus primarily on including the entire LV within the pyramidal data set. We should acquire real time or full volume images from ME view (from 0° to 120°). Temporal resolution should be maximized without compromising spatial resolution to ensure reasonably accurate identification of end-systole [1] (Fig. 3.1, Video 3.1).

If the entire LV is included in the volume data set, the left ventricular shape, the quantitative evaluation of volumes, and global and regional function can be measured by a 3D quantification software. This semiautomatic program requires the operators to determine reference points along the base and apex of the LV. An automatic endocardial border-tracking program then identifies and traces the endocardial border and the program calculates left end-systolic and end-diastolic volumes using a 3D deformable model without geometric assumptions [6] (Fig. 3.2).

Left heart contrast administration can be used to enhance border detection in patients with poor endocardial visibility.

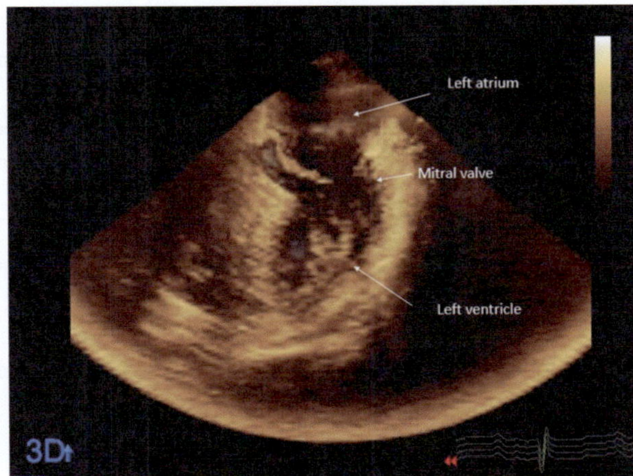


**Fig. 3.1** Full volume 3D four-chamber acquisition focus on the left ventricle for posterior analysis

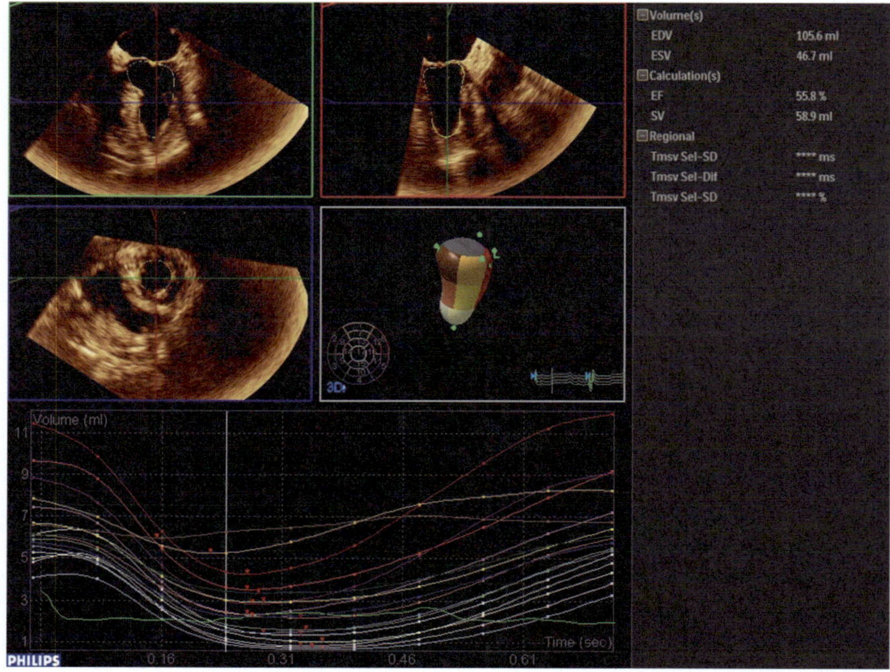



**Fig. 3.2** Full volume 3D four chamber view acquisition with off line post-processing. The program traces the end-systolic and end-diastolic endocardial borders and calculates the volumes, global and regional function without geometric assumptions

*LV measurements:*

- <u>LV volumes:</u>
- 3D echocardiographic measurements of LV volumes are recommended when feasible depending on image quality.
- Mitral annulus and LV apex are the points of reference used by the semiautomated quantification software to start the edge detection.
- Papillary muscles and LV trabeculae should be included within LV cavity for the quantification.
- LV volume is computed after the construction of a surface-rendered cavity cast of the LV.
- The distance between transducer and LV does not permit, in some cases, good images of the left ventricular trabeculae from ME. In these cases, we can try to obtain images from transgastric viewpoint.
- <u>LV global and segmentary function:</u>
- In patients with good image quality, ejection fraction measurements are reproducible and should be performed when available and feasible.
- A semiautomated endocardial interface algorithm performs the cavity contours and their changes during the cardiac cycle (manual corrections to the endocardial borders can be performed).

- 3D data allows the assessment of LV regional strain, synchrony and wall stress, but these measurements are not performed in a routine study
- 3D TEE data are complementary to 3D transthoracic data, which is the most common way to calculate LV systolic function.
- LV mass:
- Because 3D echocardiography is the only technique that measures myocardial volume in a direct way, it is an appropriate approach. However, available mass data are not sufficient to recommend normal reference values.
- It could be used in abnormally shaped ventricles or in localized or asymmetric hypertrophy, but there are no validated reference values.
- LV structural abnormalities:
- 3D TEE images can be obtained to study thrombus, inside ventricle masses or ventricular septal defect (3D Color flow mapping and visual assessment).

## *Right Ventricle (RV)*

The RV is a functionally and structurally complex cardiac chamber. The marked trabeculation, the prominent intraventricular structures and the special shape of the RV represent a challenge for the echocardiographers [1, 7].

3D TEE is a reproducible tool to provide data about RV volumes and ejection fraction with an adequate correlation to reference standards (magnetic resonance image). However, the use of 3D echo in RV measurement is not a routine in all the echocardiographic labs.

A full volume data set should be acquired from a ME or subcostal view, making sure that the entire RV is included (Fig. 3.3).

The available methods used to quantify RV function include a volumetric semi-automated border detection algorithm and the methods of discs. A semiautomated border detection algorithm determinates the RV end-diastolic and end-systolic volume and the ejection fraction.

RV segmental function can be measured from the segmental analysis of the three main portions of the chamber (apex, inlet and outflow segments).

## *Right and Left Atria*

The development of 3D TEE imaging is related to the progress of electrophysiology and the implant of percutaneous devices. 3D TEE is ideal for visualization of (LAA), pulmonary veins and the interatrial septum [2].

From ME 90° view of LAA and MV, we can obtain good images of the left pulmonary veins if we make a mild clockwise rotation. Zoom mode or narrow-angled acquisitions can be displayed [1].

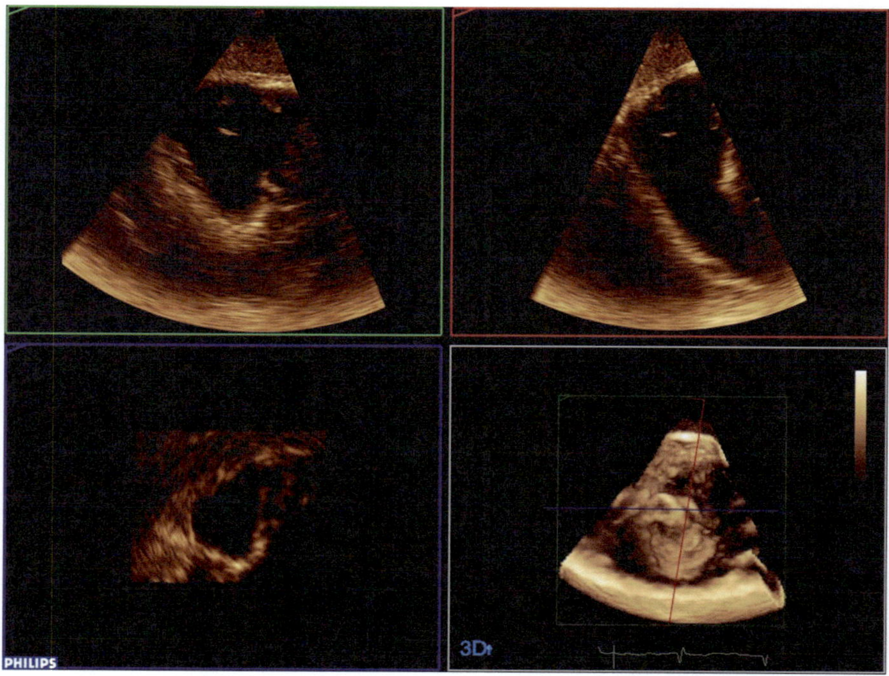


**Fig. 3.3** Multiplanar reconstruction image of the right ventricle. The 3D data set was obtained with full volume 3D from the subcostal view

Interatrial septum can be analyzed from ME view with a clockwise rotation. When viewing from the left atrium (LA), the atrial septum should be oriented with the right upper pulmonary vein at the one o'clock position; when viewing from the right atrium the superior vena cava should be located at the 11 o'clock position.

From ME (0–45–90–135°) view LAA imaging can be performed. Multiplane imaging can help to obtain information about LAA lobes. An "en face" view of the LAA orifice can be studied if we obtain a zoom mode image. 3D TEE offers an excellent estimation of LAA orifice area and useful information to choose the device's correct size (Fig. 3.4).

## *Devices*

3D TEE offers a good orientation and spatial visualization of the different cardiac structures and intracardiac devices during catheter-based percutaneous procedures.

In most patients with pacemakers or implantable cardioverter-defibrillators we can identify with this technique, the atrial or ventricular leads position inside right chambers, and the occasional tricuspid regurgitation [8]. Thrombi or vegetations can appear as complications of a pacemaker or central catheter's implantation. Usually, thrombus is positioned in the right atrium (RA) (the junction of the right atrium and the superior vena cava). To evaluate this kind of complications, images can be acquired using live

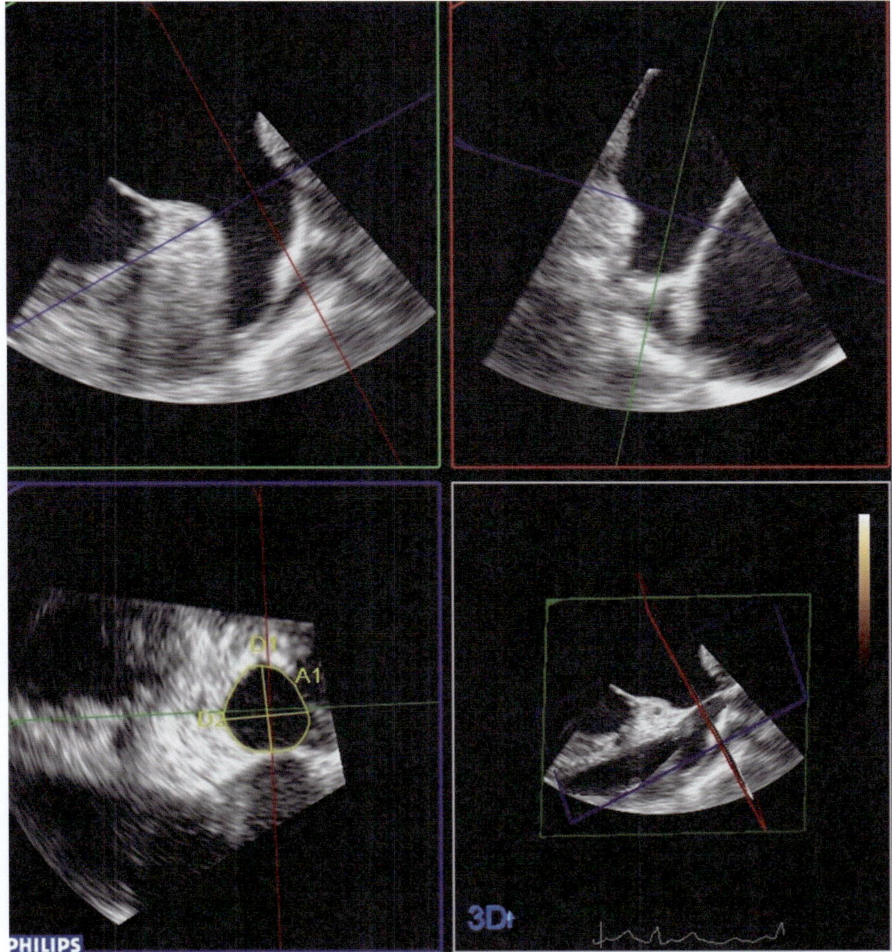

**Fig. 3.4** Multiplanar reconstruction mode used to measure left atrial appendage dimensions to choose the device correct size, from zoom 3D acquisition of the left atrial appendage

3D echocardiography and 3D zoom mode in a bicaval plane or in ME four chamber view (focused on right chambers), and we must display a simultaneous dual-plane visualization in order to obtain complete information of the spatial disposition.

As a further application, 3D echocardiography could be an available tool to guide the positioning of LV lead in coronary veins during biventricular pacemaker implantation.

# Mitral Valve

Assessment of the mitral valve (MV) primarily requires the understanding of its complex structure and function. That correct function is reliant on the integrity and coordination of each of its components: mitral leaflets, mitral annulus and subvalvular apparatus (chordae tendinae and papillary muscles). Due to that complexity, imaging of the MV valve is one of the most challenging applications of 3D echocardiography as it has the power to provide an understanding of the mechanism of valve failure and the likelihood of a successful surgical MV repair when needed [9].

## *Anatomy*

The MV comprises two leaflets, attached to the atrioventricular junction by the mitral annulus, and by the chordae tendinosus to the papillary muscles.

The mural or posterior leaflet is narrow but has a larger circumferential attachment occupying two thirds of the mitral annulus. It presents indentations (called clefts) along the elongated free edge, which divide the leaflet into three scallops. Carpentier's nomenclature organizes these scallops into P1, P2 and P3 ranging from the anterolateral to the posteromedial commissure. The anterior or aortic leaflet is broader, with a cuadrangular/semicircular shape. By its attachment to the anterior third of the mitral annulus makes continuity with left and non-coronary cusps of the aortic valve (AV), and with the interleaflet triangle between the aortic cusps that abuts onto the membranous septum, making up the fibrous trigonous of the heart. For clinical purposes, it is also divided into three scallops corresponding to the opposite regions of the mural leaflet [10].

Mitral annulus is a nonplanar saddle-shaped structure with two high points (peaks) lying anteriorly and posteriorly (at the aortic insertion and posterior left ventricular wall), and two low points (troughs) closest to the apex, located medially and laterally. Its geometry is poorly understood by 2D echocardiography as it is equivalent to a hyperbolic paraboloid [9], a geometric surface where all sections parallel to one coordinate plane are hyperbolas and all sections parallel to another coordinate plane are parabolas.

Subvalvular apparatus comprises the cordae tendinae and the papillary muscles. Papillary muscles bundles are generally described in anterolateral and posteromedial positions of the LV so any impairment on left ventricular muscle (as happens in ischaemic or dilated cardiomyopathy) may contribute to MV dysfunction.

## *Data Acquisition*

3D TEE has improved visual assessment of the MV. It provides easily understanding images without requiring probe manipulation of 2D echo, allowing a more efficient examination process.

A preliminary study of the mitral apparatus by using the 2D multiplane modality of transesophageal echocardiography is useful as a first approach to the MV. 2D images at different degrees of exploration, usually obtained at ME depth, may help us to identify the primary mechanism and aetiology of MV dysfunction.

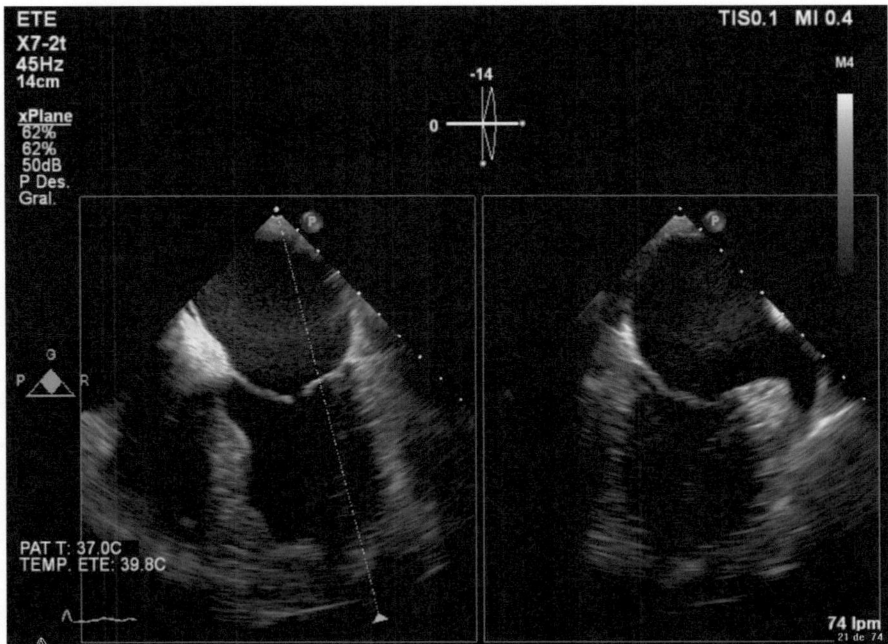

**Fig. 3.5** X plane image acquisition of the mitral valve. The left hand image displays the live image. Adjusting the cursor will alter the angle of acquisition of the second image on the right hand side

Nevertheless, 3D echocardiography probes permit the use of a dual screen to obtain two real 2D images simultaneously by simultaneous multiplane imaging (Fig. 3.5). The first image would be a reference view of the valve, typically at ME depth (so you can assess the MV and the subvalvular apparatus), while the second image or lateral plane represents a plane rotated 30–150° from the reference one [1]. This preliminary survey must be done with and without colour flow Doppler to identify the mechanism of mitral valve dysfunction if present.

Once this first approach is done, it is time for 3D images acquisition. To obtain quality 3D images, we can use the live 3D mode to optimize gain settings. Live 3D could also be useful to evaluate LV geometry and papillary muscles. In addition, it might be interesting to view the mitral apparatus in continuity with the left ventricular walls, by obtaining a real time 3D image from the entire LV after having increased depth and focus of the 2D reference image. Moreover, a real-time 3D view of the mitral apparatus could be obtained at the end of the exam from the transgastric two-chamber view to assess the papillary muscles and chordae tendineae.

Then, as we have to examine a pyramidal volume to assess the whole three-dimensional valve, we can use different acquisition modes: Live-3D, full-volume or zoom mode.

3D zoom permits a focused, wide-sector view of the MV apparatus from the annulus to the papillary muscle tips. When selected, the 3D zoom mode displays a

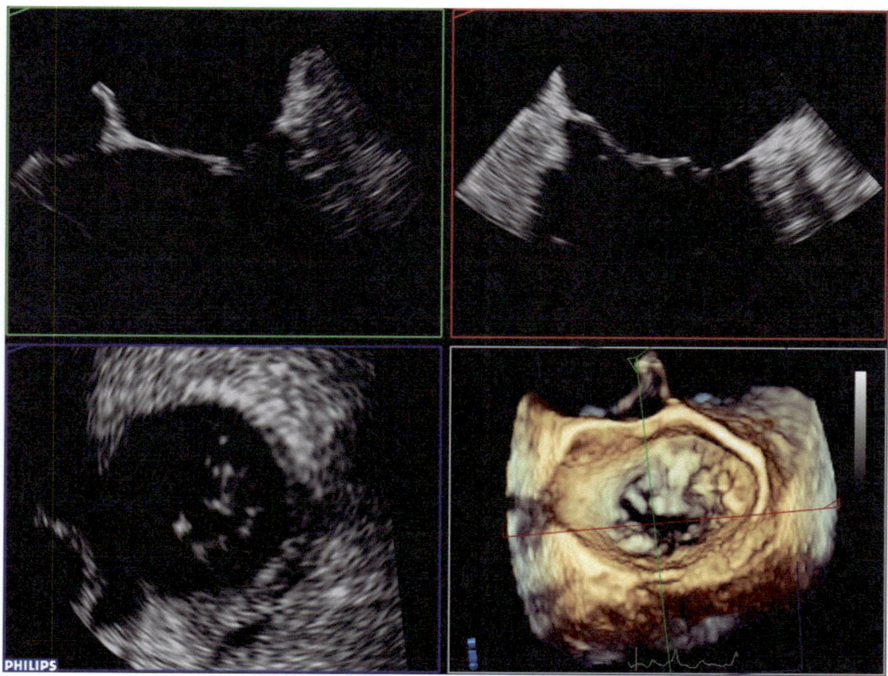

**Fig. 3.6** 3D zoom acquisition of the mitral valve and X plane display. Subsequent rotation allows visualization of the valve from the left atrium. In addition, the mitral valve should be rotated so that aortic valve is located superiorly at the 12-o'clock position

bi-plane preview screen showing the original view and the corresponding orthogonal image (as in simultaneous multiplane mode), and it displays a sector (zoom sector) over the region of interest in both planes. Zoom sector boxes should be placed carefully and sector-width minimized to obtain the leaflets and the annulus, so we can improve temporal resolution and optimize image quality. Now, acquisition can be done, so a pyramidal volume is obtained.

The obtained volume must be reoriented to be able to assess MV structure, so it should be rotated 90° counter clockwise, around the x axis to present the valve as viewed from the LA (surgeon view), or 90° clockwise, to present it as viewed from the LV. In addition, the MV should be rotated counterclockwise in the z-plane so that aortic valve is located superiorly at the 12-o'clock position (Fig. 3.6, Video 3.2).

The obtained 3D dataset can be view from multiple angles and cropped in different planes to estimate the smallest true MV orifice by planimetry.

Finally, colour flow Doppler should be added to 3D morphology to exclude the presence of regurgitant jets or stenosis [3]. 3D colour Doppler acquisition could be performed using live 3D or multiple-beat full-volume acquisition. As smaller colour Doppler volumes and lower frame rates limit live 3D mode, we recommend colour full volume acquisition for MV study. As explained before, for its preparation from a dual screen with a simultaneous colour Doppler 2D–image, zoom sectors should

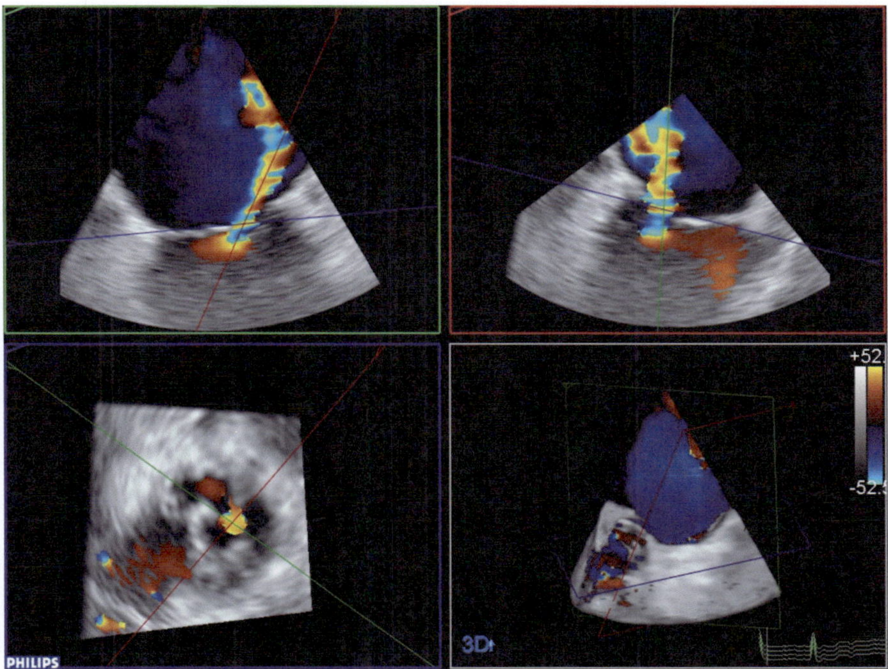

**Fig. 3.7** Two orthogonal views of the mitral valve following 3D zoom acquisition with superimposed 3D colour flow Doppler, to evaluate the origin of the regurgitant jet as well as estimate the vena contracta and regurgitant orifice area

be limited to the region of interest, placing the regurgitant jet in the center of the sector to reach a balance between the region of exploration (larger sector) and frame rate (high line density images) to obtain good and reliable images.

The 3D colour full volume data set can be rotated and cut in different planes in order to quantify the origin of the regurgitant jet as well as estimate the vena contracta and regurgitant orifice area (Fig. 3.7, Video 3.3).

As a guide to explore the mitral valve we propose the following approach:

– In the first place, use the simultaneous multiplane mode at ME depth as a starting point for the exam. Optimize 2D quality images and then use the 3D live mode to modify gain settings for a better 3D image and to assess LV anatomy and subvalvular apparatus.
– Use the dual reference view to prepare real time 3D zoom acquisition mode. This dual view can be obtained at 90° (two chambers view), and the second image would represent an orthogonal at 120°, (an aortic long axis view).
– To continue, acquire a real time 3D zoom data set by keeping the MV in the zoom sector in both the two chamber and its orthogonal plane.
– Once acquired, the image should be displayed. For that purpose, volume should be rotated around the x-axis towards the examiner, to present the valve as viewed from the LA (surgical view), or in the opposite direction if we prefer a vision

from the LV. Finally, and irrespective of perspective, the AV should be placed at 12 o'clock position.

– Finally, colour flow Doppler should be added to the region of interest to analyse regurgitant jets or valve stenosis. If present, detailed information is needed so we recommend to prepare real time 3D zoom acquisition with superimposed 3D colour flow Doppler. Now, region of interest (for example, the regurgitant jet) should be placed in the centre of the sector in both images of the simultaneous dual screen. The region of interest should be limited to the mitral apparatus and colour flow Doppler jet to optimize temporal and spatial resolution.

## *Applications*

– To assess the MV morphology and pathology.
– To plan, guide and assess the complications in the MV repair.
– To assess the prosthesis MV, allowing a detailed assessment of the valve and any coexisting pathology (dehiscence).

## **Aortic Valve, Annulus and Aortic Root**

### *Introduction*

AV imaging has gained interest during the past years probably due to the development in transcatheter valve replacement and new aortic prostheses. Visualization of the AV from transthoracic echocardiography is insufficient in many cases. 3D TEE provides superior spatial resolution and image quality for valve assessment to clarify the mechanism of pathology and also to guide the aortic valve interventional procedure [11].

The correct function of the AV is largely dependent on the integrity of each of its components: the valve itself and the aortic root. 3D data set of AV can be displayed as visualized from different angles, so its interaction with the surrounding structures can be easily understood without the need of mental reconstruction from multiple 2D views.

### *Anatomy*

The anatomy and function of the AV have always triggered scientific curiosity. As it has been said before, AV is more than just a three semilunar cusps valve. Its attachment to the aortic root and the LV plays an ineluctable role in its function. Aortic root comprises both the Valsalva sinuses and the sinotubular junction, so any dilatation of these structures will lead to valve dysfunction.

An ellipse can be used to represent the ventriculo-anatomic junction of the AV. Approximately one-third of the ellipse is connected to the anterior mitral leaflet via the fibrous continuity or aortic-mitral curtain, and the remaining two thirds to the interventricular septum. Aortic cusps insertion in the aortic root takes a crown-like shape with three highest points at the sinotubular junction and three lowest points below the anatomic ventriculo-aortic junction, making up the virtual basal ring at this basal plane. It must be notice that the true anatomic aortic ring would rather be the whole crown-like structure located between the sinotubular junction and the virtual basal ring, not only this last one [12]. Nevertheless, in clinical practice, virtual basal ring is the area of interest measured in echo-labs and labeled as aortic ring.

## *Data Acquisition*

A preliminary survey of the AV by using the 2D multiplane modality of transesophageal probe is useful as a first approach. For AV, biplane images must be obtained from upper esophageal views at different degrees of exploration, typically at 30° and 120°. In fact, this survey can be simplified with the use of simultaneous multiplane mode of 3D echo. It displays in a dual screen both the reference view (usually at 30°) and its orthogonal plane (at 120°). So the AV can be examined from its short and long axis at the same time. Then, colour flow Doppler should be added to rule out the presence of aortic valve dysfunction and to identify the mechanism, if present (Fig. 3.8).

Once these orthogonal 2D views are optimized, we can use live 3D mode to optimize gain settings. Then, a pyramidal volume must be obtained to be able to analyse the whole valve and not just the near field offered by live 3D mode.

Real-time 3D zoom permits a focused, wide-sector view of the AV and the aortic root. When selected, 3D–zoom mode displays a bi-plane preview screen showing the original view and the corresponding orthogonal image (as in simultaneous multiplane mode), and it displays a sector (zoom sector) over the region of interest in both planes. To have these zoom sectors centred in the selected structure, you might need to displace the zoom sector in the orthogonal plane (the one on the left) by using the control buttons available in the equipment. Zoom sector-width should be minimized to obtain the leaflets, the aortic ring, and usually the aortic root with its coronary ostia (of particular interest in transcatheter aortic valve replacement (TAVR) studies) [13]. These minimized sectors offer better temporal resolution and optimize image quality. Now, acquisition can be done, so a pyramidal volume is obtained.

After acquisition, image should be rotated clockwise around the y-axis, to present the valve as viewed from the ascending aorta, or counter-clockwise if we prefer a vision from the left ventricular outflow tract. In any case, the valve should be displayed with the right coronary cusp located inferiorly, regardless of perspective [1] (Fig. 3.9, Video 3.4).

 

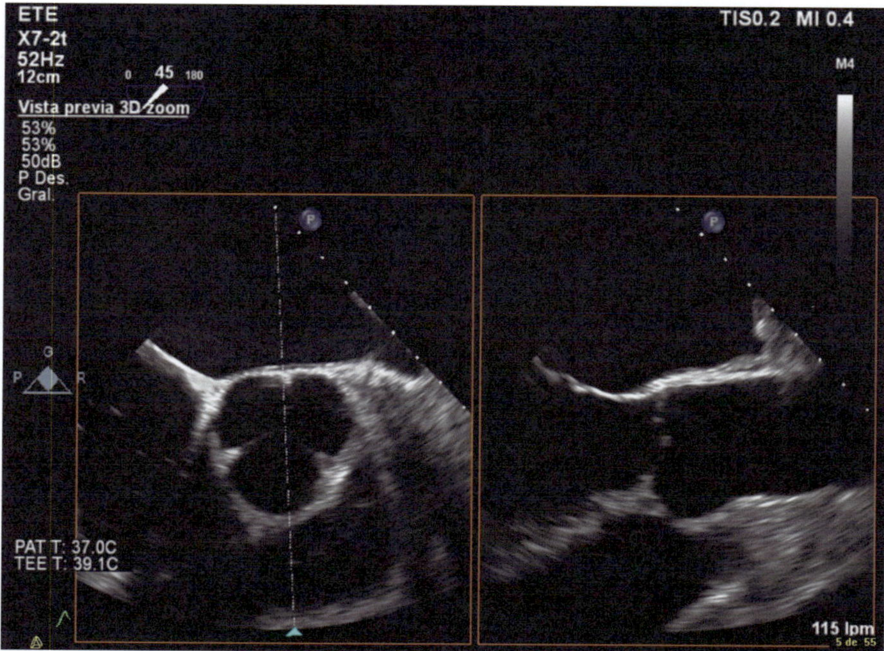

**Fig. 3.8** X plane image acquisition of the aortic valve. The left hand image displays the live image. Adjusting the cursor will alter the angle of acquisition of the second image on the right hand side

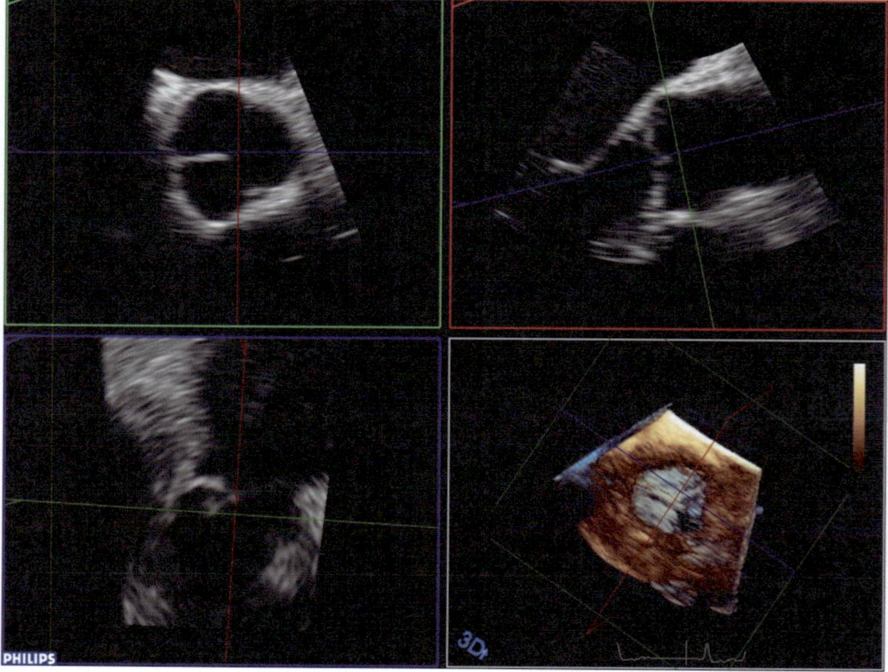

**Fig. 3.9** Two orthogonal views of the aortic valve following 3D zoom acquisition. After correct alignment of the axes, aortic valve area and annulus area can be traced and quantify

3D datasets of the AV can be post-processed so that it can be analysed from multiple angles and cropped at different planes to estimate the anatomical aortic valve area by planimetry, the aortic ring the left ventricle outflow tract and the proximal aorta.

3D flow assessment might be needed for echocardiography diagnosis. 3D colour Doppler acquisition could be done by superimposing colour Doppler to live 3D or to multiple-beat full-volume acquisition modes. As detailed data might be needed to quantify valve dysfunction, multiple-beat full-volume acquisition modes are recommended. As explained for real time 3D zoom acquisition mode, its preparation starts from a dual screen with simultaneous colour Doppler 2D–images. Again, zoom sectors should be limited to the region of interest, placing the regurgitant jet or jets in the centre of the sector. These colour Doppler signals can be cropped at the valve level to planimeter the vena contracta width [14] (Fig. 3.10, Video 3.5).

To sum up, as a guide to explore the aortic valve we propose the following approach:

- In the first place, use the simultaneous multiplane mode at upper-esophageal depth as a starting point for the exam. The reference view can be taken at 30° (short axis view), so the second image would represent the orthogonal at 120° (representing the long axis view). Optimize 2D quality images and then use the 3D live mode to modify gain settings for a better 3D image and to assess the

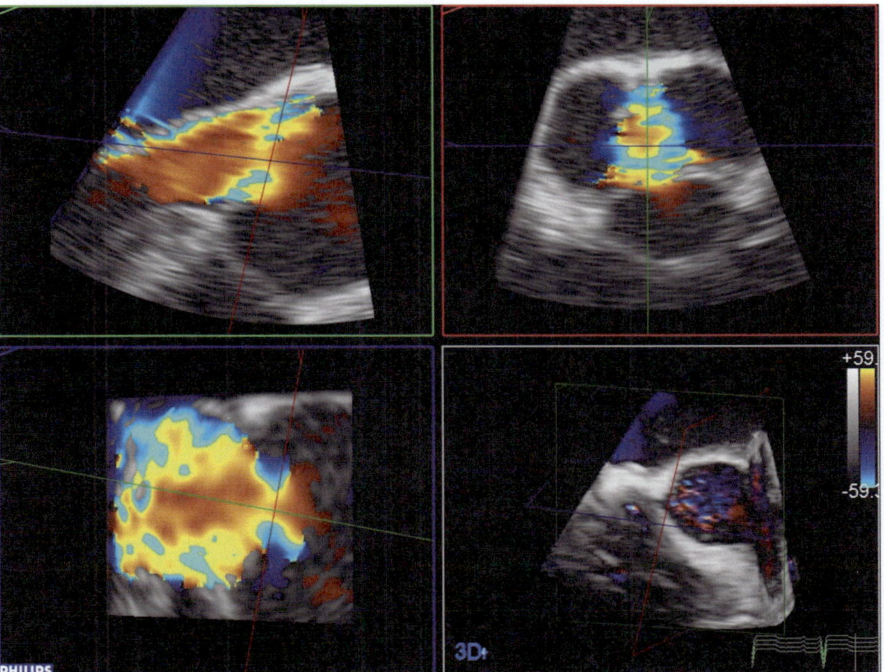


**Fig. 3.10** Two orthogonal views of the aortic valve following 3D zoom acquisition with superimposed 3D colour flow Doppler, to evaluate the origin of the regurgitant jet as well as estimate the vena contracta width

valve and its interaction with surrounding structures (aortic root and mitro-aortic continuity).

- To continue, from these images, acquire a real time 3D zoom data set by keeping the AV in the zoom sector in both the short axis and its orthogonal plane. You might need to displace the zoom sector in the orthogonal plane trough the control buttons available in the equipment.
- Once acquired, the image should be displayed. For that purpose, volume should be rotated clockwise around the y-axis, to present the valve as viewed from the ascending aorta, or counter-clockwise if we prefer a vision from the left ventricular outflow tract. Finally, and irrespective of perspective, the AV should be displayed with the right coronary cusp located inferiorly, regardless of perspective.
- Finally, blood flow should be assessed. A first approach can be done by superimposing colour flow doppler to live 3D images, but for further information, we recommend to prepare real time 3D zoom acquisition with superimposed 3D colour flow Doppler.

## *Applications*

- To assess the AV morphology and pathology.
- To plan, guide and assess the complications in the TAVR.
- To assess the prosthesis aortic valves, allowing a detailed assessment of the valve and any coexisting pathology.

## Interatrial Septum and Venous Drainage

### *Anatomy*

The left atrium (LA) has a venous component that receives the pulmonary veins, an atrial appendage, and shares the septum with the RA. The pulmonary veins drain into the LA through the ostia. There is significant variability in the branching patterns of the pulmonary veins, being the most common pattern two veins from the hilum of each lung. The right superior pulmonary vein lies behind the superior cava vein. The left pulmonary veins are separated from the left atrial appendage by the ligament of Marshall.

The RA consists of four components, the right atrial appendage, the venous part, the vestibulum and the atrial septum, which is shared with the LA.

The atrial septum is a blade-shaped structure that divides the RA and LA; due to its obliquity, RA mainly lies anterior to LA. It has a concave anterior margin that reflects the curve of the ascending aorta, a convex posterior margin, and an inferior margin along the mitral annulus.

## Data Acquisition

3D TEE is an excellent technique for the evaluation of the interatrial septum and its adjacent structures, therefore 3D imaging has become invaluable not only for confirming dimensions of atrial septal defects but also to demonstrate the spatial relationship of defects to surrounding structures and to guide percutaneous closure of the defects.

Different 3D TEE modalities can be used for its assessment because each one of them has strengths and limitations. Live 3D has high volume rate but small 3D sector size when compare with full volume. 3D zoom mode allows select a sector of the volume before off-line cropping, offering the best en face image of the septum by it is limit by slow rate [15].

Using 3D TEE zoom, imaging of the interatrial septum is usually obtained from 2D TEE bicava plane. The depth of the pyramidal data should be adjusted to acquire just the left and right sides of the atrial septum, trying to avoid surrounding structures that mask the septum. Then, 90° up-down rotation allows to visualize the interatrial septum en face from the RA (Fig. 3.11) or from the LA (Fig. 3.12).

3D colour full volume data set can be used to view the flow of blood across defects.

After acquisition, 3D datasets can be viewed from multiple angles and analyzed using multiplanar reconstruction tool and cropping to size the defect and their relationship to surround structures.

3D TEE does not allow to visualize the four pulmonary veins in the same view. Real-time 3D is probably the best tool to acquire the pulmonary veins. From 90° ME view with slight counter clockwise rotation, both left pulmonary veins can be visualized (Fig. 3.13). From the same view a clockwise rotation the entire atrial septum en face should be displayed. The right pulmonary veins should appear in the long axis orientation.

## Pulmonary Valve

### Anatomy

The pulmonary root complex is composed of the valvular leaflets, the sinuses of Valsalva, the interleaflet triangles, and the free-standing distal RV muscular infundibulum. The PV is located above the RV outflow tract, below the main pulmonary artery, and anterior, superior, and slightly to the left of the AV. In normal conditions, the PV is a semilunar valve with three cusps. The three pulmonic valve leaflets are defined by their relationship to the septum and the AV and are thus termed anterior or nonseptal, right and left leaflets.

Assessment of the PV by 2D echocardiography is difficult, because the valve cusps are hard to visualize on the short axis view, and usually only two cusps can be

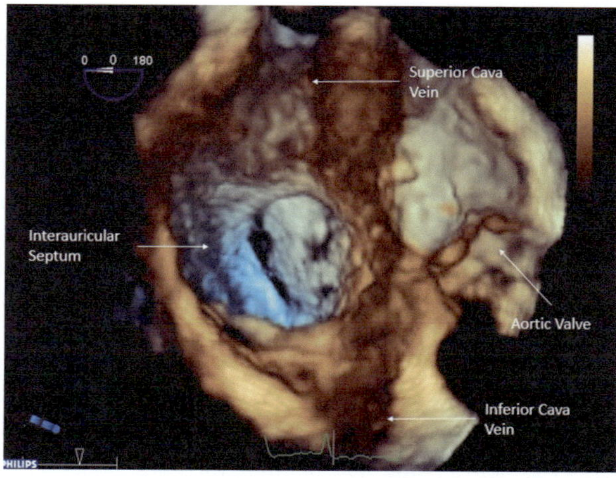



**Fig. 3.11** En face view of the interatrial septum from the right atrium following live 3D acquisition, allowing the assessment of its relationship to surround structures

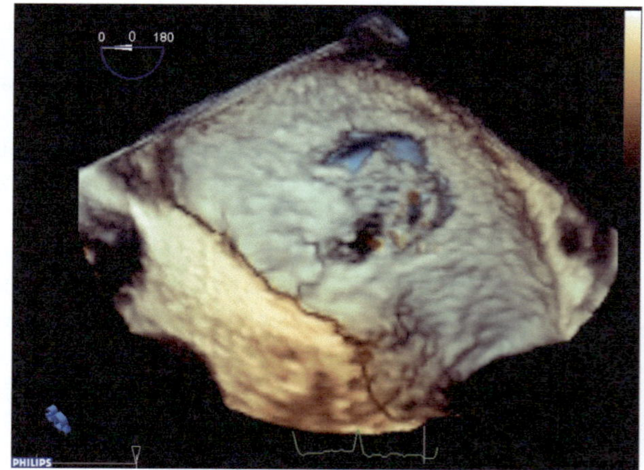



**Fig. 3.12** En face view of the interatrial septum from the left atrium following live 3D acquisition, it allows the measure of atrial defects and the assessment of its relationship to surround structures

simultaneous visualize. 3D TTE allows visualization of the entire valve structure as well as assessment of the RV outflow and main pulmonary artery. However, this technique may be limited in patients with poor acoustic windows. This is the reason why 3D TEE may allow better assessment of this structure though it is also limited because the anterior position of the PV and its thin leaflets.

## Data Acquisition

First, a primary analysis of the PV should be performed using 2D multiplane echocardiography. The TEE probe can be positioned at high esophageal position at 50° approximately. Once the valve is optimally visualized the 3D acquisition can be performed; live 3D, full-volume or zoom mode can be used. Next, the image

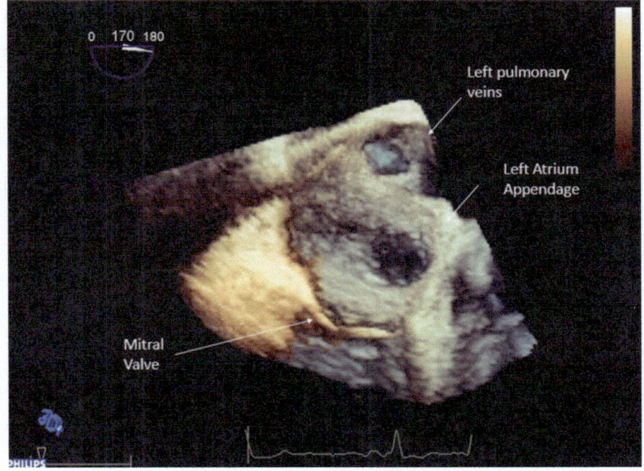

**Fig. 3.13** Live 3D acquisition of the left atrium. Subsequent rotation allows the visualization of both left pulmonary veins, left atrial appendage and its relationship with mitral valve



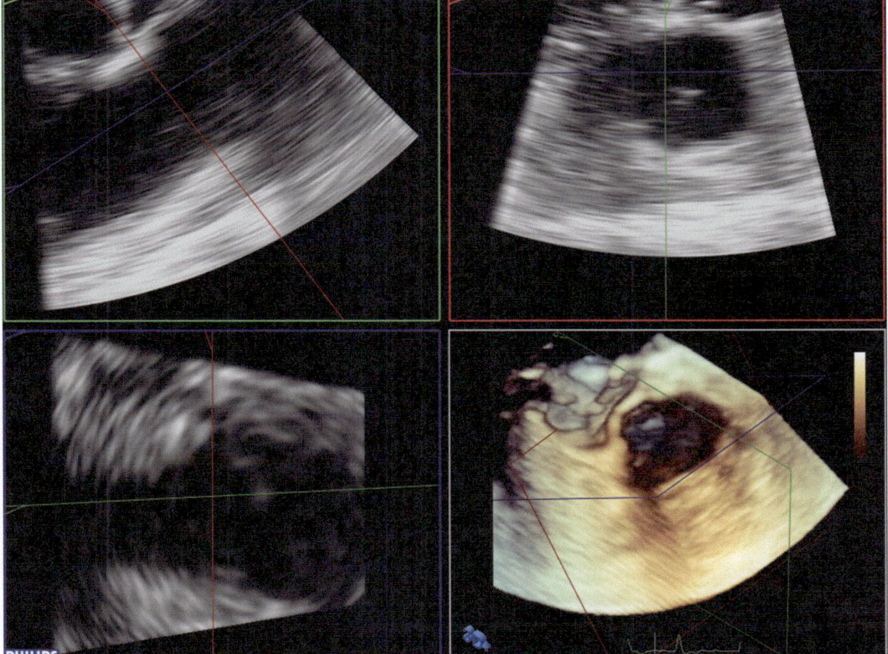

**Fig. 3.14** Two orthogonal views of the pulmonary valve following 3D zoom acquisition. After correct alignment of the axes, pulmonary valve area and annulus area can be traced and quantify

volume should be rotated around the X axis counterclockwise 90° so that the PV is displayed en face from the pulmonary artery. Finally, the anterior leaflet should be located superiorly in the 12 o'clock position, by rotating the image 180° (Fig. 3.14).

To assess the flow through the PV, color flow Doppler should be added to the full volume acquisition. The size of the region of interest should be limited to the PV and the color flow jet to optimize frame rate. 3D color data set can be analyzed using multiplanar reconstruction tool and cropping to quantify the pulmonary regurgitation and stenosis.

Although 3D echocardiography has been shown to be useful for defining the mechanism and severity of valvular dysfunction, there is no current evidence supporting the routine use of 3D TEE for the evaluation of pulmonary valve disease [1].

## Applications

–  To assess the PV morphology and pathology.

## Tricuspid Valve

### Anatomy

In normal conditions, the TV is located slightly closer to the apex than the MV. The space in between the septal insertion of the TV and the septal insertion of the anterior leaflet of MV belongs to the membranous septum that separates the LV from the right atrium (RA).

The TV is composed by the fibrous annulus, leaflets, chordae tendinae and papillary muscles.

The fibrous annulus is a saddle-shaped structure with the highest points in an antero-posterior orientation and the lowest points in a medio-lateral orientation. In patients with functional tricuspid regurgitation, the annulus dilates along the right ventricular free wall and becomes more circular and planar [16].

The valve consists of three leaflets designated by their position: anterior or superior, posterior or inferior and septal. The anterior tricuspid leaflet has the largest area and is attached along the anterolateral surface of the tricuspid annulus. The septal leaflet attaches along the interventricular surface and the posterior leaflet along the posterior portion of the annulus.

The variability of the papillary muscles is a normal characteristic of the TV, usually two papillary muscle can be seen: the anterior, which is the most prominent, and the posterior. Chords from each papillary muscle attach to the three leaflets.

### Data Acquisition

3D imaging of the TV can be difficult because of the valve's thin leaflets and also its anterior position.

First, a primary analysis of the TV should be performed using 2D multiplane echocardiography. The TEE probe can be positioned at ME position focus in the

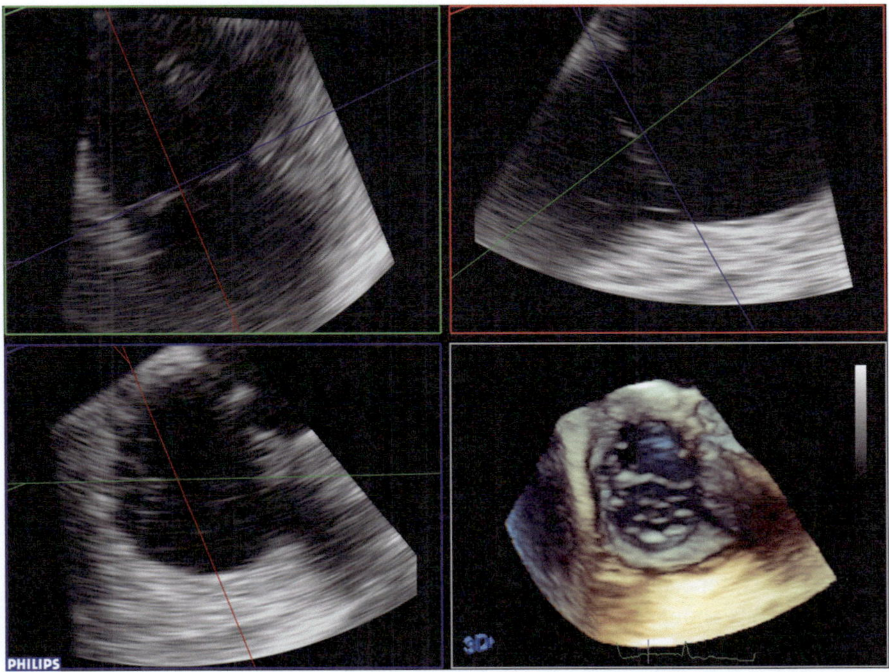

**Fig. 3.15** Two orthogonal views of the tricuspid valve following 3D zoom acquisition. After correct alignment of the axes, the smallest true tricuspid valve orifice and the annulus can be quantify by planimetry

right cavities, selecting the angle at which the TV is best visualized, which was usually 0°, so that 3D images of the TV can be optimally recorded. During the acquisition, care must be taken to include the entire annulus throughout the cardiac cycle. Next, the image volume should be rotated around the X axis counterclockwise 90° so that the TV is displayed en face. Finally, the TV, whether presented as viewed from the RA or the RV, should be orientated with the interatrial septum located inferiorly, by rotating the image 45° [1]. 3D dataset can be view from multiple angles and cropped in different planes to estimate the smallest true TV orifice by planimetry (Fig. 3.15).

To assess the flow through the TV, color flow Doppler should be added to the full volume acquisition. The size of the region of interest should be limited to the TV and the color flow jet to optimize frame rate. 3D color data set can be analyzed using multiplanar reconstruction tool and cropping to quantify the origin of the regurgitation jet as well as estimate the vena contracta and regurgitant orifice area. There are few data for quantification the tricuspid regurgitation by 3D TEE.

In the recommendations for image acquisition and display using 3D echocardiography [1] they affirm that there is evidence supporting the routine use of 3D TTE and TEE for the evaluation of TV disease.

## *Applications*

- To assess the TV and annulus morphology and pathology.
- To assess its relationship with implantable device, such as pacemakers.
- To assess the TV prosthesis.

## General Aspects of Congenital Diseases from 3D TEE

Congenital heart disease requires a detailed analysis of the spatial relationships of the cardiac structures to understand the anatomy and physiology of the cardiomyopathy and in order to plan the correct treatment. 3D TEE has become an attractive alternative for this purpose; the 3D dataset can be displayed as rendered 3D views, as a series of multiplanar images or from different projections due to the ability to alter the plane of interrogation without limitation. In addition, the general advantages of the echocardiography are present: no radiation, no need of ionic contrast, repeatability and portability. By contrast, some specific limitations of this patients should be taken into account such as severe pulmonary hypertension, severe hypoxemia, congenital or acquired oesophageal or bronchial disease, oropharyngeal pathology or cervical anomalies that may interfere with probe introduction [17].

Suitable cardiac lesions to be studied by 3D TEE include abnormalities in the atrioventricular valves, atrial septal defects, ventricular septal defects and more complex abnormalities of cardiac connections. In addition, guidance of catheter or surgical intervention is other important utility of the 3D TEE in congenital heart disease [18].

## *Atrioventricular Valves*

Understanding of valve morphology and mechanism of valvular closure and opening is essential. 3D TEE provides en face views from the ventricle or from the atrium (surgical view) that may help the surgeons in planning the surgery. In addition, full volume data allow to analyze associated atrioventricular septal defects.

For the MV, 3D TEE provides additional information for the analysis of the mechanism of mitral regurgitation, localizing the prolapsed scallops and the mitral valve cleft (Fig. 3.16). For the TV, it can be full visualized including deficiency of leaflets and, in complex cases such as Ebstein's anomaly, 3D TEE cross-sectional imaging can demonstrate the abnormal rotation of the axis of the TV.

With respect to semilunar valve, 3D TEE can be useful in identifying the mechanism of the lesion, such as leaflet tear or perforation and in quantifying the regurgitation or stenosis.

**Fig. 3.16** Live 3D acquisition of the mitral valve in a patient with P2 prolapse. The mitral valve is orientated with the aortic valve in 12 o'clock position

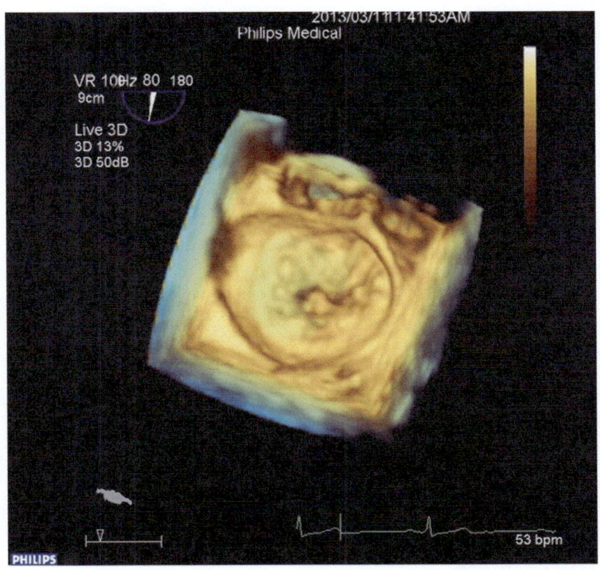


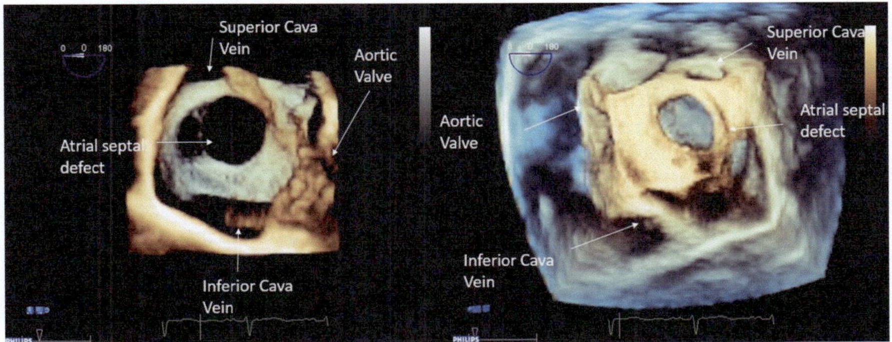


**Fig. 3.17** Live 3D acquisition of secundum atrial septal defect. *Left*: Right atrial view of secundum atrial septal defect. The superior cava vein, inferior cava vein and aortic margins of the defect should be noticed. *Right*: Left atrial view of the secundum atrial septal defect

## *Atrial Septal Defects*

One of the most common indication for TEE is the evaluation of interatrial communication. First of all, to define the type of atrial septal defect: (secundum defect, primun defect, superior/inferior vena cava defect, defect involving coronary sinus). The description of secundum atrial septal defect should include the suitability for percutaneous closure, including the size, location, shape and rims to the defect after off line analysis. In sinus venosus atrial septal defects, 3D TEE may also help in demonstrating partial abnormal drainage of the pulmonary veins (Fig. 3.17).

## *Ventricular Septal Defects*

The size, number, shape and precise location of the ventricular septal defect can be analyzed by 3D TEE. This technique can help in planning the correct treatment for the defect and guide the surgical or catheter intervention.

## *Complex Lessions*

3D TEE with novel views of intracardiac relations, can offer unique and useful information in the evaluation of patients with complex congenital heart disease, such as atrioventricular septal defect and double outlet of the RV. In addition, the information obtained by 3D TEE may assist in surgical planning.

# References


1. Lang RM, Badano LP, Tsang W, Adams DH, Agricola E, Buck T, American Society of Echocardiography, European Association of Echocardiography, et al. EAE/ASE recommendations for image acquisition and display using three-dimensional echocardiography. Eur Heart J Cardiovasc Imaging. 2012;13(1):1–46.
2. Sudhakar S, Khairnar P, Nanda N. Live/real time three-dimensional transesophageal echocardiography. Echocardiography. 2012;29:103–11.
3. Hahn RT, Abraham T, Adams MS, Bruce CJ, Glas KE, Lang RM. Guidelines for performing a comprehensive transesophageal echocardiographic examination: recommendations from the American Society of Echocardiography and the Society of Cardiovascular Anesthesiologists. J Am Soc Echocardiogr. 2013;26:921–64.
4. Hung J, Lang R, Flachskampf F, Shernan SK, McCulloch ML, Adams DB, et al. 3D echocardiography: a review of the current status and future directions. J Am Soc Echocardiogr. 2007;20:213–33.
5. Shimada YJ, Shiota T. A meta-analysis and investigation for the source of bias of left ventricular volumes and function by three-dimensional echocardiography in comparison with magnetic resonance imaging. Am J Cardiol. 2011;107:126–38.
6. Monaghan MJ. Role of real time 3D echocardiography in evaluating the left ventricle. Heart. 2006;92:131–6.
7. Lang RM, Badano LP, Mor-Avi V, Afilalo J, Armstrong A, Ernande L, et al. Recommendations for cardiac chamber quantification by echocardiography in adults: an update from the American Society of Echocardiography and the European Association of Cardiovascular Imaging. Eur Heart J Cardiovasc Imaging. 2015;16(3):233–70.
8. Seo Y, Ishizu T, Nakajima H, Sekiguchi Y, Watanabe S, Aonuma K. Clinical utility of 3-dimensional echocardiography in the evaluation of tricuspid regurgitation caused by pacemaker leads. Circ J. 2008;72:1465–70.
9. Valocik G, Kamp O, Visser C. Three-dimensional echocardiography in mitral valve disease. Eur J Echocardiogr. 2005;6:443e454.
10. McCarthy K, Ring L, Rana B. Anatomy of the mitral valve: understanding the mitral valve complex in mitral regurgitation. Eur Heart J Cardiovasc Imaging. 2010;11:i3–9.
11. Lang RM, Tsang W, Weinert L, Mor-Avi V, Chandra S. Valvular heart disease: the value of 3-dimensional echocardiography. J Am Coll Cardiol. 2011;58(19):1933–44.

12. Muraru D, Badano L, Vannan M, Iliceto S. Assessment of aortic valve complex by three-dimensional echocardiography: a framework for its effective application in clinical practice. Eur Heart J Cardiovasc Imaging. 2012;13:541–55.
13. Jánosi R, Plicht B, Kahler P, Eißmann M, Wendt D, Jakob H, et al. Quantitative analysis of aortic valve stenosis and aortic root dimensions by three-dimensional echocardiography in patients scheduled for transcutaneous aortic valve implantation. Curr Cardiovasc Imaging Rep. 2014;7:9296.
14. Patrizio L, Christophe T, AndreCas H, Luis M, Bogdan A, Popescu BA, et al. European Association of Echocardiography recommendations for the assessment of valvular regurgitation. Part 1: aortic and pulmonary regurgitation (native valve disease). Eur J Echocardiogr. 2010;11:230–2.
15. Roberson DA, Cui W, Patel D, Tsang W, Sugeng L, Weinert L, et al. Three-dimensional transesophageal echocardiography of atrial septal defect: a qualitative and quantitative anatomic study. J Am Soc Echocardiogr. 2011;24(6):600–10.
16. Ton-Nu TT, Levine RA, Handschumacher MD, Dorer DJ, Yosefy C, Fan D, et al. Geometric determinants of functional tricuspid regurgitation: insights from 3-dimensional echocardiography. Circulation. 2006;114(2):143–9.
17. Flachskampf FA, Wouters PF, Edvardsen T, Evangelista A, Habib G, Hoffman P, European Association of Cardiovascular Imaging Document Reviewers: Erwan Donal and Fausto Rigo, et al. Recommendations for transoesophageal echocardiography: EACVI update 2014. Eur Heart J Cardiovasc Imaging. 2014;15(4):353–65.
18. Simpson JM, Miller O. Three-dimensional echocardiography in congenital heart disease. Arch Cardiovasc Dis. 2011;104(1):45–56.

# Chapter 4
# 3D-ECHO Protocols for the Diagnosis of Valvular Diseases

José Luis Moya Mur and Derly Carlos Becker Filho

## Abbreviations

| | |
|---|---|
| AV | Aortic valve |
| EROA | Effective regurgitant orifice area |
| LA | Left atrium |
| LAA | Left atrial appendage |
| LV | Left ventricle |
| LVOT | Left ventricular out flow tract |
| MR | Mitral valve regurgitation |
| MS | Mitral valve stenosis |
| MV | Mitral valve |
| PV | Pulmonary valve |
| RA | Right atrium |
| RV | Right ventricle |
| TAVI | Transcatheter Aortic Valve Implantation |
| TEE | Transesophageal echocardiography |
| TTE | Transthoracic echocardiography |
| TV | Tricuspid valve |

**Electronic supplementary material** The online version of this chapter (doi:10.1007/978-3-319-50335-6_4) contains supplementary material, which is available to authorized users.

J.L. Moya Mur (✉) • D.C. Becker Filho
Cardiology Department, University Hospital Ramón y Cajal,
Carretera de Colmenar Km 9,100, 28034 Madrid, Spain
e-mail: joseluis.moya@salud.madrid.org

© Springer International Publishing AG 2017
E. Casas Rojo et al. (eds.), *Manual of 3D Echocardiography*,
DOI 10.1007/978-3-319-50335-6_4

## Introduction

Valvular heart diseases are among the most frequent heart diseases. 2D echocardiography is the preferred method to study them. However, It is well known that two-dimensional (2D) echocardiography has several limitations studying valvular heart diseases. Three-dimensional (3D) echocardiography solves same of this limitation and aport important additional diagnostic information about the valve pathology, function, and severity of valvular diseases.

## Aortic Valve

3D echocardiography, in the evaluation of the aortic valve and aortic root, represents a real and detailed view of the anatomy of the "valve complex". This consists of the sinuses of Valsalva, leaflets and the fibrous interleaflet triangles [1]. The aortic cusps are identified by the absence or presence of coronary artery: left coronary cusp, right coronary cusp and non-coronary cusp (Fig. 4.1). The aortic root is the portion of the left ventricular outflow tract (LVOT) that supports the aortic valves, bounded inferiorly by the ring and superiorly by sinotubular junction. The sinuses of Valsalva are the expansion of the root extending from the leaflets insertion to the sinotubular junction [2].

The study with 3D TTE or 3D TEE is very similar except for the unquestionable best quality of 3D TEE.

**Acquisition** The main ways to approach the aortic valve by 3D TTE echocardiography are the parasternal views and to a lesser extent apical views. With 3D TEE the high esophagus plane is used. With either of the two modes, based on a 2D short or

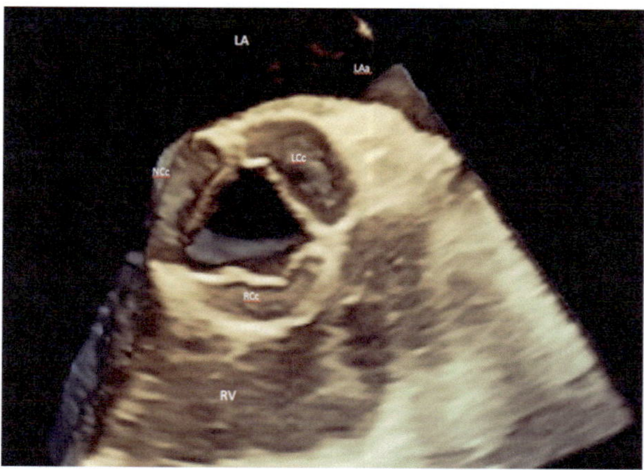


**Fig. 4.1** 3D TEE in a normal aortic valve. *En face* view from the aorta in systole. *LA* left atrium, *RV* right ventricle, *LAa* left atrial appendage, *LCc, NCc, RCc* left, non coronary and right cusps

long axis views a good image of the aortic valve can be obtained using the real-time (live) 3D or Zoom or Full Volume methods (see Chap. 3).

For a detailed study we select in the biplane study a zoomed volume including the whole valve (increasing the spacial resolution), and we use multi-beat imaging if it is possible (increasing temporal resolution). Displacement and cropping tools should be used to ensure that an appropriate volume recording the entire whole aorta is obtained and then record the volume. It is important to ensure that anatomical landmarks, such as interatrial septum, are acquired and ensure that the frame rate is high enough before recording. Record several times and then analyze the best acquisitions.

Keep in mind that using 3D Color Doppler studies a lower temporal resolution is obtained. To locate the position of the color jet in the valve we must use a volume (usually a big volume) that includes the entire valve. We can see the jet position but we will not be able to make an accurate analysis of the jet due to low frame rate. Once located the jet, a small 3D volume (focused on the jet) will allow us greater temporal resolution and a more detailed analysis of the vena contracta and PISA.

**Analysis and Measurements** On the computer or on the workstation we must use cropping and displacement tools to display successive levels of the aorta in short axis views. The aortic valve can be seen from two perspectives, aortic and ventricular. The view from the aorta is better to evaluate the valve morphology and the view from the ventricle to see vegetation and subvalvar obstructions [3]. 3D echocardiography allows for better analysis of hearts with pathological aortic root, and provides additional information of the spatial relationship with other structures such as the LVOT and the mitral annulus [3]. Two-dimensional echocardiography underestimates the area of the LVOT, therefore assuming a circular area, whereas the 3D echocardiography allows for a multi-plane image of the aortic valve (the long axis and the short axis), showing a true representation of the LVOT [3]. The analysis of the aortic valve by three-dimensional transthoracic echocardiography can be difficult even in normal individuals, those with a limited acoustic window. The analysis of the aortic valve can be further improved by color-coded Doppler in both transthoracic and transesophageal studies [3].

## Aortic Stenosis

**Anatomy** The main causes of aortic stenosis are congenital (bicuspid aortic valve) and degenerative. With an aging population, degenerative aortic stenosis is the cause most commonly found [4]. The three-dimensional evaluation of the aortic allows better appreciate the anatomy, etiology, size and location of lesions of the aortic stenosis than two-dimensional echocardiography.

**Severity** The calculation of valve area is one of the key parameters in the analysis of aortic stenosis. 3D eco gives no additional information for measuring velocities and gradients, whose criteria of severity are reflected in the guidelines [5].

However, the 3D TTE and TEE allows a better estimation of the severity [6] based on the estimation of the systolic aortic orifice area either through direct estimate of the area of the orifice or by estimating the area by the continuity equation. In any case, it is considered severe when the area is less than 1 cms$^2$.

It can be done:

– by direct measurement or planimetry. Using 3D TTE or TEE, a zoomed volume focused on aorta is acquired (if possible multi-beat). For their analysis the cropping tools are used selecting the short axis aortic plane having the smallest area in systole (Fig. 4.2, Video 4.1). You can also use the multi-slice tool selecting the plane with smaller systolic area (Fig. 4.3). Then, the aortic area is measured with the specific tool of the equipment or workstation (Figs. 4.2 and 4.3). With 3D TTE, an image achieved. 3D TEE contributes to more accurate evaluations of valve morphology and allows access to this smaller orifice [7]. 3D ETE acquisition, analysis and measurement is as with 3D TTE.

– by calculation from the continuity equation. A big advantage of 3D echocardiography in the calculation of aortic stenosis is through the continuity equation, which is the most accurate measure of the LVOT area. Two-dimensional echocardiography gives a misrepresentation of the area, assuming its shape is circular [8]. The methodology to acquire and measure LVOT area is similar to that used to estimate the area of the aortic valve, but using lower planes (Fig. 4.4).

– The aortic valve area can also be calculated using the stroke volume measured by TT 3D, divided by velocity integral (continuous Doppler through the aortic valve). The accuracy of this measurement is superior to other two-dimensional methods.

3D TEE demonstrates further increases in accuracy of these aortic valve area ratings and is particularly important for guiding percutaneous procedures when selected as the treatment for severe stenosis. Other additional assessments can also be made by 3D echocardiography such as the sphericity index of the left ventricle, left ventricular mass, three-dimensional strain of the LV. In the near future, all of these analyses may help us identify the best time for the therapeutic approach in aortic stenosis.

## *Aortic Insufficiency*

**Anatomy** It is caused by abnormalities such as bicuspid aortic valve, senile (calcification), rheumatic and also by the expansion of the ring as Marfan syndrome and annuloaortic ectasia. A new type of aortic valve insufficiency has emerged which is periprosthetic insufficiency. This occurs after surgical and percutaneous procedures [9].

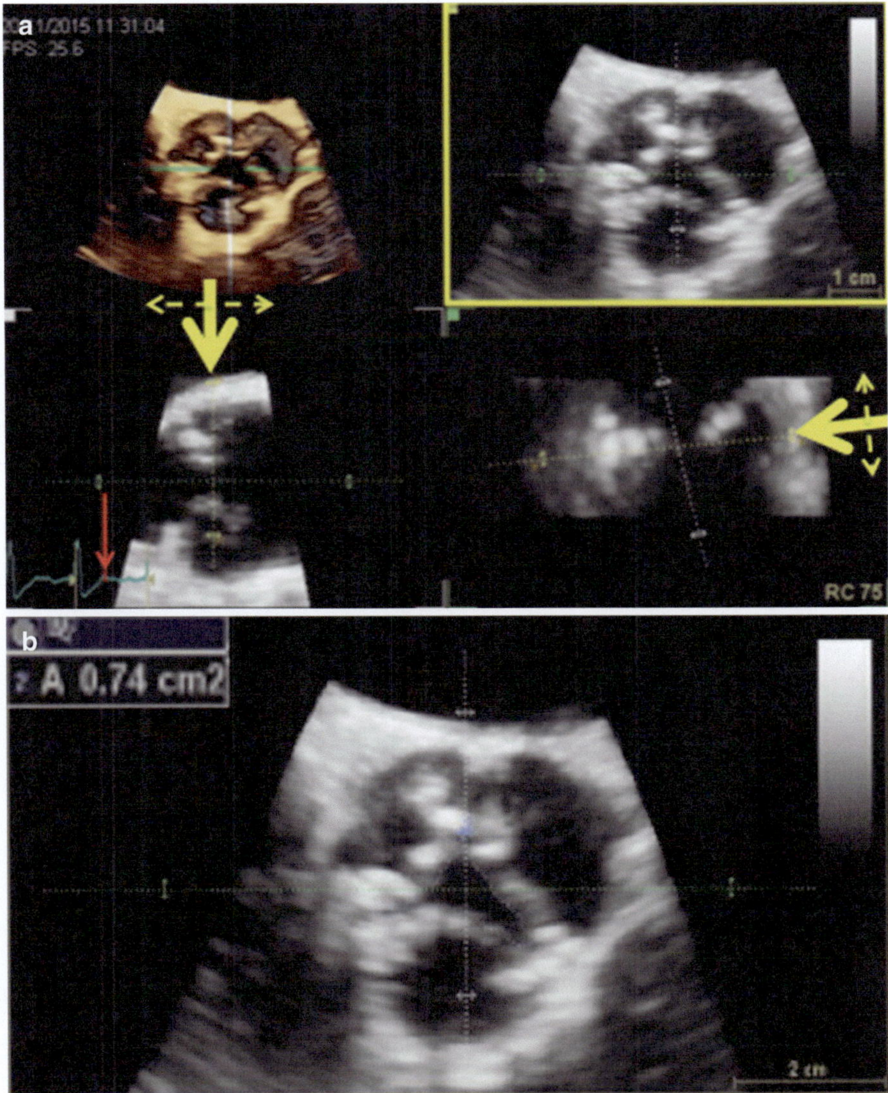

**Fig. 4.2** 3D TEE showing the estimation of aortic stenotic orifice area with cropping. Step 1. (**a**): Using cropping and displacement tools the cutting plane should be moved (*yellow*) to obtain a good image of the aortic valve in short axis and frozen in systole. Step 2. Next, the cutting plane must be carefully displaced up and down (*dashed arrows*) to select the plane with the smallest aortic orifice area. Step 3. Measure the area (**b**). In this case the area is 0.74 cm². We recommend measuring on the 2D planes obtained from the 3D study and not directly on the 3D image. 2D estimated areas are less affected by changes in gain

**Severity** The Role of three-dimensional echocardiography in the evaluation of aortic insufficiency severity lies in the anatomical details, calculation of EROA, regurgitant volume (especially in eccentric jets), regurgitant fraction and **vena contracta**.

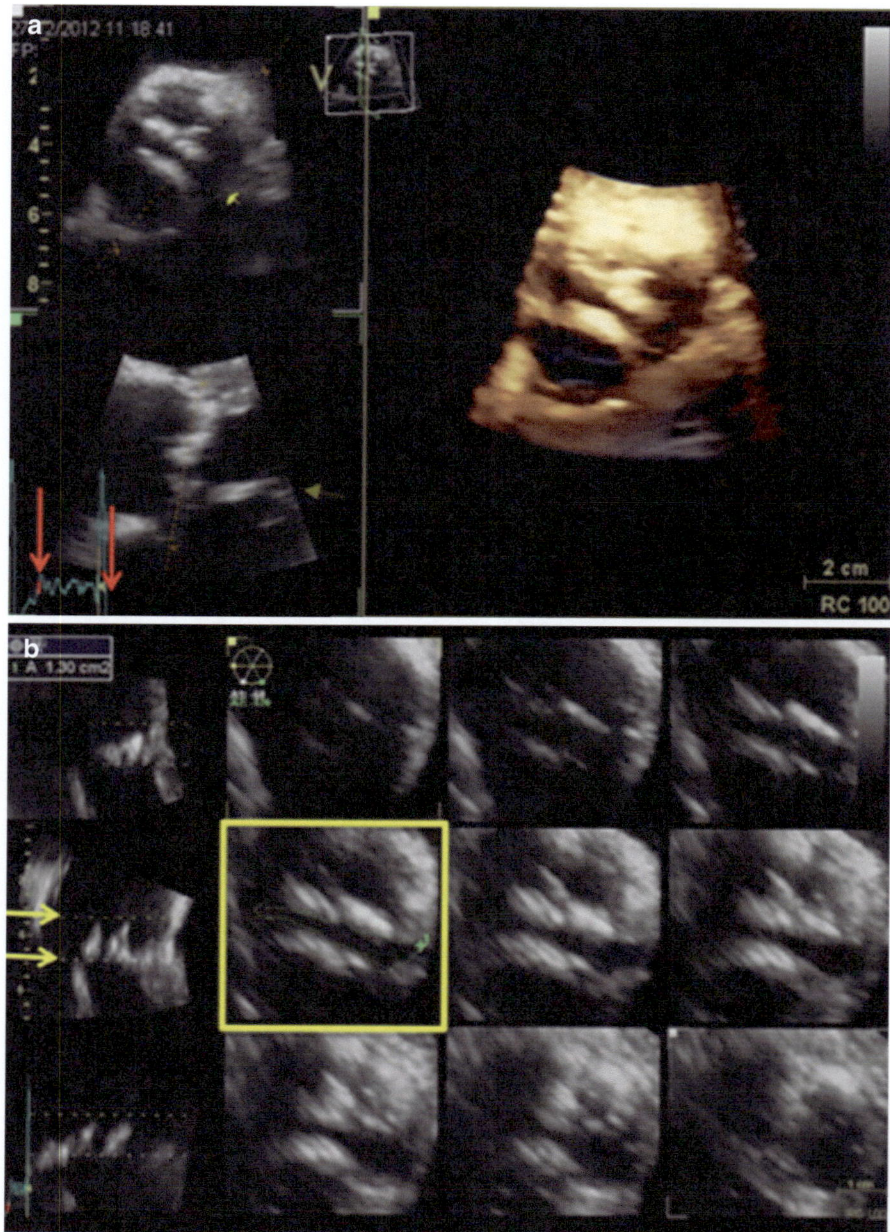

**Fig. 4.3** 3D TTE estimating the stenotic orifice area in a bicuspid aortic stenosis with the multislice tool. Step 1. (**a**) Is as in Fig. 4.3. Step 2. We must now use the "multislice" tool to delineate only the valvular region (*arrows*) in such a way that successive planes of short axis (*9 planes*) of the valve are obtained (**b**). Step 3. Among these 9 planes, select the one with smallest valve area (*frame*) and Step 4. Measure the area (**b**)

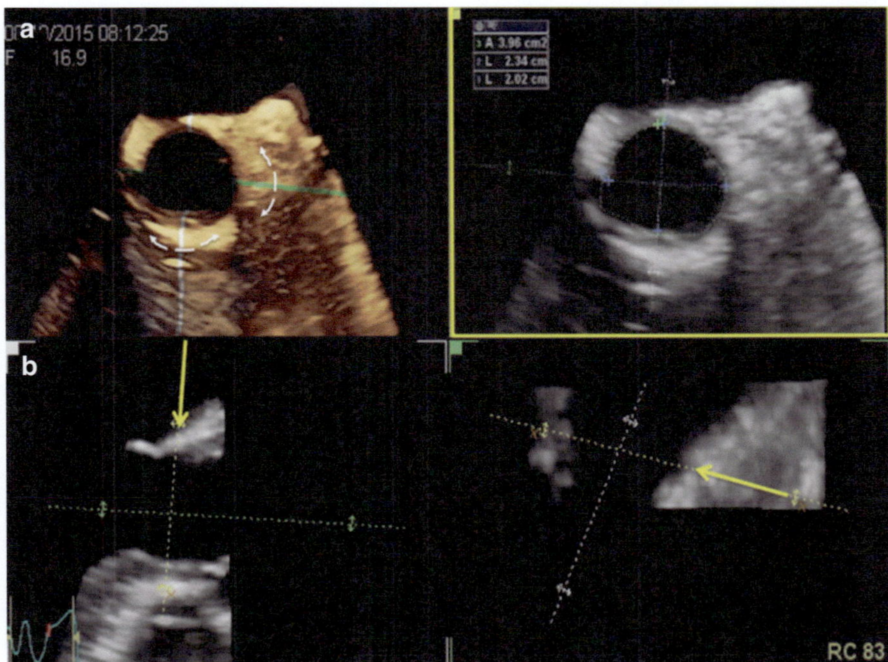

**Fig. 4.4** 3D TEE estimating the left ventricle outflow tract dimension (*LVOT*) using the cropping. Step 1.- (**a**) As in figure 4.2 but focused on an image of the LVOT in short axis in systole. Step 2.- (a) As in Fig. 4.2. Step 3 – We have to measure antero-posterior diameter, latero-lateral diameter and LVOT area (*below*). We recommend turning the orthogonal planes (*white* and *green*, *curved arrows*) to accurately define the position of valve insertion

– Sometimes RO in diastole can be estimated similarly to stenotic orifice (Fig. 4.5)

– Recent studies indicate that the cross-sectional area of the vena contracta can also be a predictor of severity. This is the narrowest part of the distal jet to regurgitation orifice, just below the flow convergence zone. The limitations of the method are the existence of multiple jets or jets with irregular shapes. The evaluation of vena contracta by two-dimensional echocardiography leads to errors, while the three-dimensional echo enables the detailed reconstruction of the region of the vena contracta (Fig. 4.6) with greater accuracy [10].

To measure the area of the VC must be careful to align the crooping tool in the direction of the jet and not in the anatomical direction of the aorta and measure the orifice as in aortic stenosis but in diastole.

EROA is obtained through the area of convergence flow. An EROA > 0.30 cm$^2$ is considered significant aortic insufficiency [10, 11]. A wide vena contracta >0.6 cm is considered important insufficiency [11]. The area of the vena contracta can be measured by three-dimensional echocardiography. A Value > 0.32 cms$^2$ suggests severe aortic insufficiency [10].

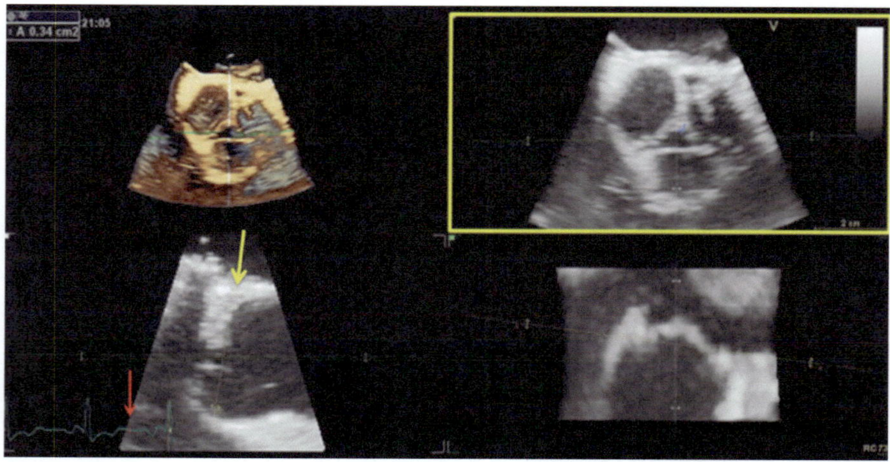

**Fig. 4.5** 3D TEE anatomic study estimating the regurgitant orifice area in aortic regurgitation. The Protocol is the same as described for the estimation of the area of aortic stenosis, but freezing the image in diastole (*red arrow*). In this case the OR is 0.34 cms$^2$

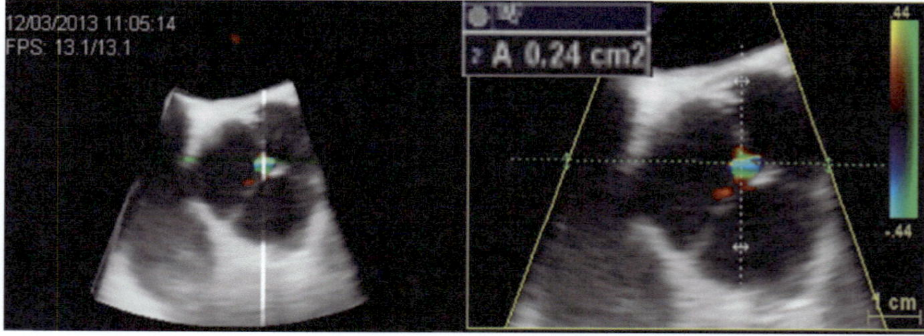

**Fig. 4.6** 3D TTE color study of aortic regurgitation severity through analysis of the Vena Contracta. Steps to follow are similar to those in Figs. 4.3 and 4.6 but the cropping planes must follow the direction of the color jet and not the anatomical orientation

## Mitral Valve

Mitral valve (MV) pathology is one of the most prevalent valve diseases. 3D echocardiography allows a complete and comprehensive understanding of valvular anatomy, avoiding some of the problems derived from 2D echocardiography [12, 13].

**Acquisition [3]** The main ways to approach the MV by 3D TT echocardiography are the apical views and to lesser stent parasternal views, and by 3D TEE echocardiography the high esophagus plane. The best image is obtained with the ultrasonic volume directed perpendicular to the mitral annulus. A good 3D study can be obtained using real-time, Zoom (Fig. 4.7) or Full-Volume. For an anatomic study follow the same recommendations used for the study of the aortic valve.

For 3D color Doppler analysis we will use a volume that includes the entire valve to locate the MR. However, a smaller volume should be selected (including the regurgitant jet) to achieve greater time resolution and a more detailed analysis of vena contrata and PISA.

**Analysis and Measurements**  The image is generally positioned en face view from the atrium, "surgeons view", with the aortic valve in the upper part of the image, the left atrial appendage in the left and the MV in the middle (Fig. 4.7). Using the displacement and cropping tools we will be able to analyze the leaflets, specify the location of pathological findings, and to quantify the severity of the valve dysfunction.

## Mitral Valve Stenosis

Mitral valve stenosis (MS) represents a still frequent clinical challenge. Most cases were due to rheumatic valve disease. Nowadays it is most often degenerative and due to calcification of the mitral annulus.

**Anatomy**  3D TTE and 3D TEE (Fig. 4.8, Video 4.2) allow an excellent anatomical study of the entire mitral valve apparatus. 3D analysis provides a better evaluation

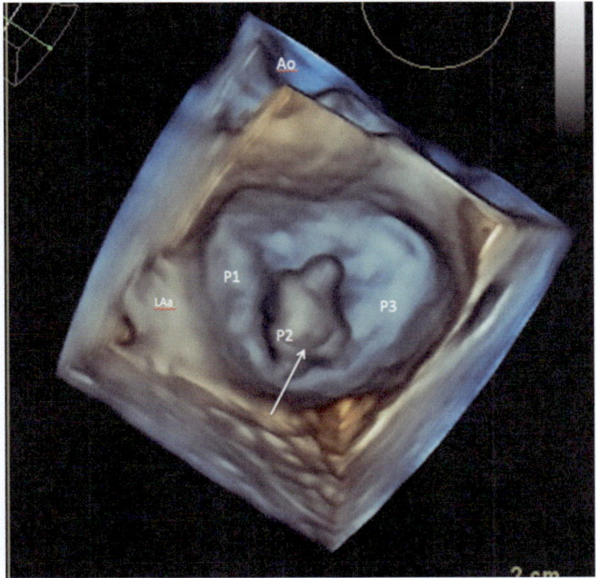


**Fig. 4.7**  3DTEE study of the mitral valve. *En face* view from the atrium. A prolapse in P2 can be seen. *Ao* aorta, *LAa* left atrial appendage

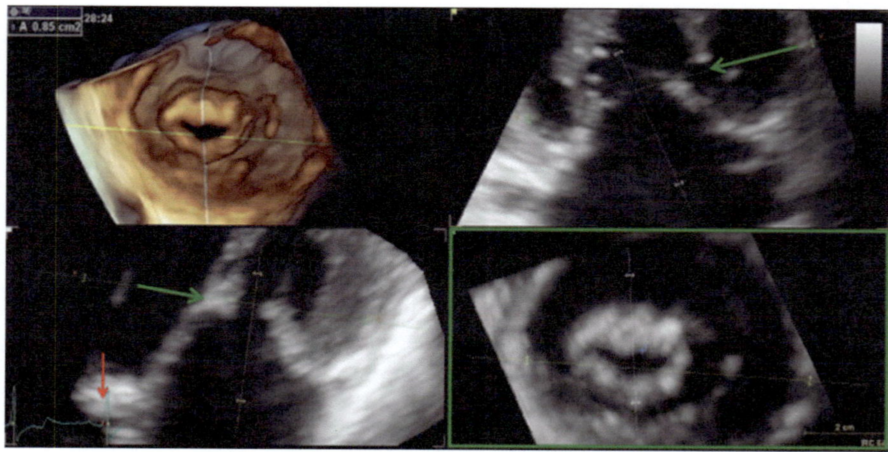

**Fig. 4.8** 3D TTE showing the estimation of mitral stenotic orifice area with cropping. Step 1. Using cropping and displacement tools the cutting plane should be moved (*green arrow*) to obtain a good image of the mitral valve in short axis with freezing in diastole. Step 2. Now the cutting plane must be carefully moved up and down to select the plane with the smallest mitral orifice area. Step 3. Measure the area. In this case the area is 0.85 cm$^2$

of the location and extent of affected/calcified areas [14], both at the level of the annulus or at the leaflets and valvular cords, when compared to 2D analysis. This is of paramount importance to plan MV valvuloplasty and surgery. Wilkins score, using 3D image, has showed high intra and interobserver agreement in the evaluation of valve's morphology.

**Severity** 2D evaluation of MS lacks some limitations: MV area estimation based on pressure half-time method is largely dependent upon hemodynamic status; planimetry of the MV orifice is limited by the orientation of the plane. MS severity by 3D echocardiography depends mainly in MV area measurement. 3D reconstruction using cropping tools (Fig. 4.8, Video 4.2) or multislide tool (Fig. 4.9, Video 4.3) makes it possible to choose the optimal plane of the smallest MV orifice, at the tip of the mitral leaflets in rheumatic stenosis or in the annulus in degenerative stenosis [14, 15]. According to current guidelines, MV intervention is indicated in case of symptomatic MS and a MV area <1.5 cm$^2$.

## *Mitral Valve Regurgitation*

The knowledge and understanding of anatomic structure and the mitral valve regurgitation (MR) mechanism [16], as well as the regurgitation severity, are crucial elements in the indication and choice of therapeutic strategies.

**Anatomy** Annular diameters can be directly measured. Leaflet morphology must be evaluated, looking for an excess of tissue and motion, chordae tendinae rup-

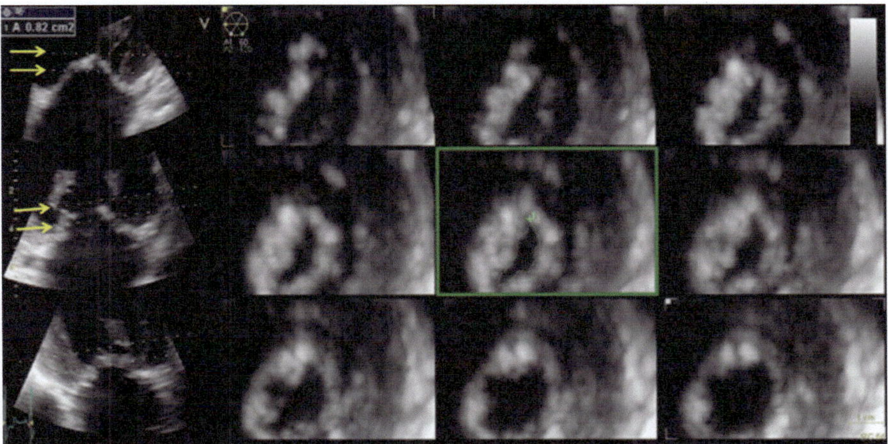

**Fig. 4.9** 3D TTE estimating the mitral stenotic orifice area with the multislice tool. Step 1. Is as in Fig. 4.8. Step 2. We must now use the "multislice" tool delimiting only the valvular region (*yellow arrows*) in such a way that successive planes of short axis (*9 plans*) are obtained. Step 3. Among these 9 planes we have to select the one with the smallest valve area (*green frame*) and Step 4. Measure the area

ture, restricted leaflet movement, leaflet perforation or presence of leaflet-associated masses or vegetations. Subvalvular apparatus state can be precisely observed from the ventricular view. Papillary muscle insertion and systolic displacement must be addressed to exclude alterations in myocardial contractility. Three-dimensional echocardiography is superior to multiplane transoesophageal echo in the assessment of regurgitant mitral valve morphology [12].

The mechanism of the MR must be determined. An initial approach should distinguish organic versus functional MR, the former being caused by intrinsic anatomical abnormalities and the latter occurring in morphologically normal valves by dilation of the annulus or tethering of one or both papillary muscles. Carpentier's classification is widely spread and divides the mitral regurgitation into four groups (Table 4.1).

En face view from LA (Fig. 4.7) allows a precise location of the anatomical and functional alterations [3] (Fig. 4.10, Video 4.4). To get a better location and quantification we recommend following the protocol presented in the Fig. 4.11.

**Severity** Owing to several studies, 3D TEE represents a more accurate and reproducible tool for the quantification of MR severity when compared with 2D analysis [17, 18], and its measure has a high correlation with cardiac magnetic resonance data. 2D analysis by PISA measurement or direct planimetry usually underestimates the severity of MR, as it needs some geometrical assumptions, including the round shape of the effective regurgitant orifice, which has been demonstrated to be, in fact, ovoid. That limitation is even more important when quantifying functional MR (Fig. 4.12).

**Table 4.1** Carpentier's classification of mitral regurgitation mechanism

| Leaflet motion | Type | Mechanism | Functional/organic |
| --- | --- | --- | --- |
| Normal | IA | Annular dilation | Functional |
| | IB | Leaflet defect | Organic |
| Increased | IIA | Cordae elongation | Organic |
| | IIB | Cordae rupture | Organic |
| | IIC | Papillary elongation | Organic |
| | IID | Papillary rupture | Organic |
| Reduced | IIIA | Commisural and cordal fusion | Organic |
| | IIIB | Leaflet tethering | Functional |

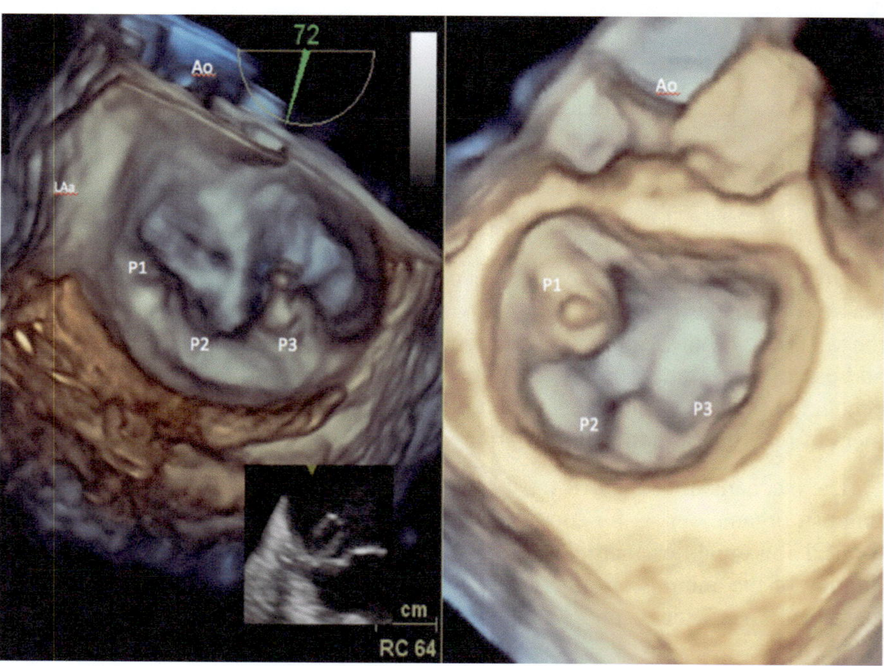


**Fig. 4.10** 3D TEE studies of two mitral valves *en face* views from the atrium in systole. (**a**) A ruptured aneurysm can be seen at level of P3. (**b**) An aneurysm at P1 level next to the anterior commissure can be seen

3D TEE image with color-Doppler allows manual measurement of the effective regurgitant orifice area by direct planimetry, as well as 3D PISA quantification. 3D image with color Doppler allows the echocardiographer to choose the optimal plane to measure the true effective regurgitant orifice, by orienting two orthogonal planes across the valve regurgitant jet (not the anatomical orientation) (Fig. 4.13, Video 4.5). Once the correct plane is selected, the area of color Doppler corresponds with the regurgitant orifice, so no geometrical assumptions are needed. This measure has

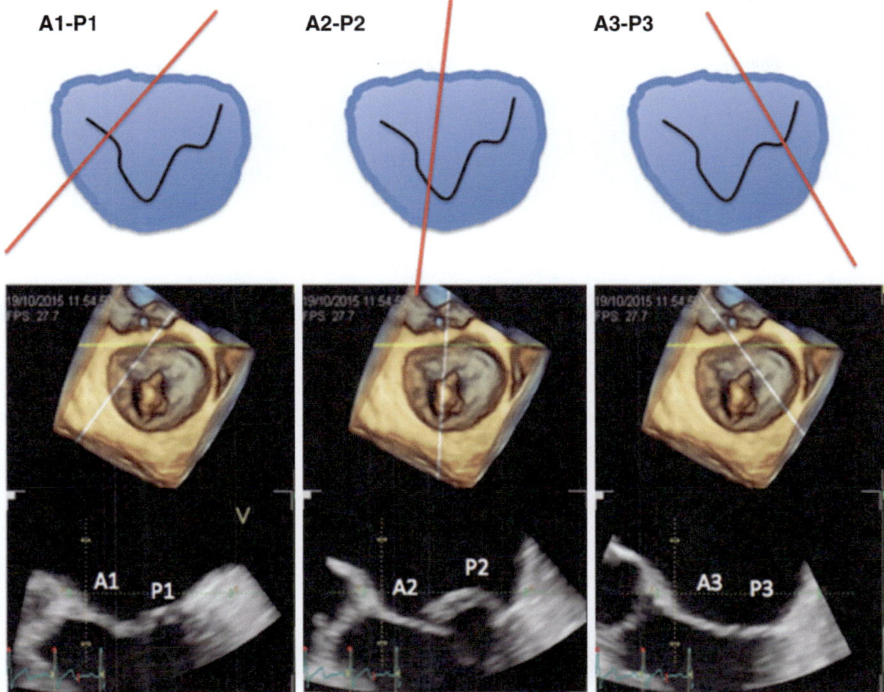


**Fig. 4.11**  3D TEE. Protocol for a detailed analysis of the morphology and function of mitral scallops: Step 1.- The firs step is to obtain an *en face* view of the mitral valve from the left atrium. Steps 2 to 4.- 2D planes must be obtained perpendicular to the line of valve closure. Between A1-P1, A2-P2 and A3-P3. As seen in the image, these planes are not parallel. This study allows definition of morphology and function of all scallops one by one

been demonstrated to be more precise and reproducible than 2D indirect quantification. There is no agreement about which area of VC correlates better with severity but a value of >0.4 cm$^2$ is assumed as indicative of severity.

## Tricuspid Valve

The tricuspid valve has some differential considerations respect to the mitral valve.

**Acquisition**  Unlike the Mitral valve, tricuspid valve is better studied with 3D TTE than with 3D TEE. If 2D TTE image quality is not bad you can get very good result studying the tricuspid valve with 3D TTE (Fig. 4.14). Using 3D TEE, the tricuspid valve is located more remote than the mitral valve and is not possible to get a plane in which tricuspid valve is perpendicular to the ultrasound volume. Therefore, 3D TEE results are sometimes suboptimal.

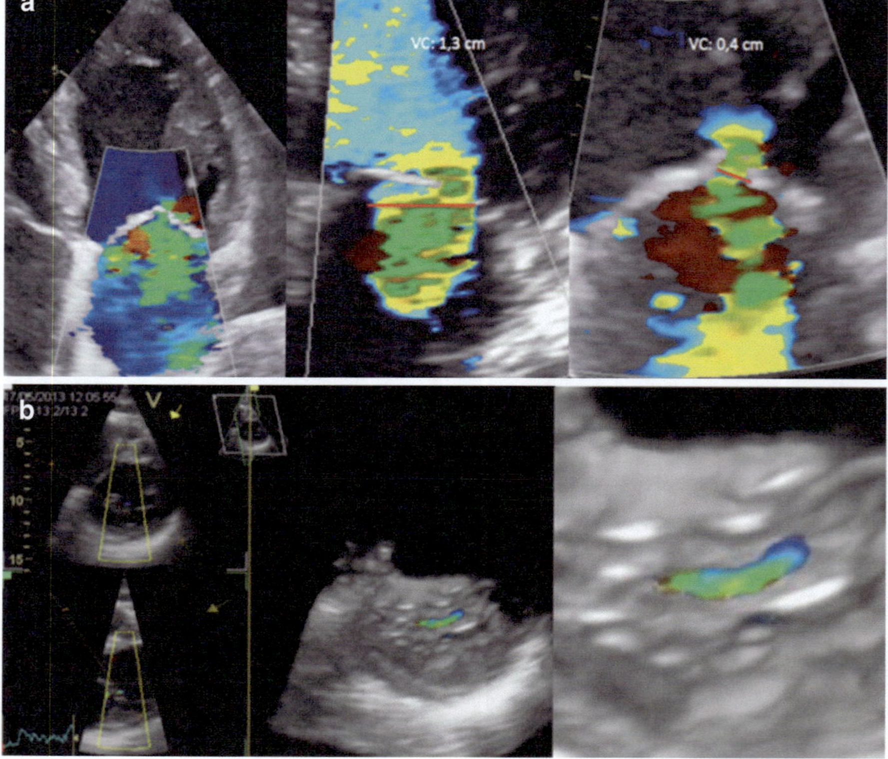

**Fig. 4.12** 2D and 3D TTE of a functional mitral regurgitation. (**a**) with 2D echocardiography the VC dimensions vary depending on the plane used. (**b**). 3D echo allows visualization of the regurgitant orifice *en face* view from left ventricle. This orifice is not circular and depends on the lack of coaptation along the edges of the valve. 3D TTE allows estimation of the VC area in a non-circular orifice without relying on geometric assumptions

In 3D TTE [3], tricuspid valve can be studied from parasternal, apical and subcostal view. We recommend using the access that best picture quality is obtained by 2D echo. The Protocol of analysis and measurements in tricuspids stenosis and tricuspid regurgitation will be similar to the one used for the mitral valve (Figs. 4.15 and 4.16). However, there is less information about severity parameters.

## Prosthetic Valve

3D TTE and TEE represent the most accurate and complete tools for the examination of normal and dysfunctional valve prosthesis [19, 20]. The protocol to study a valve prosthesis with 3D echo is similar to the protocol described for native valves, taking into account two major aspects: (1) TEE is necessary to show the auricular

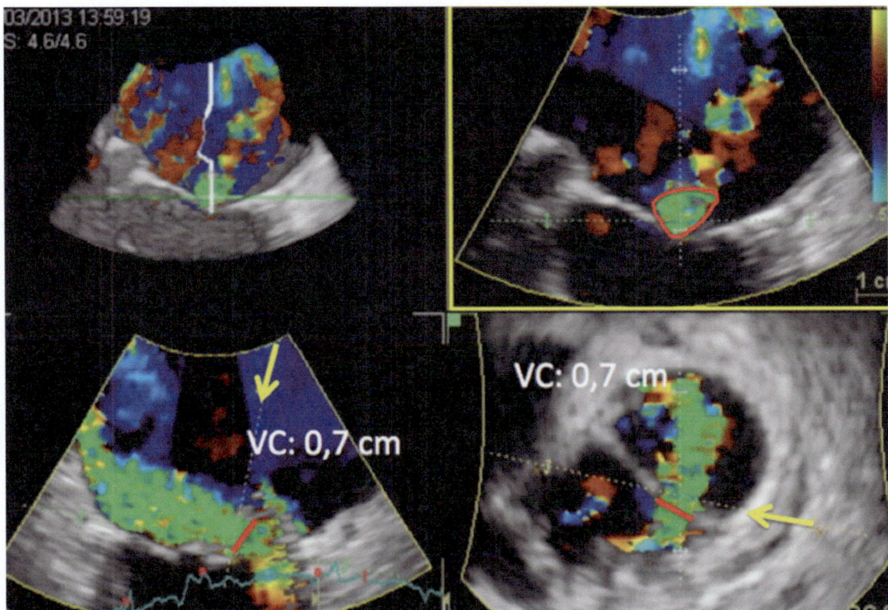

**Fig. 4.13** 3D TEE analyzing the VC in an organic mitral regurgitation. Steps to follow are similar to those in Fig. 4.12 but the cropping planes must be frozen in systole and following the color jet and not the anatomical orientation

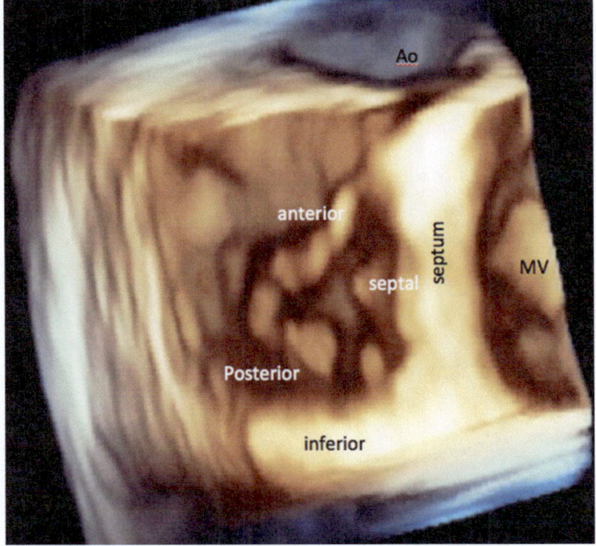


**Fig. 4.14** 3D TTE of a normal tricuspid valve. *En face* view from right ventricle

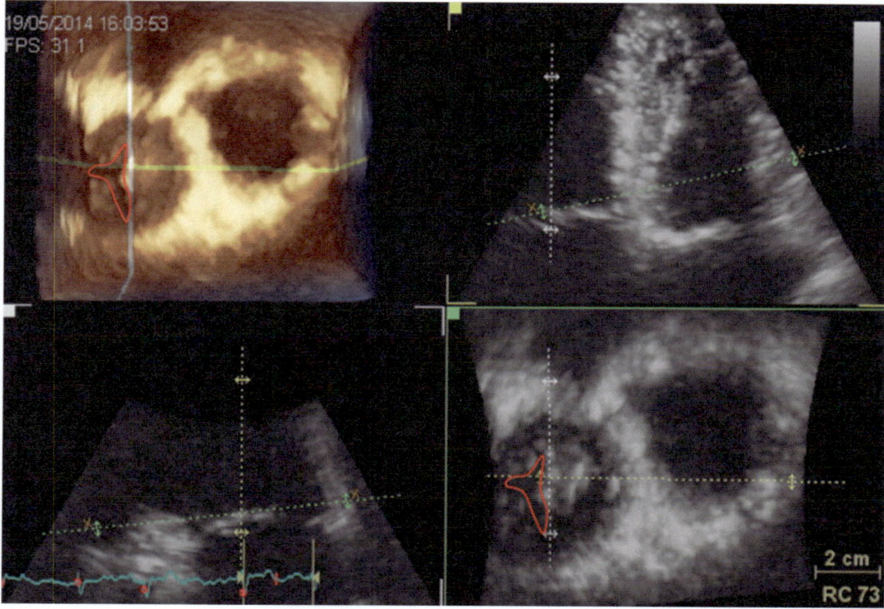

**Fig. 4.15** 3D anatomic study of the regurgitant orifice in functional TR. The Study Protocol follows the same scheme than for the estimation of the area of mitral stenosis or mitral regurgitation

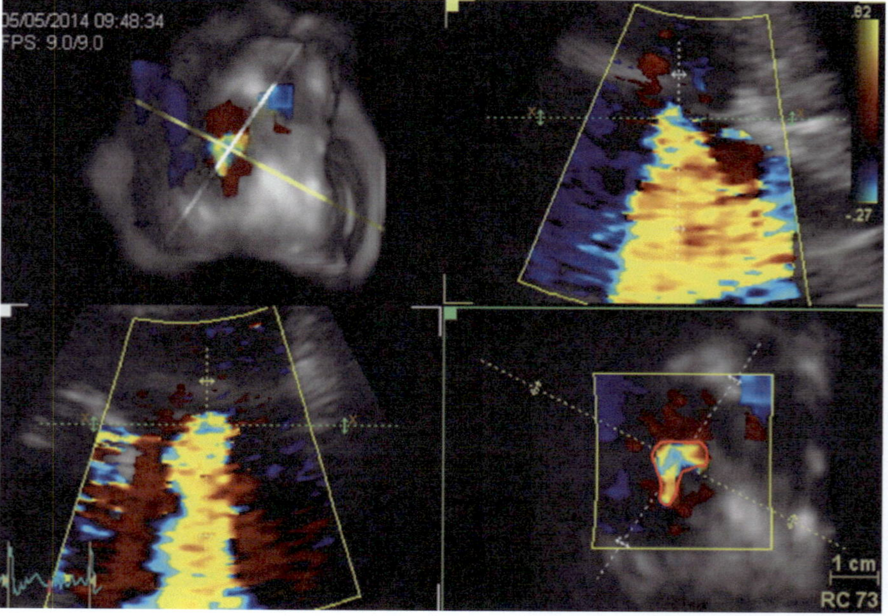

**Fig. 4.16** 3D TTE color Doppler to evaluate the severity of the functional TR through the analysis of the VC. Similar to the study of Fig. 4.19, but following the direction of the color jet, not the anatomical orientation

face of the auriculo-ventricular prosthesis and (2) the interior components of an aortic valve are difficult to analyze even with TEE.

Normal diastolic and systolic movements of the leaflets can be confirmed by 3D TTE or TEE. Physiologic intraprosthetic regurgitation can be seen by 3D color Doppler image. No paravalvular regurgitation must be present in normal prosthesis.

**Prosthetic stenosis** Prosthetic stenosis has different causes. First, prosthetic mismatch consists in the implantation of a too small prosthesis for the heart's size and body surface area. Secondary causes of stenotic prosthetic behavior are the progressive accumulation of fibrinous tissue (pannus), the formation of thrombus (especially, in mechanical prosthesis) and, rarely, prosthetic valve endocarditis.

3D TTE and 3D TEE can easily detect the limitation of leaflet movement in stenotic mitral mechanical prosthesis (Fig. 4.17), but it can be a difficult task in aortic prosthesis. It is difficult to see what happens inside the aortic prosthesis due to the masking produced by the prosthetic ring. Therefore, despite using 3D TEE, it is sometimes difficult to ensure the normal or abnormal prosthetic movement (Fig. 4.18). In these cases it is useful to resort to fluoroscopy or CT.

The presence of thrombosis is seen as a localized mass with variable degrees of mobility. Pannus is addressed as a more echogenic mass that surrounds the ring and generally obscures the stitched points. (Fig. 4.19). Again, identifying a small mass within an aortic prosthesis and confirming the presence of an intraprotsthetic mass only by analyzing image of 2D or 3D echo is more difficult. In these cases we recommend 2D and 3D TEE with Color Doppler. The location of the color jet allows

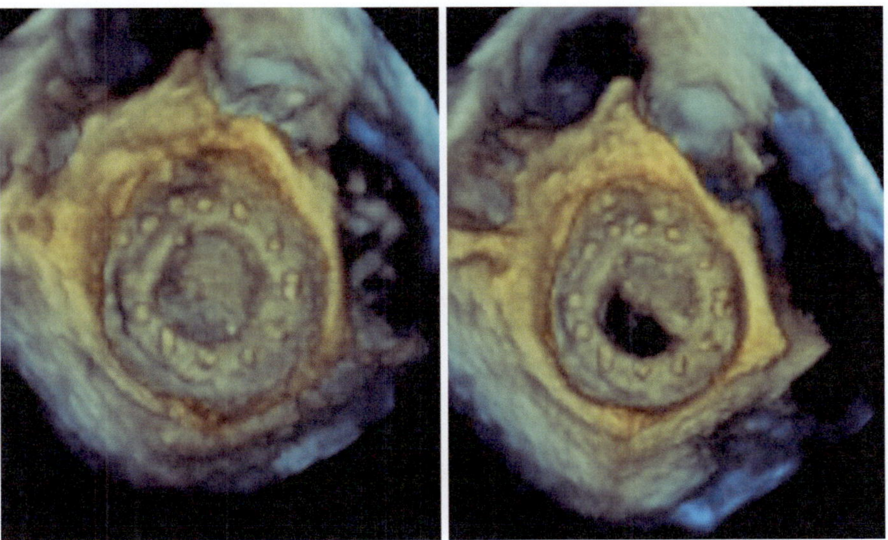

**Fig. 4.17** 3D TEE in a disfunctional mitral prosthesis. *En face* view from the LA in diastole and systole. Lack of opening of a disc is clearly seen

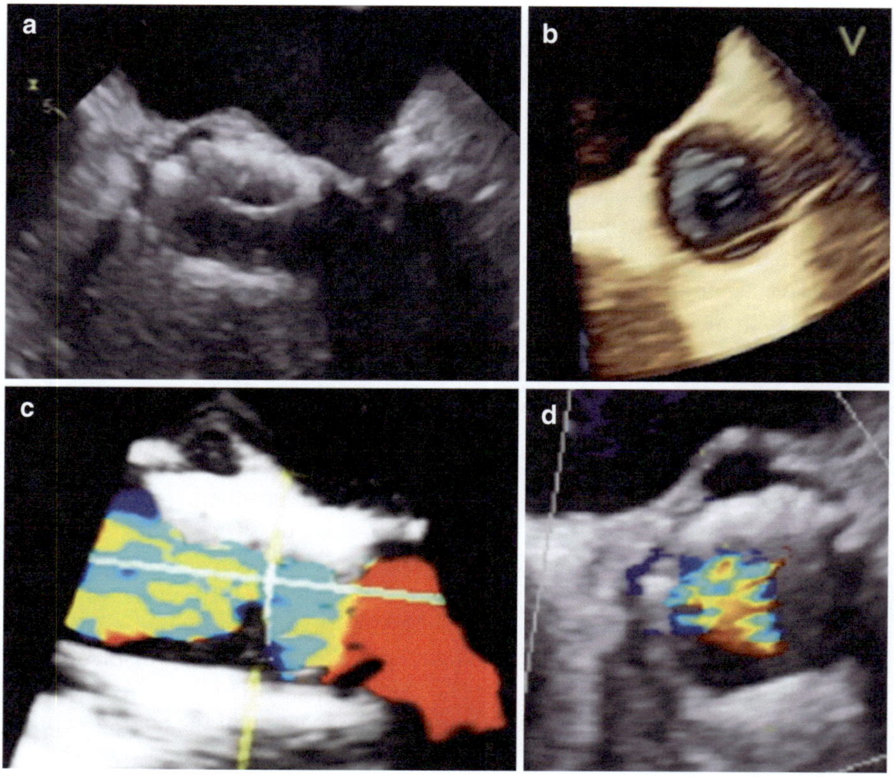

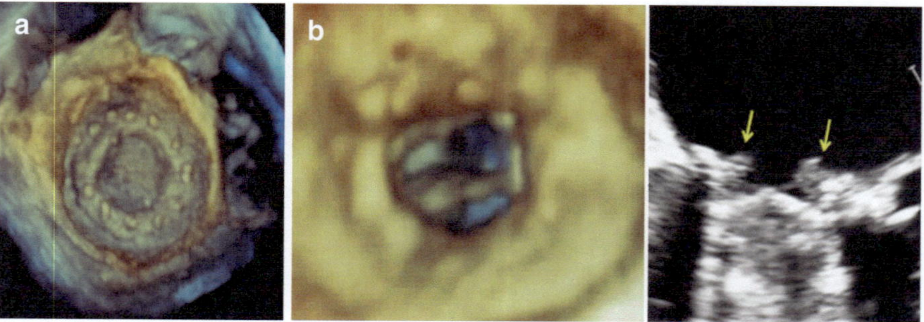

**Fig. 4.18** 3D TTE in a biological stenotic aortic prosthesis: 2D TEE (**a**) and 3D TEE (**b**) imaging gives little information of the interior of the prosthesis and even less information about the cause of stenosis. 3D TEE Color Doppler in long (**c**) and short axis (**d**) can be useful in this aspect. The color area defines the area of valve opening and delimits an area of low signal that coincides with the location of the thrombosis in CT scan

**Fig. 4.19** 3D TEE in two different mitral prostheses. *En face* view from the LA. (**a**) Normal mitral prosthesis. Stitches are clearly seen. (**b**) Mitral prosthesis with pannus. There is a small orifice and disappearance of the points of suture. Successive 2D planes show an echo-dense material covering the entire prosthetic ring (courtesy: Dr. F. Dominguez Melcón. Hospital La Paz. Madrid)

defining the area of valve opening. Moreover, distribution of color delineates areas of low signal that matches with regions of thrombosis detected on CT (Fig. 4.18).

**Prosthetic Regurgitation** Pathologic prosthetic regurgitation can be divided into intraprosthetic (secondary to degeneration, thrombus or endocarditis) or paravalvular leak, normally due to spontaneous or infective-related dehiscence of a surgical stitch (Fig. 4.20).

3DTEE provides excellent images to understand the underlying mechanism and is useful in the quantification of the paravalvular regurgitation [20], measuring the anatomical orifice, the vena contracta dimensions (Fig. 4.21) and effective regurgitant orifice by PISA. A task that may be challenging using other classical techniques. Moreover, it is not unusual to find more than one paravalvular leak; in this case, no 2D tools have been validated. When performing 3DTEE, paravalvular regurgitation can also be measured in a semi-cuantitative method, by the proportion of the regurgitant area to the circumference of the prosthesis, being mild if it occupies less than 10 % and severe when it occupies more than 20 %.

For these reasons, 3DTEE represents the diagnostic test of choice to assess paravalvular leakage and is of paramount usefulness to plan and guide surgical or percutaneous interventions.

**Acknowledgements**   Thanks to Pablo Pastor and Alejandra Carbonell for their collaboration.

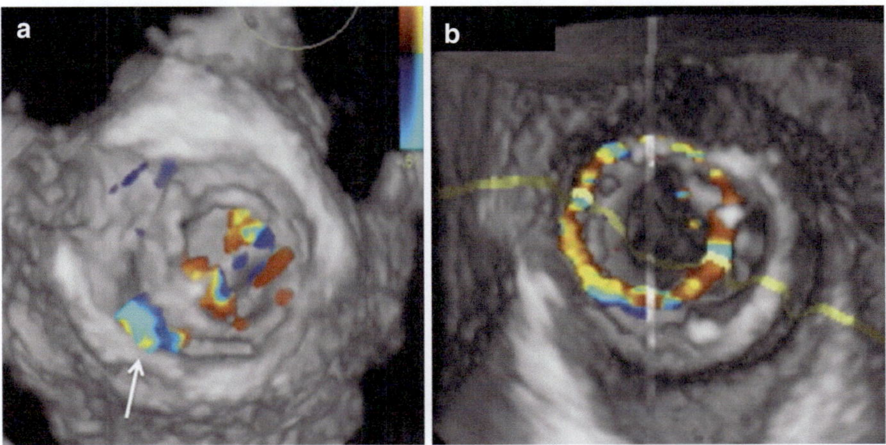

**Fig. 4.20** 3D TEE color Doppler in two different mitral prostheses in systole. (**a**) A periprosthetic leak is seen in a posterior location. (**b**) Intraprosthetic MR around the ring in a case with pannus

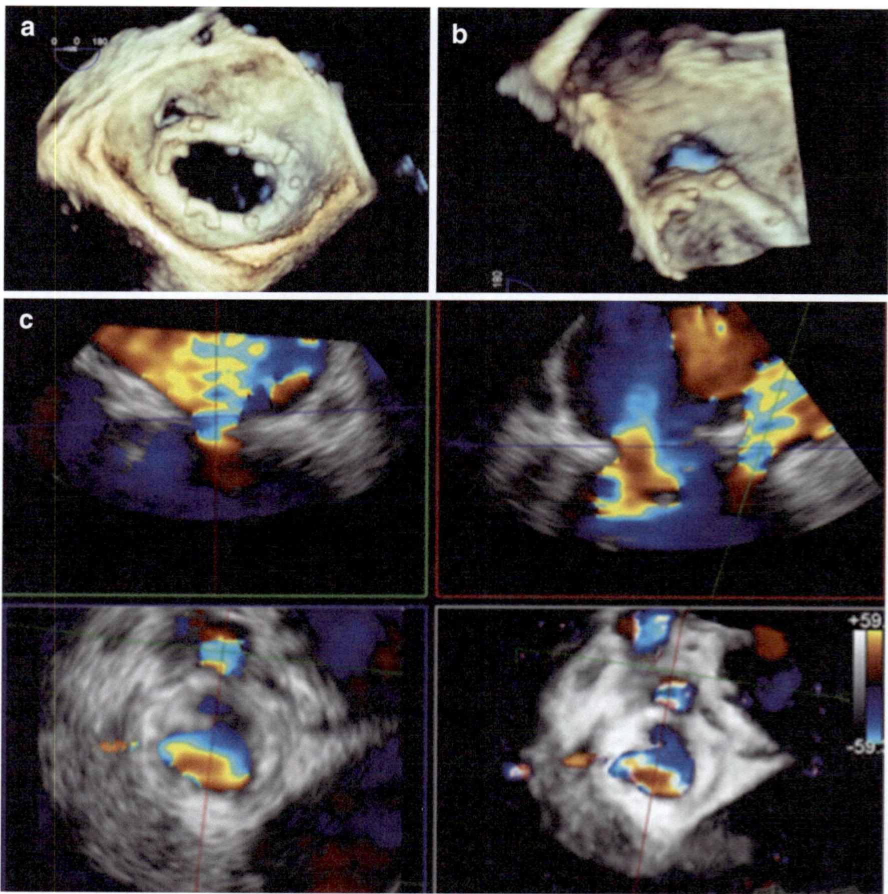

**Fig. 4.21** 3D TEE in a prosthetic ring. (**a**) A Zoom study shows a leak next to the left atrial appendage. (**b**) A focused 3D study shows the orifice with higher spatial resolution. (**c**) A study with Color Doppler allows to measure of the area of VC at that level

# References

1. Veronesi F, Corsi C, Sugeng L, et al. A study of functional anatomy of aortic – mitral valve coupling using 3D matrix transesophageal echocardiography. Circ Cardiovasc Imaging. 2009;2:24–31.
2. Messika-Zeitoun D, Serfaty JM, Brochet E, et al. Multimodal assessment of the aortic annulus diameter: Implications for transcatheter aortic valve implantation. J Am Coll Cardiol. 2010;55:186–94.
3. Lang RM, Badano LP, Tsang W, et al. Guidelines and standards EAE/ASE Recommendations for image acquisition and display using three-dimensional echocardiography. J Am Soc Echocardiogr. 2012;25:3–46.
4. Roberts WC, Ko JM. Frequency by decades of unicuspid, bicuspid, and tricuspid aortic valves in adults having isolated aortic valve replacement for aortic stenosis, with or without associated aortic regurgitation. Circulation. 2005;111:920–5.

5. Vahanian A, Alfieri O, Andreotti F, Antunes MJ, Barón-Esquivias G, Baumgartner H, Borger M, et al. Guidelines on the management of valvular heart disease. Eur Heart J. 2012;33:2451–96.

6. Gutierrez-Chico JL, Zamorano JL, Prietro-Moriche E, et al. Real-time three-dimensional echocardiography in aortic stenosis: a novel, simple, and reliable method to improve accuracy in area calculation. Eur Heart J. 2008;29:1296–306.

7. Goland S, Trento A, Iida K, et al. Assessment of aortic stenosis by three-dimensional echocardiography: an accurate and novel approach. Heart. 2007;93:801–7.

8. Khaw AV, Von Bardeleben RS, Strasser C, et al. Direct measurement of left ventricular outflow tract by transthoracic real time 3D-echocardiography increases accuracy in assessment of aortic valve stenosis. Int J Cardiol. 2009;136:64–71.

9. Mihara H, Shibayama K, Jilaihawi H, Itabashi Y, Berdejo J, Utsunomiya H, et al. Assessment of post-procedural aortic regurgitation after TAVR: a intraprocedural TEE study. JACC Cardiovasc Imaging. 2015;8:993–100.

10. Sato H, Ohta T, et al. Severity of aortic regurgitation assessed by área of vena contracta: a clinical two-dimensional and three-dimensional color Doppler imaging study. Cardiovasc Ultrasound. 2015;13:24.

11. Lancellotti P, Tribouilloy C, Hagendorff A, et al. Recommendations for the echocardiographic assessment of native valvular regurgitation: an executive summary from the European association of cardiovascular imaging. Eur Heart J Cardiovasc Imaging. 2013;14:611–44.

12. Macnab A, Jenkins NP, Bridgewater BJ, et al. Three-dimensional echocardiography is superior to multiplane transoesophageal echo in the assessment of regurgitant mitral valve morphology. Eur J Echocardiogr. 2004;5:212–22.

13. Faletra FF, Demertzis S, Pedrazzini G, Murzilli R, Pasotti E, Muzzarelli S, Siclari F, Moccetti T. Three-dimensional transesophageal echocardiography in degenerative mitral regurgitation. J Am Soc Echocardiogr. 2015;28:437–48.

14. Chu J, Levine R, Chua S, et al. Assesing mitral valve area and orifice geometry in calcific mitral stenosis. A new solution by realtime three-dimensional echocardiography. J Am Soc Echocardiogr. 2008;21:1006–9.

15. Schlosshan D, Aggarwal G, Mathur G, Allan R, Cranney G. Real-time 3D transesophageal echocardiography for the evaluation of rheumatic mitral stenosis. JACC Cardiovasc Imaging. 2011;4:580–8.

16. Zamorano J, Fernandez-Golfin C. Comprehensive 3D echocardiography assessment of mitro-aortic valvular physiology. Are we ready? Eur Heart J Cardiovasc Imaging. 2013;14:1021–2.

17. Little SH. Three-dimensional echocardiography to quantify mitral valve regurgitation. Curr Opin Cardiol. 2012;27:477–84.

18. Plicht B, Kahlert P, Goldwasser R, Janosi RA, Hunold P, Erbel R, Buck T. Direct quantification of mitral regurgitant flow volume by real-time three-dimensional echocardiography using dealiasing of color Doppler flow at the vena contracta. J Am Soc Echocardiogr. 2008;21:1337–46.

19. Lazaro C, Hinojar R, Zamorano JL. Cardiac imaging in prosthetic paravalvular leaks. Cardiovas Diagn Ther. 2014;4:307–13.

20. Arribas-Jimenez A, Rama-Merchan JC, Barreiro-Pérez M, Merchan-Gómez S, Iscar-Galán A, Martín-García A, Nieto-Ballestero F, Sánchez-Corral E, Rodriguez-Collado J, Cruz-González I, Sanchez PL. Utility of Real-Time 3-Dimensional Transesophageal Echocardiography in the Assessment of Mitral Paravalvular Leak. Circ J. 2016;80:738–44.

# Chapter 5
# 3D-Echo Protocols for Assesing Cardiac Chambers, Volume and Function


Alejandra Carbonell San Román, Rocío Hinojar Baydés, and Covadonga Fernández-Golfín Lobán


## Introduction

The assessment of size and function of cardiac chambers is determinant in every echocardiographic evaluation. Left ventricular ejection fraction (LVEF) as a surrogate of LV function (LVF) has been established as an important prognostic parameter, determinant in clinical management basic in cardiac diagnostics. Hence, an accurate measurement of these parameters is of paramount importance in order to establish LVF. Although two-dimensional (2D) echocardiography continues to be a valuable tool and remains an essential part of the standard evaluation, it continues to have numerous pitfalls in the accurate determination of cardiac volumes and function. Emerging technologies with 3-dimensional (3D) imaging have revolutionized ultrasound techniques in the last decades. The constant improvements in technology have led to real-time volumetric imaging, avoiding geometric assumptions inherent to 2D imaging which have significantly improved the accuracy of the echocardiographic evaluation of cardiac chambers size and function. Progressively, the ease of data acquisition, the ability to image the entire heart in real time, in addition to the cumulative evidence of its superiority in selected clinical scenarios have brought 3D echocardiography closer to clinical routine.


**Electronic supplementary material** The online version of this chapter (doi:10.1007/978-3-319-50335-6_5) contains supplementary material, which is available to authorized users.



A.C.S. Román • R.H. Baydés (✉) • C.F.-G. Lobán
Cardiology Department, University Hospital Ramón y Cajal, Carretera de Colmenar Km 9,100, 28034 Madrid, Spain
e-mail: rociohinojar@gmail.com



© Springer International Publishing AG 2017
E. Casas Rojo et al. (eds.), *Manual of 3D Echocardiography*,
DOI 10.1007/978-3-319-50335-6_5

# Assessing Left Ventricular Volume and Ejection Fraction

3D echocardiography has become the method of choice for the evaluation of LVF. 3D techniques avoid geometric assumptions, providing higher diagnostic accuracy compared to 2D echocardiography and similar to cardiac magnetic resonance (CMR) for determining LV volumes, mass, and LVEF with high inter and intra-observer reproducibility [1–3]. Geometric assumptions in 2D echocardiography may be feasible when assessing normally shaped ventricles but become inaccurate when dealing with severely deteriorated ventricles [4, 5], scenario in which a precise estimation of LVF is of upmost importance. It has been demonstrated that quantification of LV volumes and LVEF by 3D echocardiography is more accurate, reproducible and reliable than 2D, particularly in deformed ventricles. Another handicap encountered with 2D evaluation is the poor reproducibility and reliability related to probe positioning-dependency for image acquisition and analysis [6]; slight differences in the position of the probe resulting in different 2D planes affects consecutive measurements, with poor test-retest reliability. The development of software that enables semi-automated endocardial border detection with automatic calculation of volumes and EF provides an extra tool which potentially reduces inter-observer variability [7]. However, improvement of these algorithms is still required to avoid the need for corrections of the endocardial border by the observer, as this error would be reintroduced. Both manual and semi-automated contour detection have shown an underestimation of 3D derived LV volumes when compared to CMR [8]. Nonetheless, it is essentially considered the echocardiographic method of choice [3] for LV function assessment as it is a reproducible, fast and reliable technique [9–11]. These conditions also determine its utility in serial assessments of LV volumes and ejection fraction [12]. Fully-automated detection of endocardial border and ultimate quantification of LV volumes and EF has been developed, capable of detecting the four heart chambers in an apical transthoracic 3D data set.

3D evaluation may find limitations in subjects with poor image quality with poor acoustic windows or in atrial fibrillation. The size of 3D transducers can also limit image quality because of interference from the ribs, although rapid development of smaller sized probes aids in this technical pitfall [13]. The use of contrast in 3D echocardiographic evaluation may help determination of LV volumes and reduced inter-reader variability [14] although poor acoustic windows can still be limiting [15].

## *Acquisition Protocol*

It has been established that 3D transthoracic echocardiography is a valid and reliable evaluation tool for assessment of LV volumes and ejection fraction. It was initially based of ECG-gated full volume acquisition as the standard approach to capture the entire LV volume over several heartbeats. This method assembles together different subvolumes in sequential acquisitions in order to provide a large pyramidal volume, which integrates the complete LV volumetric information. However, this method is hampered when dealing with irregular cardiac cycles in cases of atrial fibrillation or ectopic beats, and particularly in patients that cannot perform transient apnoea where stitch artefacts are appreciated. Acquisition can be performed in an only cardiac cycle integrating the full LV volume [16, 17] with accurate results in smaller acquisition times and reducing artefacts. Acquisition of data in the full volume method must ensure complete caption of the entire ventricle, with simultaneous comparison of two orthogonal planes of 2D echocardiography previous to 3D acquisition (Figure. In severely dilated or distorted ventricles this may be difficult, requiring acquisition using multiple-beat datasets with wider angles to ensure complete caption with satisfactory temporal and spatial resolution (Fig. 5.1, Video 5.1). After optimal data acquisition, it is processed by vendor specific software for quantitative analysis of LV function; being either built-in for immediate analysis or for posterior off-line analysis at the workstation.

Post-processing of data is fast and easy to use, taking around 1–2 min. Depending on the different vendors, specific software analysis has been developed. First ones (QLab on Phillips 3D systems, or EchoView version 5.4 TomTec) required the operator to establish the end diastolic and end systolic frame as well as to define the endocardial; this is done by depicting landmark points that define the location of the mitral valve plane and the apex (Figs. 5.2 and 5.3). This must be done ensuring correct alignment of the two orthogonal anterior-posterior and medial-lateral LV

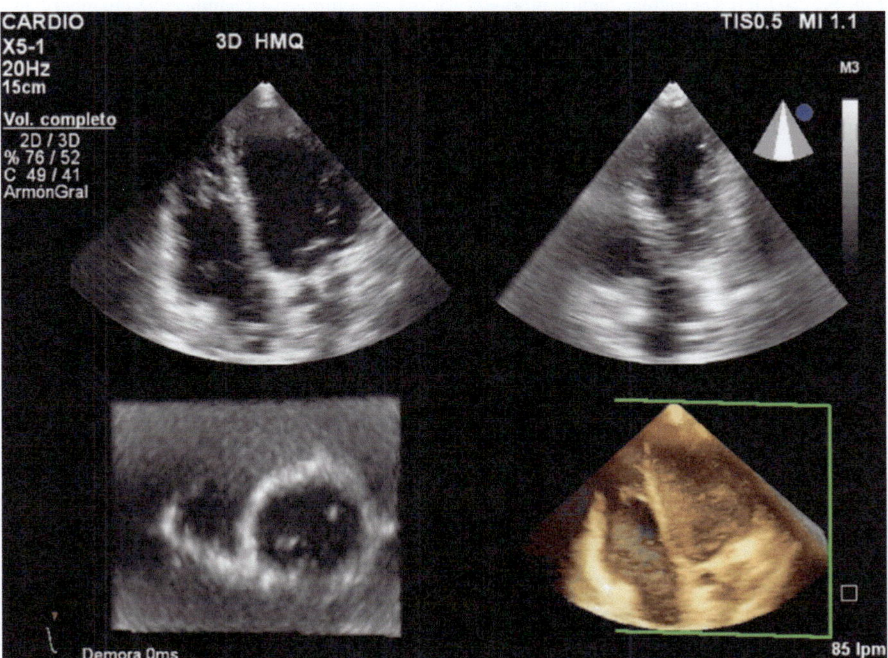


**Fig. 5.1** Image acquisition for 3D left ventricular volume and ejection fraction quantitation. 4 chambers, 2 chambers and short axis view along with 3D volume are displayed

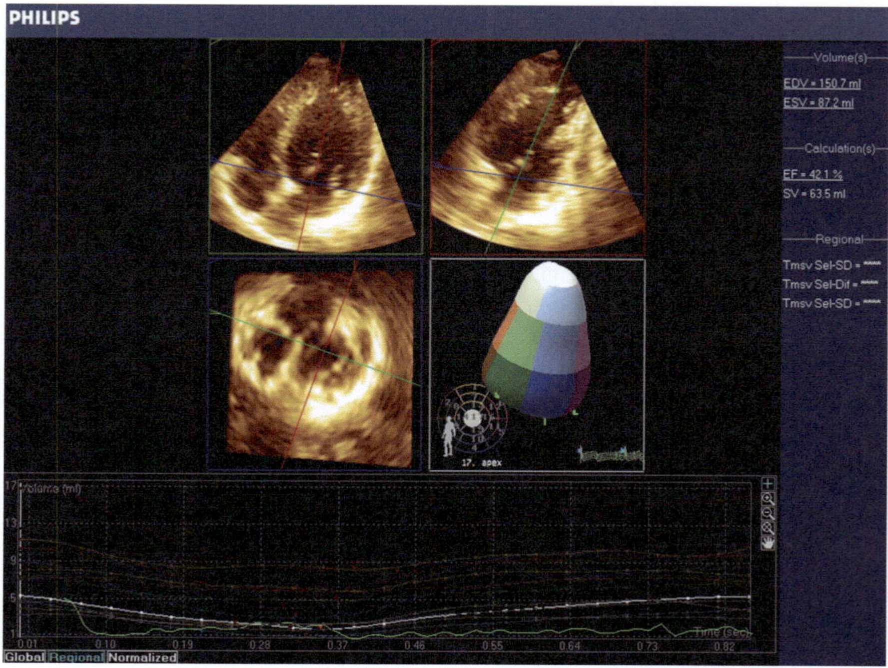

**Fig. 5.2** 3D left ventricular quantitation software (Lab, Philips). 4 chambers, 2 chambers and short axis planes obtained from the 3D volume through multiplane reconstructions are displayed

planes, along the LV longest axis thus avoiding foreshortening. A total of 10 point must be set which define the inferior and anterior walls, the medial and lateral mitral annulus and finally the apex. The system then automatically tracks the endocardial border in the 3D data set for each acquired frame. This provides a global volume-time curve displaying the dynamic course of the global volume change during the cardiac cycle with end-diastolic maximum and end-systolic minimum, and an automatic calculation of LV ejection fraction (Video 5.2). When compared to CMR, LV volumes are consistently underestimated, particularly due to tracing of the endocardial border which includes the trabeculae in CMR and excludes them in 3D imaging [8, 10, 11]. Nonetheless, when calculating EF there have been no differences in neither over or underestimation when comparing both methods [10, 11]. However, due to continuous technological development, automatic quantitation of LV volumes and EF is possible without any operator interaction in latest softwares (Figs. 5.4 and 5.5, Video 5.3). However, contour editing is still possible if needed (Fig. 5.6).

All protocol depends upon a good image quality; therefore care should be taken to clearly visualize the endocardial border before 3D dataset acquisition. Visualization may be difficult of the basal lateral segment and basal and mid-ventricular anterior myocardial segments in simultaneous 4 and 2-chamber views; when at least two myocardial segments cannot be adequately visualized, correction of the probe position or breath-holding manoeuvres must be considered to ensure a complete caption. It may be helpful to ask the patient to slowly breathe in and out to find a breath-

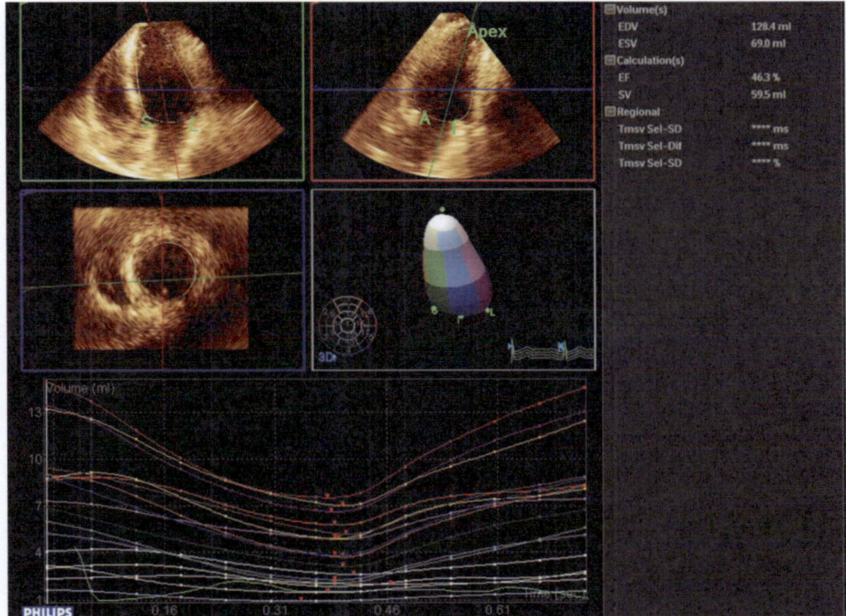

**Fig. 5.3** Same image as Fig. 5.2 with endocardial tracing and mitral and apex references points displayed

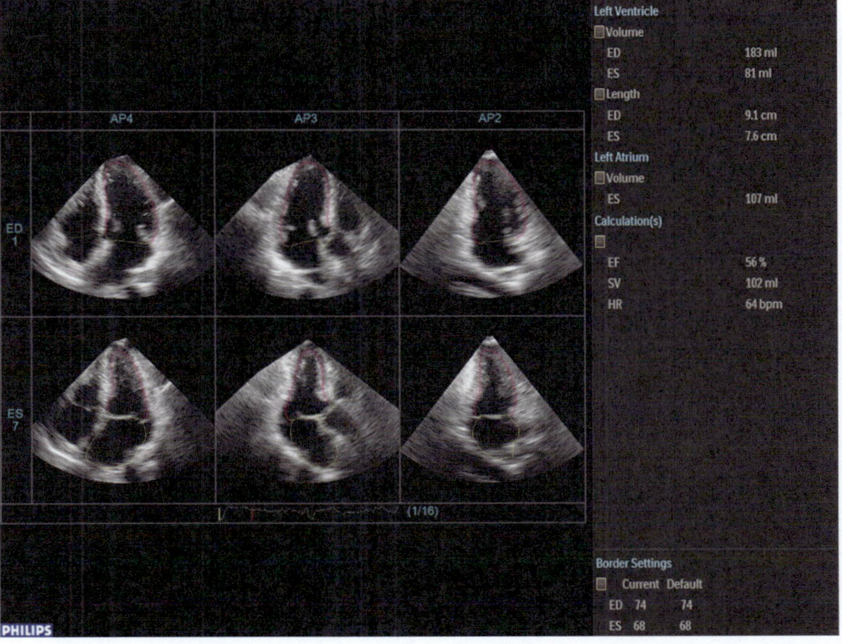

**Fig. 5.4** From a 3D volume acquisition, automatic selection of end diastolic and end systolic phase along with endocardial detection is performed. 4, 2 and 3 chambers view in both phases along with quantitative data are shown (Heart Model, Philips)

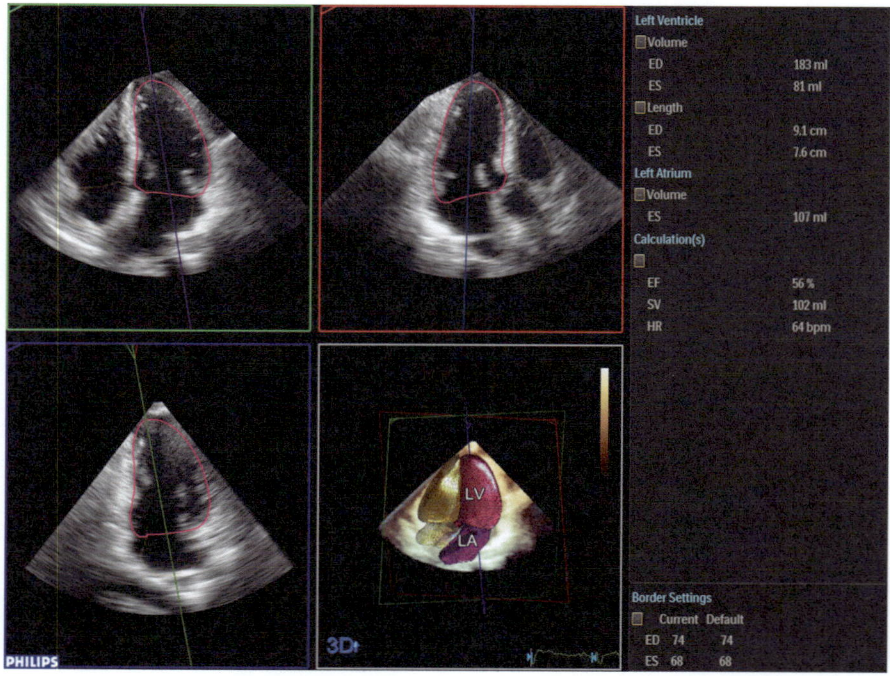


**Fig. 5.5** Final results of automatic left ventricular and left atrium volume and ejection fraction calculation with 2D planes and 3D volume shown

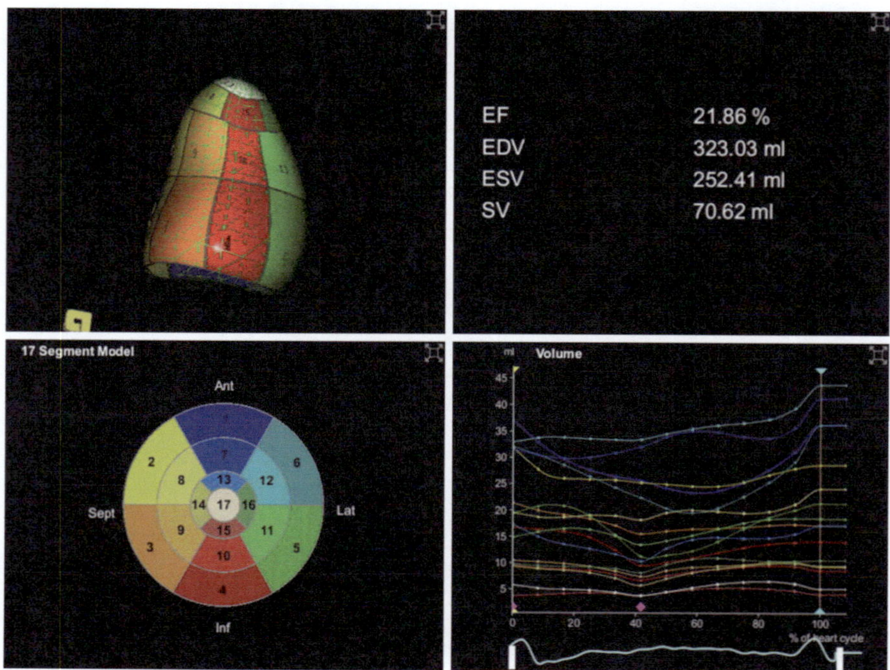


**Fig. 5.6** 3D left ventricular automatic quantitation of volume and ejection fraction, final result (Siemens). 3D volume, bull's eye, quantitative data and segmental volume/time curves are shown

holding position in which the endocardial border is best delineated, and immediately after its identification acquire the 3D data set. When despite this, the endocardial border has not been adequately traced; manual corrections can be introduced in the 2D sections extracted from the 3D data set. This is a time consuming process but ensures accurate and reproducible 3D information. Contrast can be used to enhance imaging in real-time 3D echocardiography being superior to non-contrast 3DE and both 2D modalities when compared to CMR [14, 15].

## Assessing Right Ventricular Volume and Ejection Fraction

The particular shape of the right ventricle (RV) does not allow geometric assumptions in order to accurately measure volumes and function with 2D echocardiography. This is due to the absence of a simple 3D geometrical model that represents its shape, thus clearly favouring the advantages of 3D echocardiography in this scenario. Nonetheless, the quantification of RV size and function has been proven of paramount importance in diagnosis and prognosis [18, 19]. Once more, significant pressure or volume over-load conditions markedly affect geometry, volume and wall thickness.

Evaluation with 2D echocardiography only estimates the true volume of the RV from an apical 4-chamber view [3]. The development of 3D echocardiography (3DE) provides an anatomically realistic reconstructive model of the right ventricle. Its complex size and geometry can be observed with the possibility of unlimited orientation cut-planes to appreciate its three main compartments: the inflow tract with the tricuspid valve, the trabeculated apex and the right outflow tract.

Regardless of the advantages in anatomical assessment, 3DE improves quantitative RV size and function assessment compared with 2D echocardiography [20]. Although RV EF does not directly reflect RV contractile function per se, it provides an integrated view of the interaction between RV contractility and load. Real-time 3D echocardiography provides a reproducible and accurate alternative to CMR [21] with good correlation values [22] particularly in dilated RV cavities [23, 24]. Slight underestimation of RV volumes was observed with 3D estimation, but with excellent EF agreement with CMR-derived measurements. Image quality, however remains an important limitation in transthoracic assessment, as an adequate acoustic window may be challenging given its retrosternal position. Transeosophageal echocardiographic views, including transgastric may provide views with added value to its evaluation, for a more precise determination of right chambers.

Analysis may also be challenging [23], requiring an important learning curve that might affect inter-study reproducibility in serial exams [23, 25]. Single-beat full volume capture 3DE is a valid method [26] and fully automated algorithms have been developed to optimize endocardial border detection [27]. A source of error is the intense trabeculation in the apical region of the RV in both manually and auto-mated endocardial border delineation. Two different approaches exist to quantify RV volumes using either a 3D summation-of-disk-method based on manual tracing of six to ten parallel cross-sectional RV planes [28] or specific commercially designed software for RV analysis. The latter is based on semi-automated contour detection algorithms using border delineation in the three main cut planes at end-

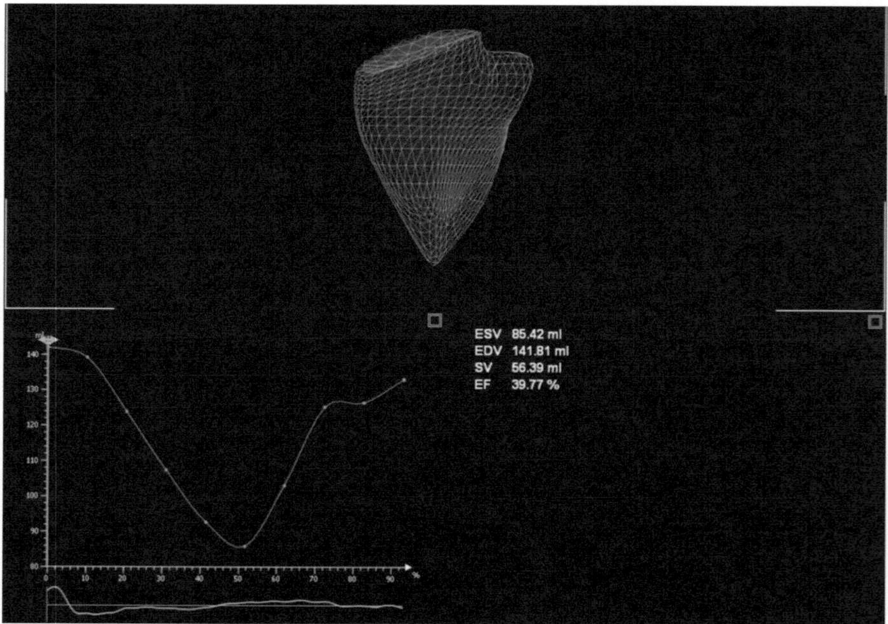


**Fig. 5.7** Right ventricular volume and ejection fraction quantitation from a 3D volume acquisition. 3D volume, quantitative data and volume/time curve is shown

diastole and end-systole. The RV endocardial border is followed throughout systole so that a 3D model is created which provides end-diastolic and end-systolic volumes, with dynamic RV volume-time curves and EF (Fig. 5.7 and Video 5.4) [29]. This method has been validated against reference values as established by CMR [30], but consistently underestimates RV volumes and EF [31] particularly when dealing with larger volumes. The 3D summation-of-disk method grossly reconstructs the right ventricular shape, but is limited by potential measurement errors particularly in the basal inflow and outflow tracts as the tricuspid valve and RV outflow tract rarely lie in the same plane. Nevertheless, real-time 3DE has demonstrated improved accuracy and reproducibility and has established normal reference values base upon on large datasets, being the volumetric semiautomated border detection approach the recommended method for the assessment of RV EF [3]. Limitations of 3D assessment of RV EF include load dependency, interventricular changes affecting septal motion, poor acoustic windows and irregular rhythms.

## Assessing of the Atria and Septal Defects

### Assessment of Atrial Volume and Function

Determination of left atrial (LA) size and function is key in clinical decision-making and has proved to be an independent predictor of long-term prognosis and survival in several cardiovascular conditions [32, 33]. Volume determinations hold higher accuracy

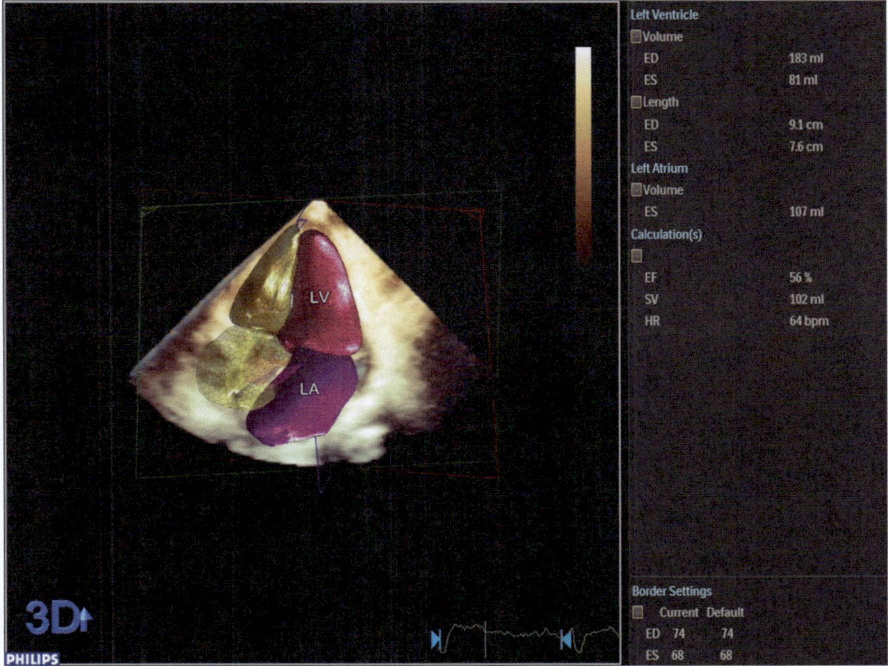


**Fig. 5.8** Left atrium 3D volume automatic quantitation with a dedicated left atrium 3D software from a 3D volume acquisition (Heart Model, Philips)

than linear dimensions to assess LA size given the frequent asymmetrical morphology of LA enlargement and remodelling [34]. 2D echocardiographic assessment of LA volumes relies on geometric assumptions, underestimating LA size compared to CMR and cardiac computed tomography. Novel 3D imaging has shown to overcome the limitations of 2D techniques, allowing robust LA calculations with high reproducibility, comparable to CMR [35, 36]. Furthermore, RT3DE has demonstrated to be more accurate [37] and reproducible method for assessment of active and passive LA function compared to 2DE given its higher sensitivity to volume changes [38]. The same semiautomated algorithm previously described can be used to obtain LA volumes, even in atrial fibrillation [39].Recent software development allows automatic specific quantitation of LA volumes as it does for the left ventricle (Fig. 5.8). Moreover, 3D echocardiography provides functional information of LA atrium by temporal analysis of LA volumes throughout the cardiac cycle [40] with significant differences throughout.

Transesophageal echocardiography (TEE) is the main imaging modality for evaluation of the left atrial appendage (Figs. 5.9 and 5.10). Its particular 3D shape can be characterised by 3D TEE. 3D TEE is helpful in differentiating a thrombus from LAA pectinate muscles [41]. Several studies validate that RT 3D TEE more accurately assesses the true LAA orifice size (Fig. 5.11). RT 3D TEE was found to be closely related to CT measurements [42, 43], whereas 2D TEE tends to underestimate the LAA orifice area [44]. Prior percutaneous device closure of the LAA several, specific measurements by 2D and particularly 3D imaging must be obtained as described in a later chapter [45].

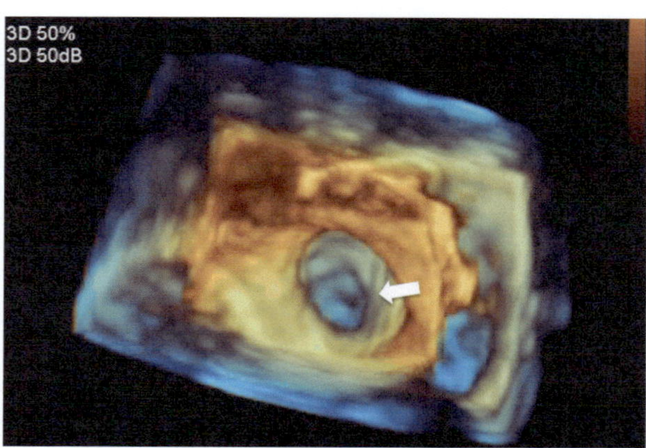

**Fig. 5.9** 3D TEE zoom 3D image showing left atrial appendage (*arrow*)

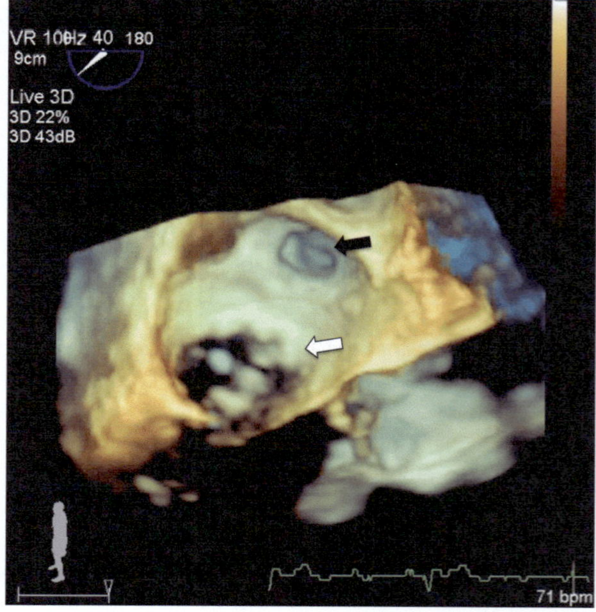

**Fig. 5.10** Live 3D TEE image showing left atrial appendage (*black arrow*) and mitral valve (*white arrow*)

The anatomy of the right atrium by 3DTEE provides key information in the planning and guidance of transcatheter ablation of arrhythmias [46]. Given the proximity of the transducer to the right atrium, this technique provides high-quality images of those atrial structures involved in ablation procedures. The acquisition of a zoom 3D image must be obtained from the 2-dimensional 4-chamber view, using a pyramidal dataset large enough to include the entire right atrium. By using the auto-crop function, the anterior half of the atrium is removed. Moreover, an arbitrary crop can be used to remove further remaining structures of less interest. Real-time 3D TEE enables consistent visualization of right atrial structures, provided proper image

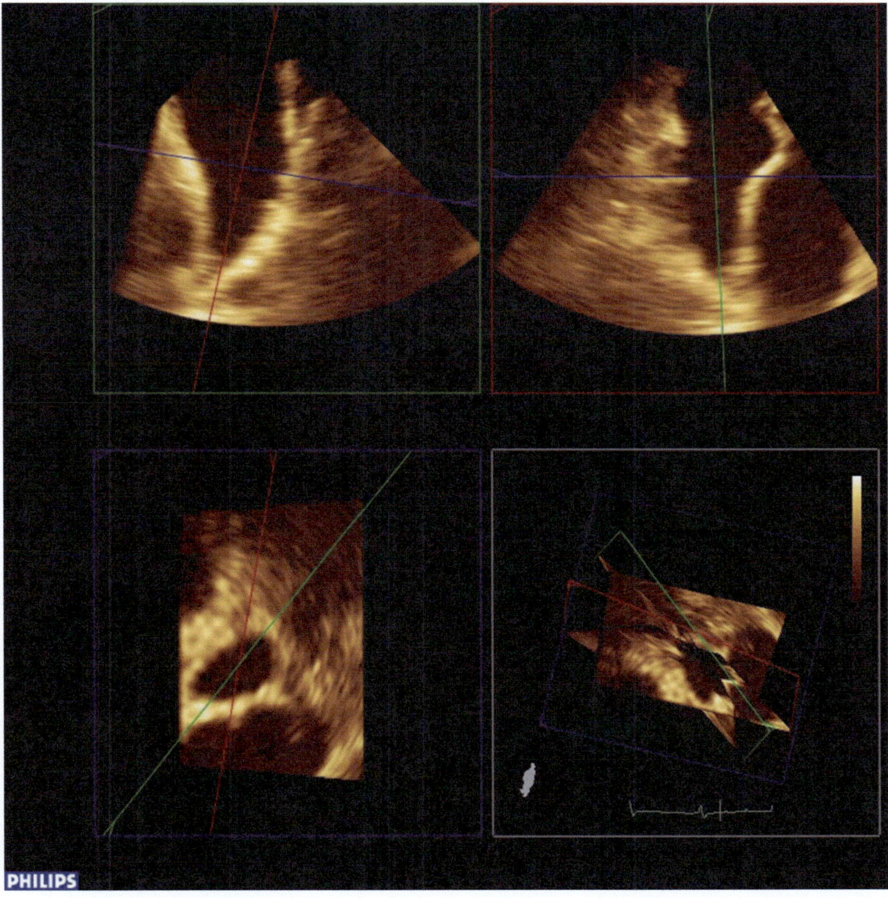

**Fig. 5.11** Multiplanar reconstruction of left atrial appendage from TEE 3D zoom image acquisition

acquisition and image rendering process have been used [46]. Sizing of the right atrium by 3DE has also been established as accurate and reproducible when compared to CMR imaging [47].

## *Assessment of Interatrial Septum*

Three- dimensional transesophageal echocardiography (3DTEE) offers the unique advantage by providing "en face" view of the interatrial septum from the left atrium for assessment of its integrity and other important surrounding structures in a single live 3D echo view using 3D zoom, live 3D and 3D full volume with iCrop modalities.

It may contribute to assess the exact anatomy of the interatrial septum, including the functionality of a patent foramen ovale and the extent of the fossa ovalis membranous aneurysm. The assessment of interatrial septum defects will be described in detail in another chapter.

## Abnormal Masses and Findings

The differential diagnosis uncovered by the finding of a cardiac mass is extensive, being primary and secondary cardiac tumors infrequent while intracardiac thrombi or vegetations are common findings. A major advantage of 3D imaging is the manipulation to provide "en face" views of cardiac structures, but also RT 3D TEE has demonstrated to be more accurate compared with 2D TEE in characterizing diameters and real size, types, surface features, mobility, and sites of intracardiac masses, and its spatial relationship to surrounding structures [48–50], so that they can be displayed in a more anatomically realistic manner [51]. Particular features such as mobility, surface structure and deformation may aid in the identification of its aetiology. The benefit of this added value has been largely recognised and is currently endorsed by current American Society of Echocardiography guidelines when evaluating intracardiac tumors [52].

## *Spontaneous Echocontrast and Cardiac Thrombi*

The presence of spontaneous echocontrast (SEC) implies an increased risk for thrombus formation, particularly in the LAA. Live 3DE is able to illustrate this phenomenon although its advantage over 2DTEE in this scenario is still undetermined.

On the contrary, RT3DEE not only identifies the presence of intracavitary thrombi but allows its determination of its size and exact point of anchorage [53], adhered to a cardiac structure or a central venous catheter (Figs. 5.12, 5.13 and 5.14, Video 5.5). Its utility can be extended to the monitorization of the size and areas of echolucenticity as response to anticoagulant therapy [54]. Furthermore, when assessing the presence of thrombi in the LAA, 3DTEE provides a direct view of the often irregularly shaped LAA; the use of two simultaneous orthogonal planes allows acquisition of a 3D live dataset for further analysis. This is important in differentiating thrombi from muscular trabeculae, particularly when faced with a bilobar LAA.

## *Infective Endocarditis*

Standard 2D transesophageal echocardiography is the preferred approach when suspecting endocarditis, with excellent sensitivity and specifity [55]. RT3D TEE offers an added diagnostic value (Fig. 5.15) to identify multiple vegetations and to

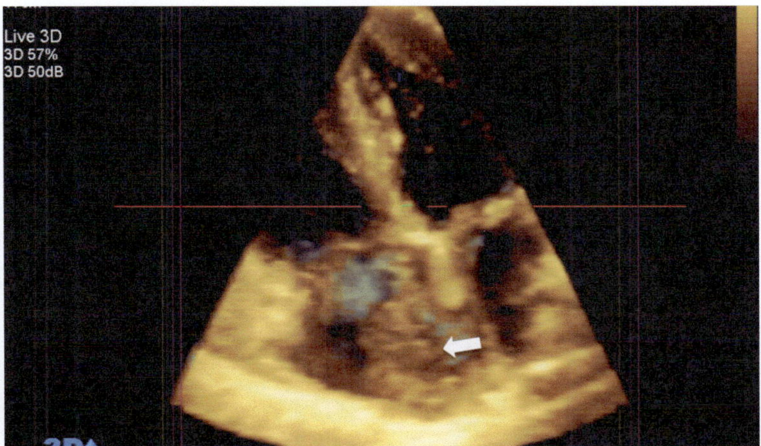

**Fig. 5.12** 4 chambers 3D image showing a large right atrial thrombus (*arrow*)

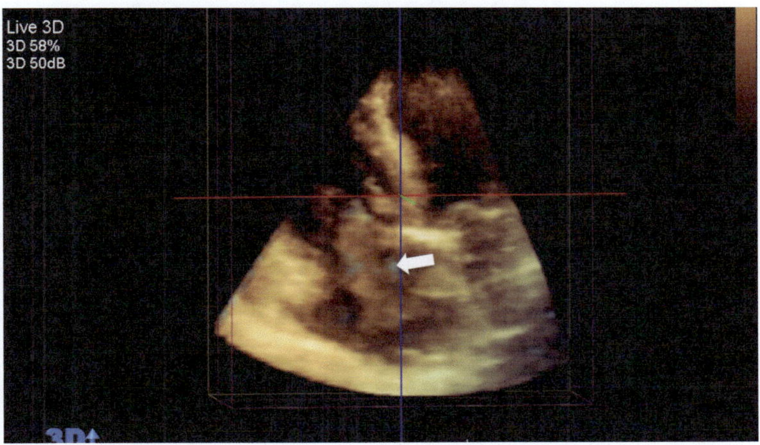

**Fig. 5.13** Same image as in Fig. 5.12 showing the right atrial thrombus protruding through the tricuspid valve.

accurately assess their size [56–58], and therefore estimating the possible embolic risk [59]. A precise diagnosis of complications can improve clinical management, such as chordal rupture, leaflet perforation or paravalvular abscess [60, 61], particularly in complex cases like prosthetic valve endocarditis in the assessment of dehiscence or paravalvular regurgitation [62, 63]. Another major advantage of RT3D compared both with TTE and TEE is the ability to acquire 'en face' views of valves and presentation in a 'surgical view' which combined with simultaneous 2D views provides detailed information for surgical planning and assessing valve reparability (Figs. 5.16 and 5.17, Video 5.6). Nonetheless, 3D echocardiography should be regarded as a supplement to standard 2D. Given the lower frame rate, it may impair detection of smaller vegetations [64]. Volume datasets acquired in the live 3D mode are recommended, given the rapid and unpredicted motion of vegetations, because

**Fig. 5.14** 3 chambers view full volume acquisition from TEE. A thin and long atrial mass protruding into the left ventricle arising from the right upper pulmonary vein is shown. Pulmonary vein thrombosis diagnosis was made

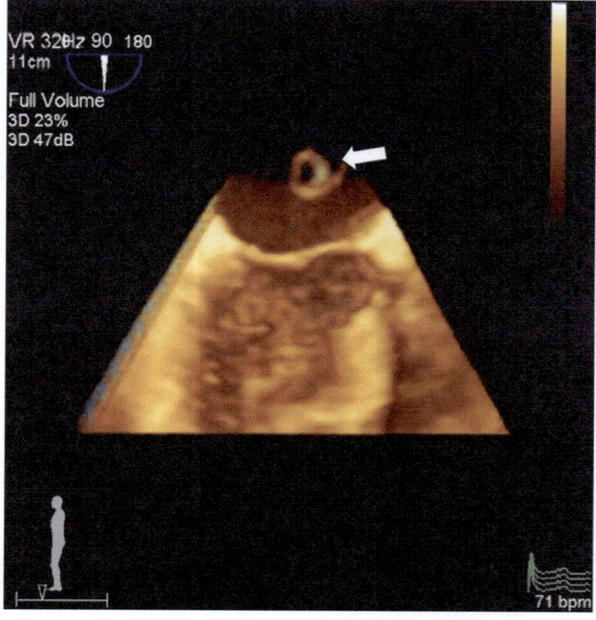

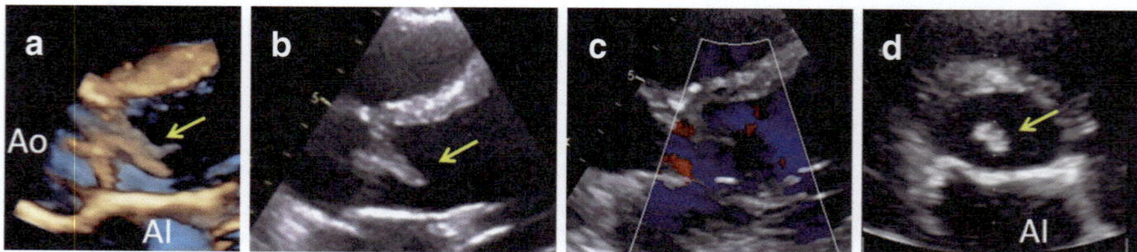

**Fig. 5.15** This series of images illustrate the aortic valve with suspicion of active infective endocarditis. Long paraesternal axis of de aortica valve in 3D (**a**), 2D (**b**), with colour Doppler (**c**) and the aortic short axis (**d**). The yellow arrow point to the adhered mass on the anterior aortic leaflet in an aortic valve, with no associated regurgitation

**Fig. 5.16** TEE 3D image of the mitral valve, zoom 3D acquisition, "en face" surgical view showing two endocarditic vegetations at the level of A1 and A3 scallops (*arrows*)

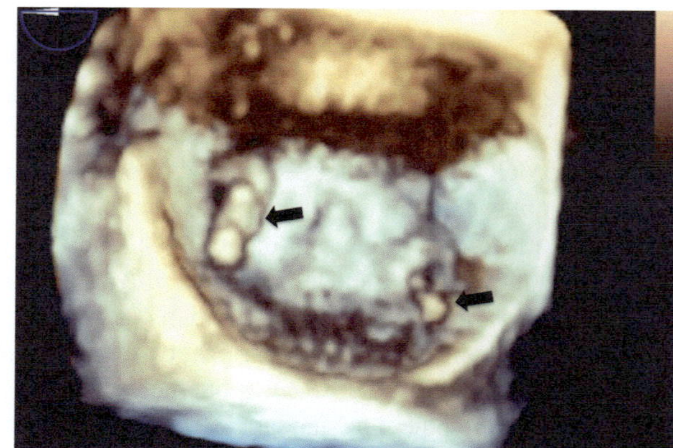

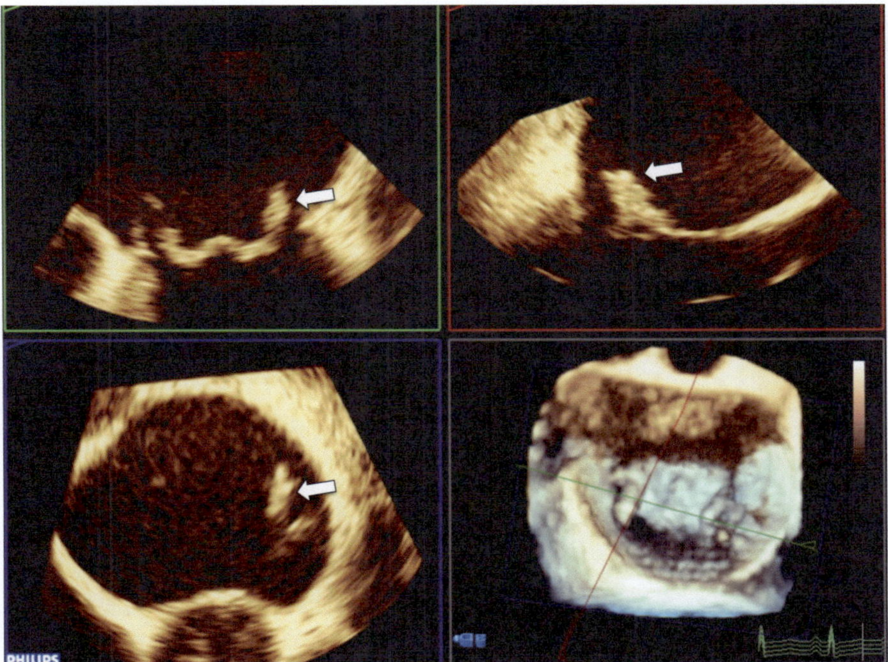

**Fig. 5.17** Same image as in Fig. 5.16, multiplanar reconstruction showing the different planes of the valve with endocarditic vegetations (*arrows*) are shown

of the relatively high spatial resolution. However, a potential limitation is the acquisition of the full area of interest, as the 3DTEE volumes might be too narrow. Intracardiac devices like pacemaker or defibrillator probes or venous central lines should follow a similar protocol.

## *Cardiac Tumors*

The diagnosis of intracardiac primary or secondary tumors is frequently incidental being the differential diagnosis challenging in many scenarios. The assessment with RT3D TEE offers advantages given its superior delineation of characteristics (Fig. 5.18) such as size, shape, mobility and location, and even the exact site and extent of adherence of the studied mass [51]. Since, the whole volume of the mass can be evaluated; the differential diagnosis of cardiac masses becomes narrower. The presence or absence of necrotic areas or echolucencies may help in the diagnosis, as the latter are consistent with thrombus lysis. The use of colour Doppler aids in evaluation of its vascularization as well as in identification of flow acceleration where the mass may cause flow obstruction.

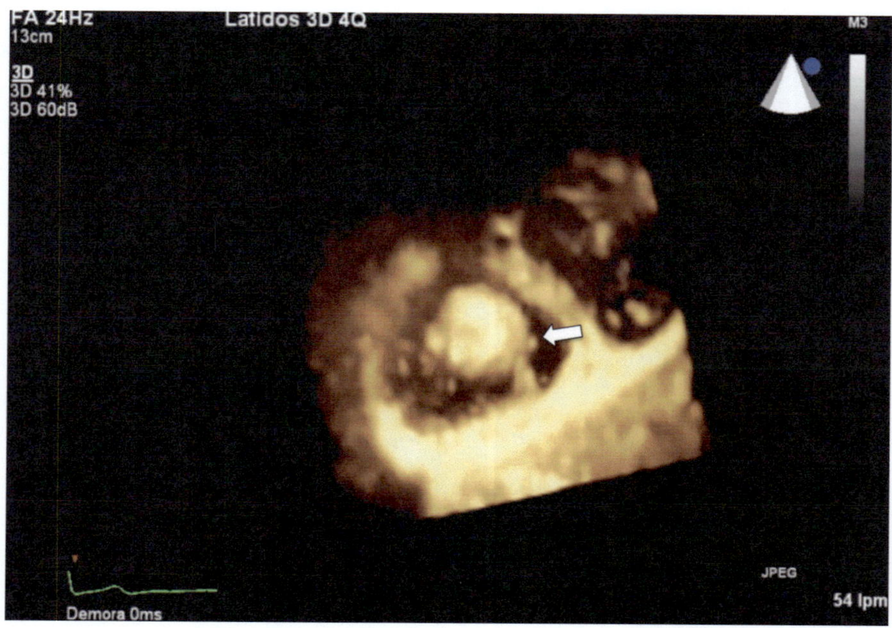

**Fig. 5.18** 3D image showing left and right ventricles, surgical view. A large left ventricular mass is depicted, anchored to the left anterolateral ventricular wall

**Myxomas** are the most common benign cardiac tumors and are usually attached to the left-sided interatrial septum and the fossa ovalis by a pedicle but can have a broad attachment base. RT3DE provides accurate anatomic visualization with high spatial resolution of the relationship of the mass with the interatrial septum [65]; the presence of an interatrial septal stalk adds evidence that the mass is a myxoma. RT3D TEE can be particularly helpful to assess mass heterogeneity by using the cropping function and carefully using digital analysis to dissect the lesion.

**Papillary fibroelastomas** are the second most frequent tumors typically affecting valve tissue with a characteristic appearance: small, mobile, vibrating masses. When affecting the aortic valve, they mimic infectious vegetations or Lambls' excrescences and the differentiation can be challenging. Evaluation with RT3DE, particularly RT3D TEE, helps to determine the attachment point to the valve surface and to discern whether resection would impede valve function [66]. Evaluation of its size and mobility is also important in regard to the risk of embolization.

In the evaluation of other primary tumors such as hemangiomas, rhabdomyoma, lypomas or fibromas, RT3DE has also offered advantages. Hemangiomas are extensively vascularized in comparison to myxomas [65] and with extensive echolucencies. Rhabdomyomas appear as multiple masses pedunculated or intramural in shape, involving the ventricular myocardium with echodense appearance, and consequently with the appearance of regional wall motion abnormalities. This can be visualized with RT3DE imaging which demonstrated an inhomogeneous echogenicity and even a dyskinetic movement during systole.

**Secondary and metastatic tumors** are the most common tumors affecting cardiac structures. The use of RT3D color Doppler datasets aids in the detection of tumoral vascularization. Also, echodense areas by 3D correlate with fibrotic areas of the tumor by pathology and similarly, echolucencies correlate with areas of necrosis. RT3DE can also be used to obtain 3D volumetry of the metastasis with definition if its size and attachment point.


# Bibliography


1. Dorosz JL, Lezotte DC, Weitzenkamp DA, Allen LA, Salcedo EE. Performance of 3-dimensional echocardiography in measuring left ventricular volumes and ejection fraction: a systematic review and meta-analysis. J Am Coll Cardiol. 2012;59(20):1799–808.
2. Lang RM, Mor-Avi V, Sugeng L, Nieman PS, Sahn DJ. Three-dimensional echocardiography: the benefits of the additional dimension. J Am Coll Cardiol. 2006;48(10):2053–69.
3. Lang RM, Badano LP, Mor-Avi V, Afilalo J, Armstrong A, Ernande L, Flachskampf FA, Foster E, Goldstein SA, Kuznetsova T, Lancellotti P, Muraru D, Picard MH, Rietzschel ER, Rudski L, Spencer KT, Tsang W, Voigt JU. Recommendations for cardiac chamber quantification by echocardiography in adults: an update from the American Society of Echocardiography and the European Association of Cardiovascular Imaging. Eur Heart J Cardiovasc Imaging. 2015;16(3):233–70.
4. Sapin PM, Schröder KM, Gopal AS, Smith MD, De Maria AN, King DL. Comparison of two- and three-dimensional echocardiography with cineventriculography for measurement of left ventricular volume in patients. J Am Coll Cardiol. 1994;24(4):1054–63.
5. Qin JX, Jones M, Shiota T, Greenberg NL, Tsujino H, Firstenberg MS, Gupta PC, Zetts AD, Xu Y, Ping Sun J, Cardon LA, Odabashian JA, Flamm SD, White RD, Panza JA, Thomas JD. Validation of real-time three-dimensional echocardiography for quantifying left ventricular volumes in the presence of a left ventricular aneurysm: in vitro and in vivo studies. J Am Coll Cardiol. 2000;36(3):900–7.
6. King DL, Harrison MR, King Jr DL, Gopal AS, Martin RP, DeMaria AN. Improved reproducibility of left atrial and left ventricular measurements by guided three-dimensional echocardiography. J Am Coll Cardiol. 1992;20(5):1238–45.77.
7. Monaghan MJ. Role of real time 3D echocardiography in evaluating the left ventricle. Heart. 2006;92(1):131–6.
8. Mor-Avi V, Jenkins C, Kühl HP, Nesser HJ, Marwick T, Franke A, Ebner C, Freed BH, Steringer-Mascherbauer R, Pollard H, Weinert L, Niel J, Sugeng L, Lang RM. Real-time 3-dimensional echocardiographic quantification of left ventricular volumes: multicenter study for validation with magnetic resonance imaging and investigation of sources of error. JACC Cardiovasc Imaging. 2008;1(4):413–23.
9. Kühl HP, Schreckenberg M, Rulands D, Katoh M, Schäfer W, Schummers G, Bücker A, Hanrath P, Franke A. High-resolution transthoracic real-time three-dimensional echocardiography: quantitation of cardiac volumes and function using semi-automatic border detection and comparison with cardiac magnetic resonance imaging. J Am Coll Cardiol. 2004;43(11):2083–90.
10. Jenkins C, Bricknell K, Hanekom L, Marwick TH. Reproducibility and accuracy of echocardiographic measurements of left ventricular parameters using real-time three-dimensional echocardiography. J Am Coll Cardiol. 2004;44(4):878–86.
11. Jacobs LD, Salgo IS, Goonewardena S, Weinert L, Coon P, Bardo D, Gerard O, Allain P, Zamorano JL, de Isla LP, Mor-Avi V, Lang RM. Rapid online quantification of left ventricular volume from real-time three-dimensional echocardiographic data. Eur Heart J. 2006;27(4):460–8.

12. Jenkins C, Bricknell K, Chan J, Hanekom L, Marwick TH. Comparison of two- and three-dimensional echocardiography with sequential magnetic resonance imaging for evaluating left ventricular volume and ejection fraction over time in patients with healed myocardial infarction. Am J Cardiol. 2007;99(3):300–6.
13. Ruddox V, Mathisen M, Bækkevar M, Aune E, Edvardsen T, Otterstad JE. Is 3D echocardiography superior to 2D echocardiography in general practice? A systematic review of studies published between 2007 and 201. Int J Cardiol. 2013;168(2):1306–15.
14. Hoffmann R, Barletta G, von Bardeleben S, Vanoverschelde JL, Kasprzak J, Greis C, Becher H. Analysis of left ventricular volumes and function: a multicenter comparison of cardiac magnetic resonance imaging, cine ventriculography, and unenhanced and contrast-enhanced two-dimensional and three-dimensional echocardiography. J Am Soc Echocardiogr. 2014;27(3):292–301.
15. Wood PW, Choy JB, Nanda NC, Becher H. Left ventricular ejection fraction and volumes: it depends on the imaging method. Echocardiography. 2014;31(1):87–100. doi:10.1111/echo.12331. Epub 2013 Nov 26.
16. Chang SA, Lee SC, Kim EY, Hahm SH, Jang SY, Park SJ, Choi JO, Park SW, Choe YH, Oh JK. Feasibility of single-beat full-volume capture real-time three-dimensional echocardiography and auto-contouring algorithm for quantification of left ventricular volume: validation with cardiac magnetic resonance imaging. J Am Soc Echocardiogr. 2011;24(8):853–9. doi:10.1016/j.echo.2011.04.015. Epub 2011 Jun 8.
17. Shibayama K, Watanabe H, Iguchi N, Sasaki S, Mahara K, Umemura J, Sumiyoshi T. Evaluation of automated measurement of left ventricular volume by novel real-time 3-dimensional echocardiographic system: validation with cardiac magnetic resonance imaging and 2-dimensional echocardiography. J Cardiol. 2013;61(4):281–8. doi:10.1016/j.jjcc.2012.11.005.
18. de Groote P, Millaire A, Foucher-Hossein C, Nugue O, Marchandise X, Ducloux G, Lablanche JM. Right ventricular ejection fraction is an independent predictor of survival in patients with moderate heart failure. J Am Coll Cardiol. 1998;32(4):948–54.
19. Gavazzi A, Berzuini C, Campana C, Inserra C, Ponzetta M, Sebastiani R, Ghio S, Recusani F. Value of right ventricular ejection fraction in predicting short-term prognosis of patients with severe chronic heart failure. J Heart Lung Transplant. 1997;16(7):774–85.
20. van der Zwaan HB, Geleijnse ML, McGhie JS, Boersma E, Helbing WA, Meijboom FJ, Roos-Hesselink JW. Right ventricular quantification in clinical practice: two-dimensional vs. three-dimensional echocardiography compared with cardiac magnetic resonance imaging. Eur J Echocardiogr. 2011;12(9):656–64.
21. Medvedofsky D, Addetia K, Patel AR, Sedlmeier A, Baumann R, Mor-Avi V, Lang RM. Novel approach to three-dimensional echocardiographic quantification of right ventricular volumes and function from focused views. J Am Soc Echocardiogr. 2015;28(10):1222–31.
22. Gopal AS, Chukwu EO, Iwuchukwu CJ, Katz AS, Toole RS, Schapiro W, Reichek N. Normal values of right ventricular size and function by real-time 3-dimensional echocardiography: comparison with cardiac magnetic resonance imaging. J Am Soc Echocardiogr. 2007;20(5):445–55.
23. Knight DS, Grasso AE, Quail MA, Muthurangu V, Taylor AM, Toumpanakis C, Caplin ME, Coghlan JG, Davar J. Accuracy and reproducibility of right ventricular quantification in patients with pressure and volume overload using single-beat three-dimensional echocardiography. J Am Soc Echocardiogr. 2015;28(3):363–74.
24. Fang F, Chan A, Lee AP, Sanderson JE, Kwong JS, Luo XX, Li S, Yu CM. Variation in right ventricular volumes assessment by real-time three-dimensional echocardiography between dilated and normal right ventricle: comparison with cardiac magnetic resonance imaging. Int J Cardiol. 2013;168(4):4391–3.
25. van der Zwaan HB, Geleijnse ML, Soliman OI, McGhie JS, Wiegers-Groeneweg EJ, Helbing WA, Roos-Hesselink JW, Meijboom FJ. Test-retest variability of volumetric right ventricular measurements using real-time three-dimensional echocardiography. J Am Soc Echocardiogr. 2011;24(6):671–9.

26. Zhang QB, Sun JP, Gao RF, Lee AP, Feng YL, Liu XR, Sheng W, Liu F, Yang XS, Fang F, Yu CM. Feasibility of single-beat full-volume capture real-time three-dimensional echocardiography for quantification of right ventricular volume: validation by cardiac magnetic resonance imaging. Int J Cardiol. 2013;168(4):3991–5.
27. Nillesen MM, van Dijk AP, Duijnhouwer AL, Thijssen JM, de Korte CL. Automated assessment of right ventricular volumes and function using three-dimensional transesophageal echocardiography. Ultrasound Med Biol. 2016;42(2):596–606.
28. Chua S, Levine RA, Yosefy C, Handschumacher MD, Chu J, Qureshi A, Neary J, Ton-Nu TT, Fu M, Wu CJ, Hung J. Assessment of right ventricular function by real-time three-dimensional echocardiography improves accuracy and decreases interobserver variability compared with conventional two-dimensional views. Eur J Echocardiogr. 2009;10(5):619–24.
29. Tamborini G, Brusoni D, Torres Molina JE, Galli CA, Maltagliati A, Muratori M, Susini F, Colombo C, Maffessanti F, Pepi M. Feasibility of a new generation three-dimensional echocardiography for right ventricular volumetric and functional measurements. Am J Cardiol. 2008;102(4):499–505.
30. Ostenfeld E, Carlsson M, Shahgaldi K, Roijer A, Holm J. Manual correction of semi-automatic three-dimensional echocardiography is needed for right ventricular assessment in adults; validation with cardiac magnetic resonance. Cardiovasc Ultrasound. 2012;10:1. doi:10.1186/1476-7120-10-1.
31. Shimada YJ, Shiota M, Siegel RJ, Shiota T. Accuracy of right ventricular volumes and function determined by three-dimensional echocardiography in comparison with magnetic resonance imaging: a meta-analysis study. J Am Soc Echocardiogr. 2010;23(9):943–53.
32. Sanfilippo AJ, Abascal VM, Sheehan M, Oertel LB, Harrigan P, Hughes RA, Weyman AE. Atrial enlargement as a consequence of atrial fibrillation. A prospective echocardiographic study. Circulation. 1990;82(3):792–7.
33. Tsang TS, Abhayaratna WP, Barnes ME, Miyasaka Y, Gersh BJ, Bailey KR, Cha SS, Seward JB. Prediction of cardiovascular outcomes with left atrial size: is volume superior to area or diameter? J Am Coll Cardiol. 2006;47(5):1018–23. Epub 2006 Feb 9.
34. Lester SJ, Ryan EW, Schiller NB, Foster E. Best method in clinical practice and in research studies to determine left atrial size. Am J Cardiol. 1999;84(7):829–32.
35. Miyasaka Y, Tsujimoto S, Maeba H, Yuasa F, Takehana K, Dote K, Iwasaka T. Left atrial volume by real-time three-dimensional echocardiography: validation by 64-slice multidetector computed tomography. J Am Soc Echocardiogr. 2011;24(6):680–6. doi:10.1016/j.echo.2011.03.009.
36. Mor-Avi V, Yodwut C, Jenkins C, Kühl H, Nesser HJ, Marwick TH, Franke A, Weinert L, Niel J, Steringer-Mascherbauer R, Freed BH, Sugeng L, Lang RM. Real-time 3D echocardiographic quantification of left atrial volume: multicenter study for validation with CMR. JACC Cardiovasc Imaging. 2012;5(8):769–77. doi:10.1016/j.jcmg.2012.05.011.
37. Artang R, Migrino RQ, Harmann L, Bowers M, Woods TD. Left atrial volume measurement with automated border detection by 3-dimensional echocardiography: comparison with Magnetic Resonance Imaging. Cardiovasc Ultrasound. 2009;7:16. doi:10.1186/1476-7120-7-16.
38. Anwar AM, Soliman O, Geleijnse ML, Nemes A, Vletter WB, ten Cate FJ. Assessment of left atrial volume and function by real-time three-dimensional echocardiography. Int J Cardiol. 2008;123(2):155–61.
39. Heo R, Hong GR, Kim YJ, Mancina J, Cho IJ, Shim CY, Chang HJ, Ha JW, Chung N. Automated quantification of left atrial size using three-beat averaging real-time three dimensional Echocardiography in patients with atrial fibrillation. Cardiovasc Ultrasound. 2015;13:38. doi:10.1186/s12947-015-0032-5.
40. Poutanen T, Ikonen A, Vainio P, Jokinen E, Tikanoja T. Left atrial volume assessed by transthoracic three dimensional echocardiography and magnetic resonance imaging: dynamic changes during the heart cycle in children. Heart. 2000;83(5):537–42.
41. Marek D, Vindis D, Kocianova E. Real time 3-dimensional transesophageal echocardiography is more specific than 2-dimensional TEE in the assessment of left atrial appendage thrombosis. Biomed Pap Med Fac Univ Palacky Olomouc Czech Repub. 2013;157:22–6.

42. Shah SJ, Bardo DM, Sugeng L, et al. Real-time three-dimensional transesophageal echocardiography of the left atrial appendage: initial experience in the clinical setting. J Am Soc Echocardiogr. 2008;21:1362–8.
43. Nucifora G, Faletra FF, Regoli F, et al. Evaluation of the left atrial appendage with real-time 3-dimensional transesophageal echocardiography: implications for catheter-based left atrial appendage closure. Circ Cardiovasc Imaging. 2011;4:514–23.
44. Ohyama H, Hosomi N, Takahashi T, et al. Comparison of magnetic resonance imaging and transesophageal echocardiography in detection of thrombus in the left atrial appendage. Stroke. 2003;34:2436–9.
45. Wunderlich NC, Beigel R, Swaans MJ, Ho SY, Siegel RJ5. Percutaneous interventions for left atrial appendage exclusion: options, assessment, and imaging using 2D and 3D echocardiography. JACC Cardiovasc Imaging. 2015;8(4):472–88. doi:10.1016/j.jcmg.2015.02.002.
46. Faletra FF, Ho SY, Auricchio A. Anatomy of right atrial structures by real-time 3D transesophageal echocardiography. JACC Cardiovasc Imaging. 2010;3(9):966–75. doi:10.1016/j.jcmg.2010.03.014.
47. Keller AM, Gopal AS, King DL. Left and right atrial volume by freehand three-dimensional echocardiography: in vivo validation using magnetic resonance imaging. Eur J Echocardiogr. 2000;1(1):55–65.
48. Anwar AM, Nosir YF, Ajam A, Chamsi-Pasha H. Central role of real-time three-dimensional echocardiography in the assessment of intracardiac thrombi. Int J Cardiovasc Imaging. 2010;26:519–26.
49. Muller S, Feuchtner G, Bonatti J, et al. Value of transesophageal 3D echocardiography as an adjunct to conventional 2D imaging in preoperative evaluation of cardiac masses. Echocardiography. 2008;25:624–31.
50. Asch FM, Bieganski SP, Panza JA, Weissman NJ. Real-time 3-dimensional echocardiography evaluation of intracardiac masses. Echocardiography. 2006;23:218–24.
51. Plana JC. Added value of real-time three-dimensional echocardiography in assessing cardiac masses. Curr Cardiol Rep. 2009;11(3):205–9.
52. Saric M, Armour AC, Arnaout MS, Chaudhry FA, Grimm RA, Kronzon I, Landeck BF, Maganti K, Michelena HI, Tolstrup K. Guidelines for the use of echocardiography in the evaluation of a cardiac source of embolism. J Am Soc Echocardiogr. 2016;29(1):1–42.
53. Duncan K, Nanda NC, Foster WA, Mehmood F, Patel V, Singh A. Incremental value of live/real time three-dimensional transthoracic echocardiography in the assessment of left ventricular thrombi. Echocardiography. 2006;23(1):68–72.
54. Sinha A, Nanda NC, Khanna D, Dod HS, Vengala S, Mehmood F, Agrawal G, Upendram S. Morphological assessment of left ventricular thrombus by live three-dimensional transthoracic echocardiography. Echocardiography. 2004;21(7):649–55.
55. Habib G, Lancellotti P, Antunes MJ, Bongiorni MG, et al. 2015 ESC Guidelines for the management of infective endocarditis: The Task Force for the Management of Infective Endocarditis of the European Society of Cardiology (ESC)Endorsed by: European Association for Cardio-Thoracic Surgery (EACTS), the European Association of Nuclear Medicine (EANM). Eur Heart J. 2015;36(44):3075–128. doi:10.1093/eurheartj/ehv319. Epub 2015 Aug 29.
56. Gulotta JC, Gaba S, Bulur S, Joson M, Sungur A, Nanda NC. Two- and live/real time three-dimensional transthoracic echocardiographic assessment of infective endocarditis of a valved pulmonary conduit. Echocardiography. 2015;32(2):361–4.
57. Sungur A, Hsiung MC, Meggo Quiroz LD, Oz TK, Haj Asaad A, Joshi D, Dönmez C, Güvenç TS, Nanda NC. The advantages of live/real time three-dimensional transesophageal echocardiography in the assessment of tricuspid valve infective endocarditis. Echocardiography. 2014;31(10):1293–309.
58. Tanis W, Teske AJ, van Herwerden LA, Chamuleau S, Meijboom F, Budde RP, Cramer MJ. The additional value of three-dimensional transesophageal echocardiography in complex aortic prosthetic heart valve endocarditis. Echocardiography. 2015;32(1):114–25.

59. Berdejo J, Shibayama K, Harada K, Tanaka J, Mihara H, Gurudevan SV, Siegel RJ, Shiota T. Evaluation of vegetation size and its relationship with embolism in infective endocarditis: a real-time 3-dimensional transesophageal echocardiography study. Circ Cardiovasc Imaging. 2014;7(1):149–54.
60. Cheng HL, Cheng YJ, Lai CH. Anterior mitral leaflet perforation identified by real time three-dimensional transesophageal echocardiography. Cardiol J. 2012;19(1):89–91.
61. Sadat K, Joshi D, Sudhakar S, Bicer EI, Ibrahim H, Nanda NC, Bhagatwala K, Karia N, Pandey A. Incremental role of three-dimensional transesophageal echocardiography in the assessment of mitral-aortic intervalvular fibrosa abscess. Echocardiography. 2012;29(6): 742–4. doi:10.1111/j.1540-8175.2012.01672.x. Epub 2012 Mar 9.
62. Singh P, Manda J, Hsiung MC, Mehta A, Kesanolla SK, Nanda NC, Tsai SK, Wei J, Yin WH. Live/real time three-dimensional transesophageal echocardiographic evaluation of mitral and aortic valve prosthetic paravalvular regurgitation. Echocardiography. 2009;26:980–7.
63. Kronzon I, Sugeng L, Perk G, Hirsh D, Weinert L, Garcia Fernandez MA, Lang RMI. Real-time 3-dimensional transesophageal echocardiography in the evaluation of post-operative mitral annuloplasty ring and prosthetic valve dehiscence. J Am Coll Cardiol. 2009;53:1543–7.
64. Lang RM, Tsang W, Weinert L, Mor-Avi V, Chandra S. Valvular heart disease. The value of 3-dimensional echocardiography. J Am Coll Cardiol. 2011;58:1933–44.
65. Khairnar P, Hsiung MC, Mishra S, Nanda NC, Daly Jr DD, Nayyar G, Patel A, Mishra J, Chuang YC, Tsai SK, Yin WH, Wei J. The ability of live three-dimensional transesophageal echocardiography to evaluate the attachment site of intracardiac tumors. Echocardiography. 2011;28(9):1041–5.
66. Le Tourneau T, Pouwels S, Gal B, Vincentelli A, Polge AS, Fayad G, Maréchaux S, Ennezat PV, Jegou B, Deklunder G. Assessment of papillary fibroelastomas with live three-dimensional transthoracic echocardiography. Echocardiography. 2008;25(5):489–95.

# Chapter 6
# 3D-Wall Motion Tracking: Measuring Myocardial Strain with 3D

Eduardo Casas Rojo

## Introduction

The routine study of ventricular function with echocardiography has been limited for years to diameter measurements, volume estimations with methods that applied geometric assumptions, and calculation of the ejection fraction (EF). The appearance of 3D Echocardiography helped to achieve more reliable methods for those estimations. However, the evaluation of regional myocardial mechanics was initially limited to a subjective assessment of myocardial thickening and shortening at every segment. A subjective wall motion score could be applied [1] but it depended on the particular experience and opinion of the operator, and inter-observer agreement was not great.

Additionally, other aspects of the cardiac motion such as rotation were not easily measurable. With the development of myocardial strain analysis, quantitative estimation of several myocardial mechanics-related parameters was possible. At the beginning, the first attempt to achieve strain analysis was through Tissue Doppler Imaging (TDI) [2]. However, angle dependence of these systems made them inaccurate in some settings. A few years later, two dimensional speckle tracking (2DST) offered an alternative approach, which was based on tracking of blocks of scatter echoes (called "speckles"). Similar patterns of speckles are identified on every frame and tracked through the cardiac cycle [3].

Strain is a measure of deformation. Applied to a myocardial segment, *"strain"* is defined as the difference in length of the segment (end-systolic length – end-

**Electronic supplementary material** The online version of this chapter (doi:10.1007/978-3-319-50335-6_6) contains supplementary material, which is available to authorized users.

E. Casas Rojo
Cardiology Department, Hospital Ramon y Cajal, Madrid, Spain
e-mail: ecasasweb@hotmail.com

© Springer International Publishing AG 2017
E. Casas Rojo et al. (eds.), *Manual of 3D Echocardiography*,
DOI 10.1007/978-3-319-50335-6_6

"

diastolic length) divided by the end-diastolic length. It is usually expressed as a percentage. It is also possible to measure the rate of change in strain with respect to time which is called "*strain rate*" and expressed as percentage divided by seconds [4].

The shortening of the left ventricle (LV) or any other chamber may be measured as longitudinal (LS) (shortening of the long axis) and circumferential strain (CS) (shortening of the circumference of the short axis). Both are negative values. The subsequent thickening in the radial direction may be expressed as radial strain (RS) which reflects the change in diameter between endocardial and epicardial layers and is a positive value; even complex parameters such as rotation, torsion and twist may be estimated from these data [5]. Many clinical papers have shown the prognostic value of these indexes in a number of different cardiac diseases [6–24]. However, there are some limitations of this approach when it is based on a two-dimensional ultrasound system.

First of all, 2D–ST can achieve direct strain measurement on a certain region of a fixed 2D plane, and these values may be useful for assessment of regional contractility, but it's desirable to evaluate all segments and get global or mean values out of these parameters, so multiple planes and views will be needed. In addition, speckle-tracking is based on matching of the same pattern of image on consecutive frames, but when certain part of a myocardial segment gets out of a fixed plane during the cardiac cycle, these speckles cannot be found on all frames, and therefore a part of the information is lost.

Second, global values of strain parameters, and rotation information are assessed through calculations based on different views that belong to different cardiac cycles with the subsequent differences in time intervals and loading conditions.

Third, some aspects of myocardial 3D mechanics are not possible to estimate from 2D views. For instance, radial strain only evaluates thickening in a transversal axis, but real 3D thickening is comprised by many different vectors of thickening in any possible direction. Also, endocardial area deformation may be calculated from longitudinal and circumferential information, but this approach requires 3D tracking of the speckles.

The appearance of 3D–Speckle Tracking (3DST) overcomes these limitations and offers a fast way to study 3D cardiac mechanics and easily obtains 3D models of the LV and other structures with several modalities (Fig. 6.1; Video 6.1).

## Technical Aspects

3DST technology is capable of tracking 3D volumes in any desired direction. Usually 3D images are acquired through a 3D matrix-array transducer with a single acquisition from apical window [25], and processed in a specifically designed ultrasound machine, providing a relevant reduction of acquisition and processing time: a complete processed study is achieved in one third of the time when compared with 2DST [26, 27]; in other cases a generic 3D echocardiography machine is used and off-line processing with an external workstation and specific software will be necessary [28].

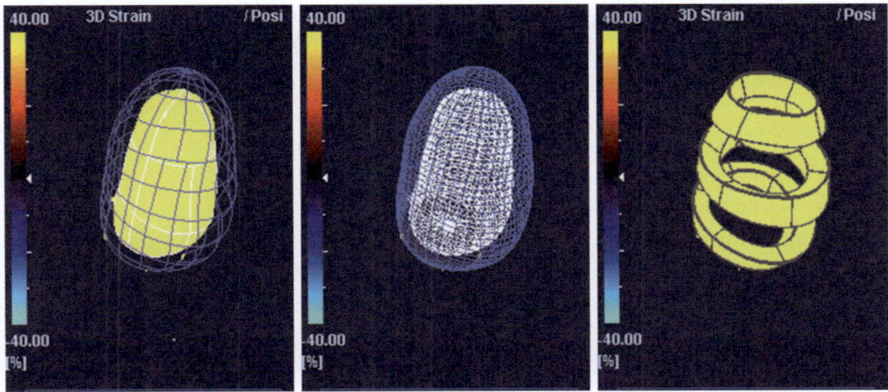

**Fig. 6.1** Different modalities of 3D Strain graphic representations. Left: Plastic Bag view; Middle: Wires view; Right: Doughnuts view. With the current settings, yellow colour indicates high values of strain for all visible segments. All these views can be rotated and tilted for assessing the contraction of segments of interest

Due to the limitations of current 3D echocardiography, these studies feature a lower frame rate than 2DST datasets. Also quality and resolution of the images are lower. At the moment, several consecutive beats [2, 6], are needed to compose the image, resulting in occasional stitching artifacts.

## Acquisition Protocol

In the following section we describe step by step the way to acquire and process a 3DST study of the LV. However, it is also possible to study other structures like the right ventricle or the atria, but commercial software is mainly optimized for LV at the moment.

The *fist step* for acquiring a 3DST study is to assess that all required conditions are OK:

- Acceptable acoustic window. Septal, lateral, inferior and anterior walls must be visible on echo image. Use the multiplane application for best assessing.
- ECG must be shown properly on screen and free from artifacts.
- No contrast can be used during acquisition.

  The *second step* is to improve the settings for acquisition.

- Adjust the depth in order to include the whole LV. The less depth needed, the more volume rate and quality of data. It is useful to select a 2 plane view (pre-full 4D mode on Toshiba Artida system) and check the good visualization of all endocardial and epicardial borders.
- If needed, adjust the scan range, by widening or shortening the pyramidal sector. Again, shortest ranges will provide better quality, but dilated LV's may need more range for avoiding loss of apical segments.

- The number of subvolumes used for composing the image usually range from 2 to 6. In the presence of irregular rhythm, lower values may help to avoid stitching, but some of the image quality will be lost.

The *third step* is the acquisition.

- Ask the patient to hold his breath.
- Start 4D protocol ("Full 4D" for Toshiba Artida)
- Wait as many cardiac cycles as the number of sub-volumes selected for composing the image, then store the resulting loop. ("Clips Store" for Artida)
- It is desirable to have several acquired loops and choose the best quality one for post-processing.

## Processing

Several vendors have developed 3DST software for processing 3D echocardiography data. This software may be included in the ultrasound system allowing an almost "on-line" analysis of the data (e.g. Toshiba Artida), or it may be loaded into a separate workstation for off-line processing (e.g. General Electric Echo-Pac). We will explain the processing protocol for both cases.

### *Toshiba Artida*

- A correct alignment of the LV axis must be checked and corrected is necessary.
- Before semi-automated detection of the endocardial and epicardial border, the system will ask for landmarks setting, usually at both sides of the mitral annulus and at the apex. Manual delineation is also possible.
- When semi-automated detection is performed, manual corrections are also possible in cases with poor automatic results.
- Perform automatic wall motion tracking process.
- Play the loop and check the tracking. Some cases may require frame by frame corrections at this stage.
- Display the tables with the individual values for each segment and the global values. The system allows selection of a number of parameters, with a different table for each one.
- The definitive processed dataset after manual corrections should be saved in order to use always the same settings for any needed data from the patient.

See Fig. 6.2 and legends for additional details.

Also see Figs. 6.3 and 6.4 for finding explanation of examples for right ventricle and left atria 3DST processing.

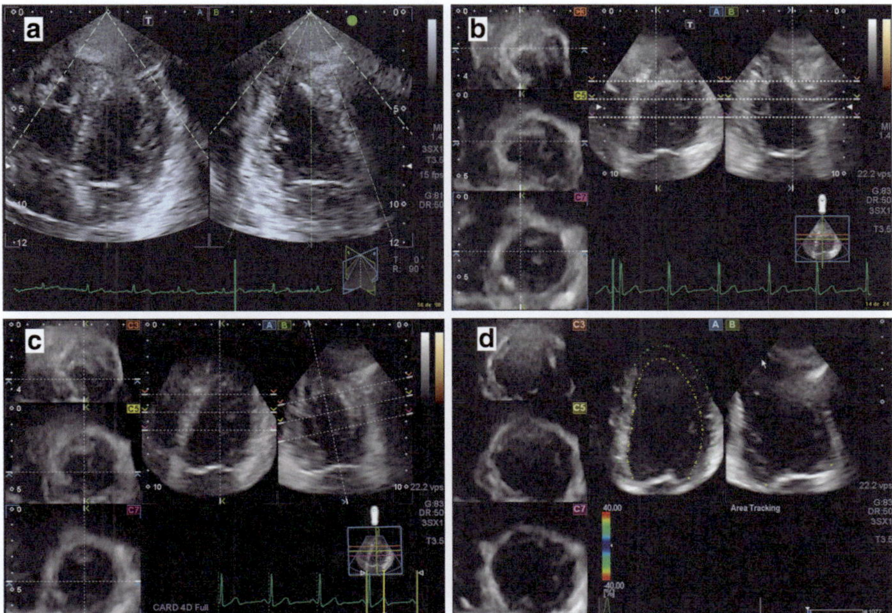

**Fig. 6.2** Protocol for 3DST on ARTIDA. 1- The "Pre-4D" screen shows a biplanar 2D view. It allows depth and azimuth adjustment and number of subvolumes (from 2 to 6) selection; 2- The "Full 4D" mode allows acquisition of a 3D echo loop. The clip should be stored. 3- The saved clips can be selected and processed by pressing again "Full 4D". Axis adjustment is performed at this stage. 4- "3DT" (3D- tracking) mode will ask for reference points at the mitral annulus and the apex. Manual corrections and even manual delineation instead of points setting are also possible. Pressing "Start" will begin the automatic tracking process

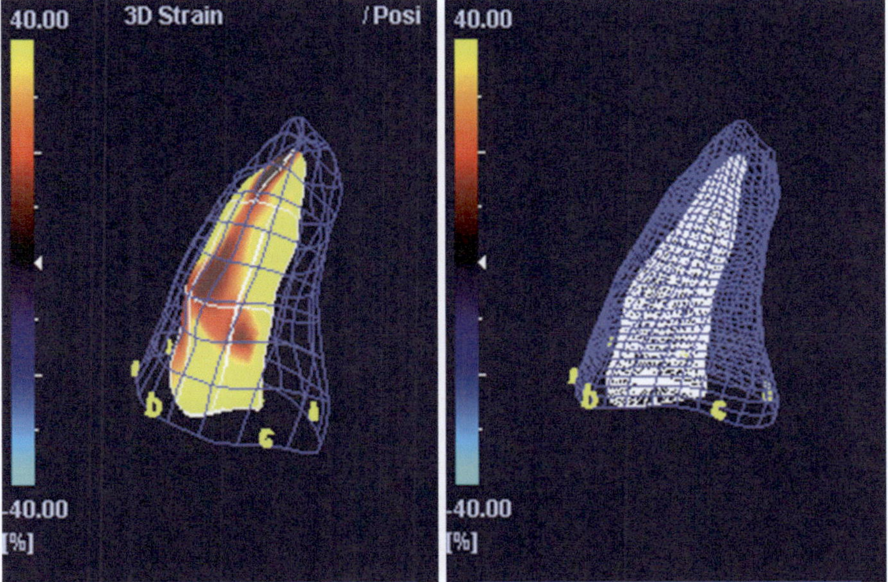



**Fig. 6.3** "Plastic Bag" and "Wires" image modalities for the right ventricle (RV) modeling. When processing chambers like the RV or the atria, the method is similar to the protocol we have described for the  LV, but the desired chamber must be properly centered in the middle of the screen during acquisition, and "Other" must be specified instead of "LV"

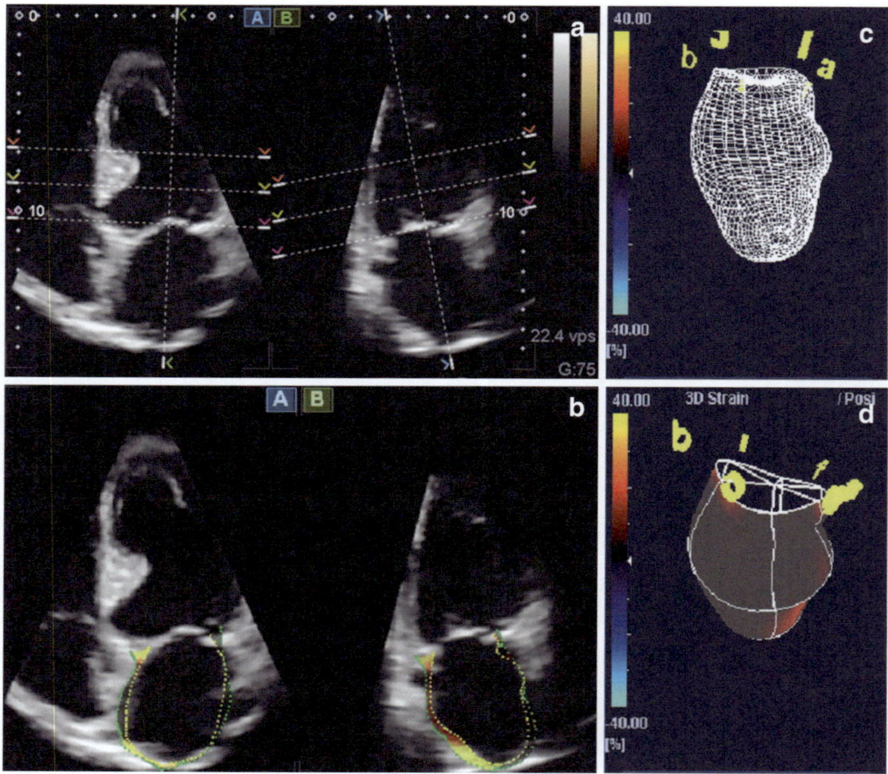

**Fig. 6.4** 3DST of the left atrium (LA). (**a**) Full 4D volume acquisition of both LV and LA with corrected alignment of the LA axis; (**b**) Multiplane images of LA 3D strain as a result of automatic tracking after drawing endocardial borders of LA; (**c**) "Wires" representation of the LA model; (**d**) "Plastic Bag" view

## GE EchoPac

Only datasets with enough volume rate (generally over 30 vps) will be available for processing. The 4D Auto Left Ventricular Quantification tool menu includes the following consecutive steps for getting at the end the 3D strain analysis.

– Aligning views (similar to Artida)
– EDV: Setting landmarks for the endocardial borders at diastole
– ESV: Same process at systole.
– Volume wave: Internal endocardial borders and LV volume data are displayed.
– LV mass: external epicardial borders and LV mass data are displayed.
– 4D Strain: Regional and global values for longitudinal, radial, circumferential and area strain may be selected for display. If any segment fails to be tracked properly, it may be excluded for analysis. More than 3 excluded segments will make not possible the global value estimations.

See Fig. 6.5 and Video 6.2 for additional details.

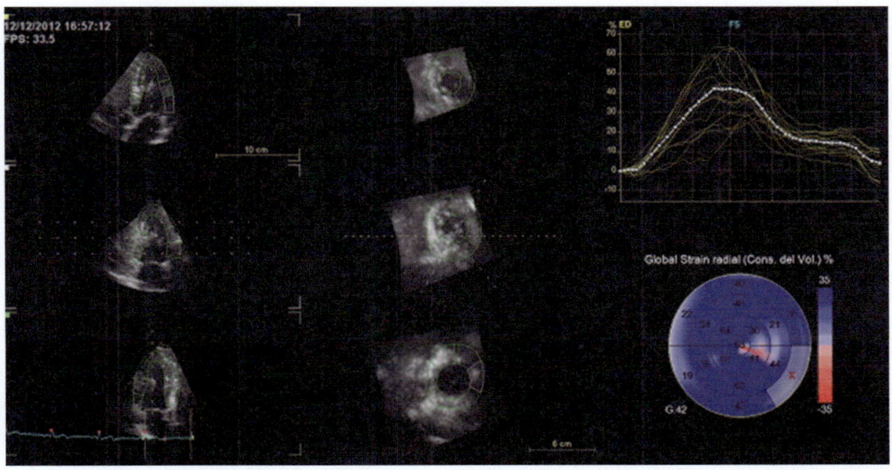

**Fig. 6.5** Radial strain 3DST analysis with GE. 3 long-axis and 3 short-axis views from 3D data are shown for assessing endocardial and epicardial tracking. Strain/time curves show the segmental strain from the 17 segments (yellow curved lines) and global strain (white line) through the cardiac cycle. The polar map displays the maximum radial strain values. One of the segments (basal lateral) has been excluded for analysis due to suboptimal quality. The global value of RS (42%) is shown as "G42" besides the polar map

## Interpretation

On Echo-PAC software, the global values and the graphic representations for the main strain parameters are displayed in a simple way when reaching the final step of the process.

On Toshiba Artida the results are displayed on a complex table (Figs. 6.6 and 6.7) including among other data the maximum and minimum value of strain (in its different modalities) for every segment (with 16 or 17 segments models) and the time to achieve this peak. Also global values are provided. It's important to know that when assessing thickening parameters such as radial strain and 3D strain, the desired peak value will be placed as maximum value (positive), whereas in the case of shortening parameters like longitudinal, circumferential or area strain, the relevant value is the minimum one (negative) (Fig. 6.6).

Data about peak twist or twist degree at a certain segment are also available, however if *untwist* values are needed, they must be calculated [29]:

Untwist (%) = (peak LV twist − Twist1*)/(Peak LV twist) × 100* Twist1= twist at a specific point along diastole, usually mitral valve opening.

Besides the numerical data, 3DST software usually offers several different modalities of graphic representation of LV 3D model (Fig. 6.1), multiplane 2D views of the 3D echocardiography with volumes and ejection fraction information (Fig. 6.8) a 16 or 17 segments polar map with regional values of strain or other parameters (Fig. 6.9 and Video 6.3) and many other features.

| | Max1 | Max1T | Max2 | Max2T | Min1 | Min1T | Min2 | Min2T |
|---|---|---|---|---|---|---|---|---|
| BA | 0.00 | 0 | -4.38 | 722 | -25.55 | 316 | -4.38 | 722 |
| BAS | 0.00 | 0 | -7.26 | 722 | -20.58 | 271 | -13.62 | 496 |
| BS | 0.86 | 45 | 0.00 | 0 | -14.06 | 406 | -11.24 | 496 |
| BI | 3.80 | 631 | 1.47 | 722 | -15.31 | 406 | 0.00 | 0 |
| BP | 2.95 | 677 | 1.66 | 722 | -14.25 | 180 | -12.93 | 361 |
| BL | 0.00 | 0 | -6.35 | 722 | -14.80 | 316 | -14.17 | 226 |
| MA | 0.00 | 0 | -3.38 | 722 | -8.38 | 271 | -4.46 | 631 |
| MAS | 0.00 | 0 | -1.18 | 677 | -10.23 | 271 | -1.22 | 722 |
| MS | 0.00 | 0 | -5.06 | 722 | -13.72 | 271 | -5.06 | 722 |
| MI | 0.00 | 0 | -6.39 | 722 | -16.21 | 361 | -6.39 | 722 |
| MP | 0.00 | 0 | -1.04 | 722 | -16.38 | 271 | -1.04 | 722 |
| ML | 0.38 | 45 | 0.07 | 677 | -12.41 | 271 | -0.03 | 722 |
| AA | 0.00 | 0 | -4.84 | 722 | -24.31 | 316 | -7.03 | 631 |
| AS | 0.00 | 0 | -5.15 | 586 | -34.65 | 361 | -8.30 | 677 |
| AI | 0.60 | 45 | 0.00 | 0 | -28.97 | 361 | -10.41 | 722 |
| AL | 0.07 | 45 | 0.00 | 0 | -22.89 | 406 | -11.52 | 586 |
| global | 0.00 | 0 | -4.23 | 722 | -17.52 | 316 | -4.23 | 722 |
| | % | msec | % | msec | % | msec | % | msec |

**Fig. 6.6** Data table for the 16 myocardial segments and global longitudinal strain. As a shortening parameter, LS is a negative value at systole and its peak value for each segment will appear on the "minimum" column (Min1), highlighted in red box. The global value for the whole left ventricle appears below them (in white). The next row (Min1T) shows the time to reach the peak. This information is useful for dyssynchrony analysis

## Old and New Parameters

3DST technology offers a number of different parameters for assessing myocardial mechanics. The basic information is "displacement" and from that data, strain and rotation parameters can be obtained. The usual 2DST parameters (RS, LS, CS, torsion, rotation, twist…) are also available from 3D to ST [4] and additionally new parameters like area tracking/area strain and 3D strain have been described. The practical definitions of these parameters are displayed on Table 6.1.

| | Max1 | Max1T | Max2 | Max2T | Min1 | Min1T | Min2 | Min2T |
|---|---|---|---|---|---|---|---|---|
| BA | 21.77 | 448 | 9.03 | 746 | 0.00 | 0 | 9.03 | 746 |
| BAS | 13.50 | 249 | 12.52 | 398 | 0.00 | 0 | 1.03 | 498 |
| BS | 32.06 | 398 | 10.41 | 746 | 0.00 | 0 | 10.41 | 746 |
| BI | 22.17 | 299 | 12.87 | 697 | 0.00 | 0 | 10.88 | 746 |
| BP | 40.79 | 398 | 3.46 | 697 | 0.00 | 0 | 1.60 | 597 |
| BL | 17.19 | 448 | 0.00 | 0 | -8.80 | 149 | -5.79 | 697 |
| MA | 8.74 | 199 | 0.00 | 0 | -10.77 | 498 | -4.38 | 746 |
| MAS | 22.47 | 199 | 2.31 | 448 | -3.15 | 547 | -1.85 | 746 |
| MS | 29.28 | 249 | 3.95 | 746 | 0.00 | 0 | 3.95 | 746 |
| MI | 17.17 | 249 | 0.00 | 0 | -2.21 | 547 | -1.57 | 746 |
| MP | 17.10 | 249 | 0.00 | 0 | -7.86 | 697 | -6.49 | 746 |
| ML | 0.00 | 0 | -0.01 | 249 | -8.74 | 597 | -6.75 | 746 |
| AA | 32.82 | 249 | 0.00 | 0 | -3.64 | 746 | -1.85 | 498 |
| AS | 28.60 | 249 | 16.72 | 448 | 0.00 | 0 | 1.58 | 746 |
| AI | 23.56 | 249 | 0.00 | 0 | -2.60 | 597 | -2.19 | 746 |
| AL | 24.48 | 249 | 3.94 | 746 | 0.00 | 0 | 3.94 | 746 |
| global | 18.11 | 249 | 0.97 | 746 | 0.00 | 0 | 0.97 | 746 |
| | % | msec | % | msec | % | msec | % | msec |

**Fig. 6.7** Data table for radial strain in a patient with an anterolateral infarction. Medium lateral and medium anterior segments show low strain values (red circles) and global radial strain is also decreased. As a thickening parameter, RS reaches positive maximum values during systole, which are displayed on the first column of the table (Max1). Time to reach peak (Max1T) and second peak value (Max 2) are also available

During systole, myocardial fibers are shortened in both longitudinal and circumferential directions [30]. *Longitudinal strain* is defined as $SL=100*(L–L_0)/L_0$ where L is the instantaneous longitudinal length of the segment and $L_0$ is the initial length at end systole. *Circumferential strain* is the same concept applied to circumferential length of the segment. As myocardial tissue is incompressible, the result of longitudinal and circumferential strain is thickening in the radial direction for conservation of the mass. *Radial strain* is a estimation of that component of myocardial deformation.

As for rotational mechanics, counter-clockwise *rotation* of the LV apex is normally observed and it can be expressed as positive degrees, and clockwise rotation

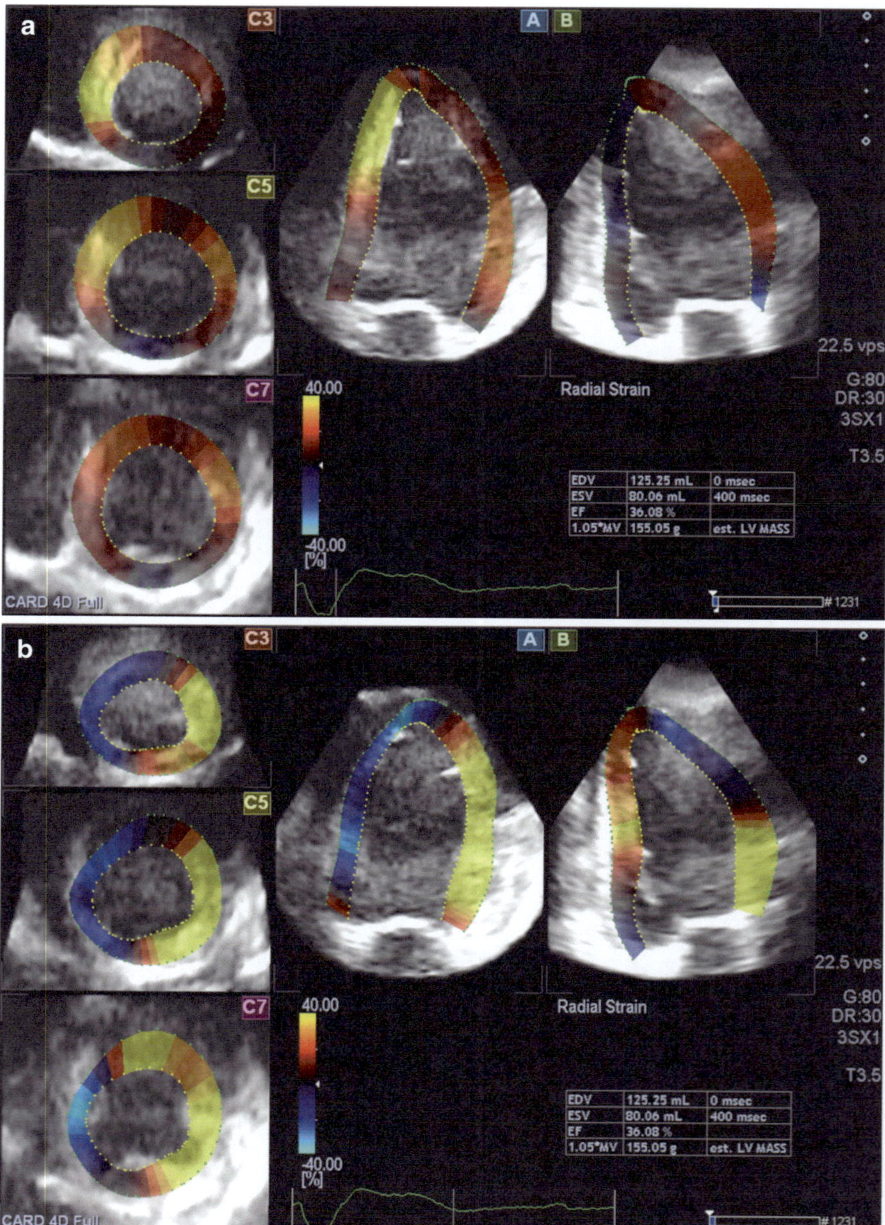



**Fig. 6.8** Multiplane representation of radial strain at early systole ("a" image) and late systole ("b" image) frames. The "Hold" function is disabled, allowing to represent both positive and negative strain. Yellow color indicates high positive strain which appears first on septal apical wall and later on lateral and anterior wall. Blue color indicates negative strain on the opposite wall in each frame. With the "Hold" function enabled, only positive strain would be coded (from black to yellow). On this screen, also LV volumes, mass and ejection fraction are shown

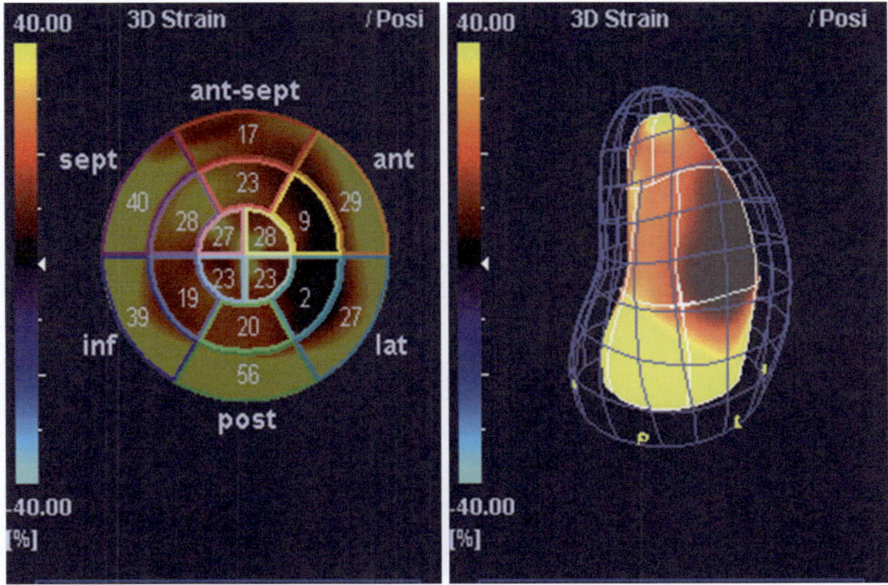



**Fig. 6.9** Polar map and Plastic Bag view in a patient with a myocardial infarction. Low values of 3D strain at peak systole are shown specially at mid- lateral (2%) and mid-anterior (9%) segments. An anterolateral 3D strain defect is evident on the 3D model. 3D Strain with "Hold" setting on (yellow/black coding) is particularly useful for visual assessment of contractility defects

**Table 6.1** Frequently used 3DST- derived parameters with their simplified definitions

| Variable | Units | Practical definition |
|---|---|---|
| Radial strain | % | Thickening (direction: normal to endocardial contour) |
| Longitudinal strain | -% | Shortening (tangential to endocardium) |
| Circumferential strain | -% | Shortening (circumferential to the endocardial contour) |
| Rotation | ° | Rotation angle (counterclockwise) of endocardium around the center |
| Twist | ° | Angle difference between apex (or a segment) and base |
| Torsion | °/cm | Twist change per distance |
| Area strain | -% | Endocardial area change |
| 3D Strain (Toshiba) | % | Thickening (in the wall thickening direction) |
| 3D Strain (Philips) | -% | Tangential shortening. Vector sum of longitudinal and circumferential components. Similar to Area Strain. |
| Area change rate | %/s | Velocity of area change |

of the LV base will result in negative degrees (Fig. 6.10, Video 6.4). We also may want to measure the degrees of difference in rotation between apex (or any segment) and the LV base, which would be called "*Twist*". If we measure the change in twist per distance we will call it "*Torsion*".

The new 3D–WMT based systems also provide some new parameters, which were not available with the 2D approach.

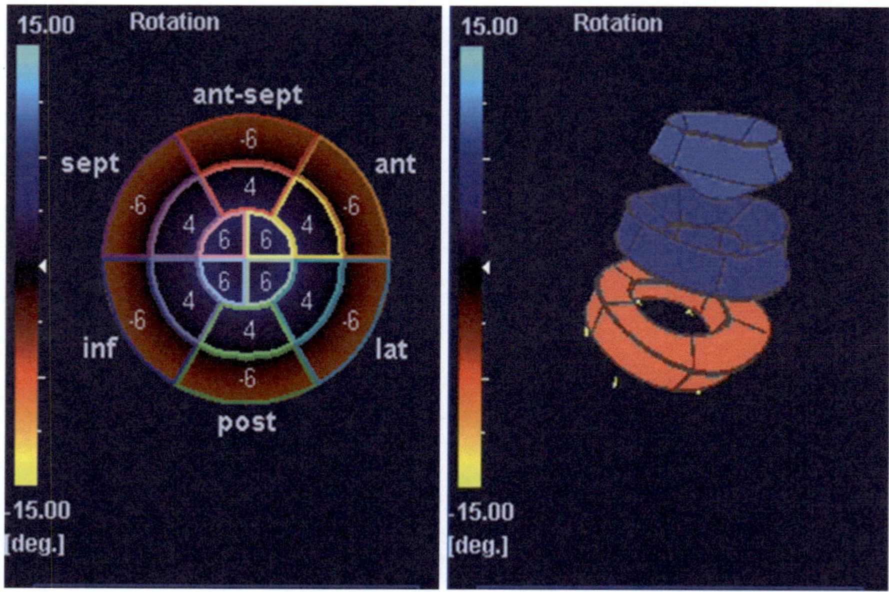


**Fig. 6.10** Physiological LV rotation. Polar map and doughnuts view, with "averaged levels" setting in a healthy subject: average values of rotation for basal, midventricular and apical segments are shown. Positive numbers on mid (4 degrees) and specially on apical segments (6 degrees) indicate counter-clockwise rotation. Negative numbers on basal segments (-6 degrees) confirm the clockwise rotation of the LV base

## *Area Strain*

This index estimates the degree of change of the sub-endocardial area (Fig. 6.11). It can be obtained from the combined information of longitudinal and circumferential shortening when both measures are obtained simultaneously from a 3D dataset. The result is a negative value which is called Area Change (Toshiba) [31, 32] or Area Strain (GE) [28], and also a similar concept is used for a parameter called "3D Strain" on Philips platforms [33]. This "3D Strain" should not be confused with 3DS from Toshiba, which is a different concept, as it will be explained below. These area change parameters are expected to be useful for detection of ischaemia, given that sub-endocardial surface is particularly sensitive in that context.

## *3D Strain*

As stated previously, on Philips platforms the denomination"3D Strain" is applied to a parameter which is equivalent to AS from other vendors. However on Toshiba systems 3D Strain (3DS) is a totally different index, with positive values like RS, and indicates strain in any wall thickening direction [34]. Its range of values is

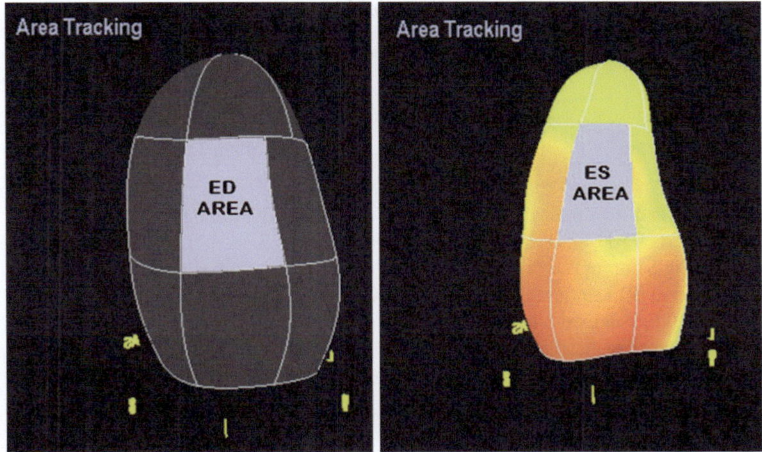



**Fig. 6.11** Area Strain or Area Tracking is obtained from 3D longitudinal and circumferential strain information. The objective is to estimate the percentage of change between end-diastolic (ED) and end-systolic (ES) endocardial areas in a segment (on this example, medium inferior wall) or in the whole left ventricle. IF ES area is 30% shorter than ED, area strain is -30% in that segment

usually similar to RS, but it is expected to overcome its limitations, as RS takes as reference the endocardial contour and 3DS takes into account the direction of thickening in 3D space. Though, few data support the possible clinical advantage of 3DS over RS at the moment.

## Reliability, Normal Values and Differences Between Vendors

Kleijn et al. described reliability data for 3DST [35]. LV volumes, EF and global CS measurements demonstrated good intra-observer, inter-observer and test-retest reliability with intraclass correlation coefficients (ICC) 0.85–0.99; however, global LS and RS, while maintaining good intra-observer ICC (0.92 and 0.88) showed lower inter-observer (0.74 and 0.58) and test-retest (0.66, 0.52) results.

It is important to mention that, as usual on 3DST studies, these results exclude patients with atrial fibrillation or insufficient image quality (23 of the 140 patients, 16%). In the real clinical practice, image quality may lower the reproducibility in some cases. Also, in our experience, depending on the need for manual adjustments of the automatic tracking this reliability may also change. The absence of manual corrections when automatic tracking is not optimal may result in better reproducibility within the same dataset, but it may not reflect the real motion and strain.

There have been a few attempts to set the normal values for some of these indexes [33, 36, 37]. As noticed on Table 6.2, discrepancies between different vendors are significant. Furthermore, Muraru et al. also compared data from the same platform

**Table 6.2** Normal values of usual 3DST parameters according to different authors

| Variable | Kleijn et al. | Kaku et al. | Muraru et al. |
|---|---|---|---|
| Radial strain | 35.6±10.3 | 47.1 ± 20.3 | Median 52 (Q1 47, Q3 59) LLN 38 |
| Longitudinal strain | -15.9±2.4 | −11.3 ± 4.4 | Median 19 (Q1 21, Q3 17) LLN15 |
| Circumferential strain | 30.6±2.6 | −19.2 ± 6.7 | Median 18 (Q1 20, Q3 17) LLN 14 |
| Area tracking | 42.0±6.7 | – | Median 33 (Q1 36, Q3 31) LLN 26 |

Kelijn et al.: Artida 4D scanner (Toshiba Medical Systems) with built-in software
Kaku et al.: Sonos 7500 or iE33 scanner (Philips Medical Systems); 4D LV analysis software (TomTec Imaging Systems)
Muraru et al.: Vivid E9 scanner (GE Vingmed Ultrasound AS); 4D AutoLVQ - EchoPAC BT12 and BT13 software (GE Vingmed Ultrasound AS)
Values are expressed as mean±standard deviation or as median values with additional data: *LLN* Lower limit of normality, *Q1* first quartile, *Q3* third quartile

processed by vendor-specific software and the same data processed with vendor-independent software, and they found also significant differences in RS and CS results [36]. Overall there seems to be a need for agreement between vendors for setting standard methods for obtaining and processing 3DST data before clinical use of these data and comparisons between studies from different platforms in the daily practice can be a reality.

Additionally, differences in normal values among individuals with different gender and age have to be considered also. On both Toshiba and GE platforms, RS and CS tend to be higher with age and LS tends to be lower. AS seem to keep similar values. However, in Philips platforms all the mentioned parameters (including AS equivalent 3D Strain) have significantly lower absolute values with aging. As for gender differences, negative LS and AS values seem to be higher on women.

## Review of Literature and Clinical Applications

### *General Strain Applications*

3D estimations of "traditional" 2D–ST parameters such as longitudinal, circumferential or radial strain promise to be more accurate and therefore they are expected to have at least the same usefulness and prognostic value as the original 2D parameters, including among others:

– Detection of subclinical diseases such as amyloidosis, chemotherapy-related myocardial disease or hypertensive disease [6, 7]
– Detection of ischaemia during stress echocardiography, and assessing of viability and prognostic information in coronary artery disease [8–12]
– Study of myocardial deformation in cardiomyopathies, and congenital heart diseases [13–16].
– Assessing changes in rotation or twist in diastolic dysfunction, coronary artery disease, cardiomyopahies and valve diseases [17–24].

## *3D Strain Applications: Brief Review of Literature*

In addition to 2DST applications, many studies suggest further value of the 3D–WMT approach; 3DST was validated against data obtained by sonomicrometry in sheeps [38], with correlations ranging from 0.84 to 0.90 for the classic strain parameters (LS, RS, CS); Pérez de Isla et al. assessed similar values for these parameters when compared with 2DST, with much lower acquisition and analysis times [26].

Nesser et al. tested the accuracy of 3DST to quantify left ventricular volumes, using cardiac magnetic resonance (CMR) as a reference [39]. Additionally 2DST measures were compared with the new method. 3DST showed better correlation and agreement with CMR, smaller biases and narrower limits of agreement.

The same paper and additional studies have stated that reliability of 3DST is good for assessing LV volumes, including high agreement for inter-observer, intraobserver and test-retest results. For strain parameters, CS seems to be the most reproducible, whereas RS and LS depend more on the particular observer. Additionally all these studies excluded certain number of patients because of poor ultrasonic quality. Furthermore, some papers have described a high intervendor variability for both volume assessment and strain parameters [40–42]. Therefore the accuracy of this technique is very dependant on the image quality, and differences are expected when comparing studies performed on different platforms. These limitations have to be taken into account when performing this kind of studies in the real clinical practice.

Yodwut et al [43] reported the effects of different frame rate settings on 3DST studies. The results suggest that, with the current technology, at least four beats, and frame rates of at least 18 fps are needed to avoid loss of important data.

Another area for 3DST is the assessment of dissynchrony in candidates for cardiac resynchronization therapy (CRT) [44–47] (See also Video 6.5). Some parameters, specially 3D–ST derived radial strain (Fig. 6.12) and area strain have been successfully tested for this purpose and may help to identify the most delayed segments in order to select the optimal position for the lead. The study of torsional mechanics with 3DST seems to be also useful for possible CRT candidates [47]. Even atrial deformation and synchrony assessment with this technology have been proposed for identifying atrial dyssynchrony and identifying patients with paroxysmal atrial fibrillation [48].

Also, 3D–ST has been shown to be useful for evaluating the effects of right ventricular pacing in the LV mechanics [49].

In patients with acute myocardial infarction, 3DST may help to assess infarct size and 3DST-derived LS predicts improvement of LV function after the acute event [50].

In valvular disease, researchers have found advantages of 3DST parameters over 2DST and conventional echocardiography. As an example, 3D global LS was the only significant predictor of MACE in an asymptomatic aortic stenosis study cohort [51]. In a study from our group, AS was the only independent predictor of heart failure in a series of 45 patients with severe mitral regurgitation and preserved ejection fraction [52].

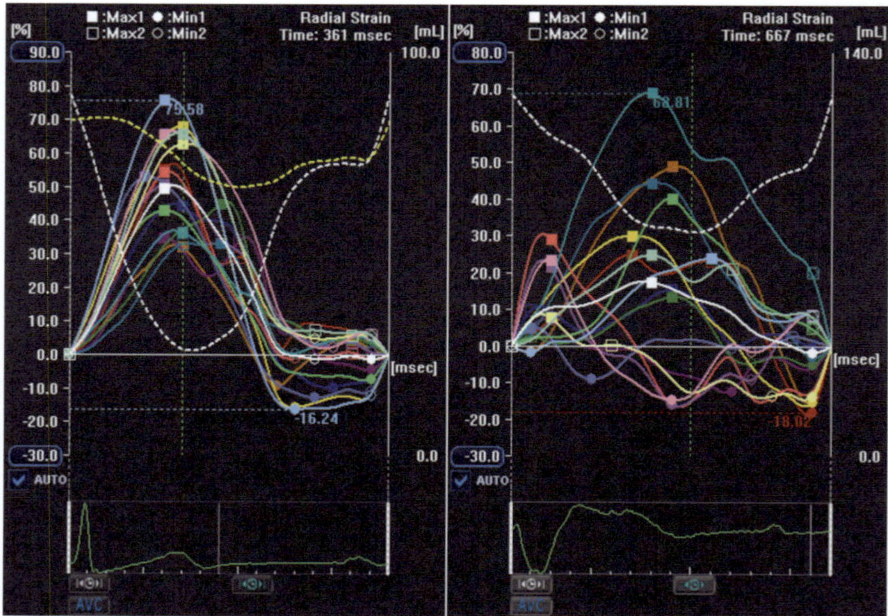

**Fig. 6.12** Strain/time curves from a healthy heart (*left*) and from a patient with intraventricular dyssynchrony (*right*). On the left, every segment reaches its peak of strain in a similar time. On the right, left bundle branch block explains the delay between early septal and late lateral segments. By checking the data provided by the system, delay of the latest segments (356 ms.) and the earliest (89 ms) allow to calculate the intraventricular delay (267 ms). Also, the segments with the latest activation (anterior, anterolateral and inferolateral wall) are identified and could be taken into account for selecting the location of the lead in resynchronization therapy

Although most investigations are based on LV mechanics, there are also some interesting papers about atria or right ventricle 3D strain analysis [53, 54].

## Limitations and Future

### *Limitations*

In this section we summarize the limitations we have mentioned previously:

#### Image Quality

As 3DST technology depends on the identification of certain shapes and patterns, it is largely dependent on the quality of the ultrasound dataset. Even when working with 2D acquisitions, in cases with poor ultrasound quality speckle-tracking analysis is either not possible or not accurate. Furthermore, 3D–ST ultrasound is limited by lower resolution than 2DST, and this issue makes more challenging the correct tracking of the endocardial and epicardial borders. As a result of this, further manual corrections are needed after the automated process of tracking, and in the daily practice greater inter-observer and intra-observer variability is expected, even when some data suggest good reproducibility.

## Frame/Volume Rate

In addition to the basic quality of the display, lower volume rates are obtained, when compared with frame rates available for 2D–ST technology. Therefore, the timing of events has to be less accurate when using this modality, and the precision of the identification of peak values of strain parameters across the cardiac cycle is also lower.

## Several Beats Needed

Current systems need ECG-gating and merge information from several cardiac sub-volumes for constructing the full 3D images. The number of beats needed may vary between 2 and 6. Beat to beat variations result in stitching artifacts, specially in patients with atrial fibrillation and other rhythm disorders. Such artefacts usually make more difficult the adequate tracking and strain measurement.

## Differences Between Vendors

Several studies have detected significant differences between parameters when using different platforms for assessing 3D–ST data on the same patients. Additionally, some new indexes with similar names may not have the same meaning in different systems (like Toshiba's "3D strain" which is a positive thickening measure, whereas Philips "3D strain" is a shortening parameter, equivalent to area strain). For the clinical application of these concepts, consensus must be reached by all companies to follow the same methodology and to offer the same tools, with independence of the vendor.

## *Future*

3DST is expected to overcome some of its limitations in the near future, when the technology of the ultrasound platforms allow higher frame rates and best resolutions, and when standardization of the methods make possible to compare studies from any vendor. Wider clinical data will be needed to reach the moment at which concepts like 3D strain and torsion will be used on a daily practice and not only as investigation concepts. Some advanced applications of this technology like 3D stress echocardiography and fusion between tomography and 3DST are beginning to arise and will be discussed in the next chapter.

CHAPTER 6 – VIDEOS

VIDEO 1 – Plastic Bag loop from 3D Strain in a healthy heart.

VIDEO 2 – Multiplane screen with polar map and radial strain curves in a healthy heart, from General Electric Eco-Pac.

VIDEO 3 – Doughnuts view from 3D Strain in a patient with Diagonal branch occlusion.

VIDEO 4 – Normal rotation of the heart on doughnuts view.

VIDEO 5 – Multiplane screen in a patient with septal and inferior hipokynesis and dissynchrony, from Toshiba Artida.

# References


1. Bjørnstad K, al Amri M, Lingamanaicker J, Oqaili I, Hatle L. Interobserver and intraobserver variation for analysis of left ventricular wall motion at baseline and during low and high-dose dobutamine stress echocardiography in patients with high prevalence of wall motion abnormalities at rest. J Am Soc Echocardiogr. 1996;9(3):320–8. PubMed PMID: 8736017.
2. Heimdal A, Støylen A, Torp H, Skjaerpe T. Real-time strain rate imaging of the left ventricle by ultrasound. J Am Soc Echocardiogr. 1998;11(11):1013–9. PubMed PMID: 9812093.
3. Leitman M, Lysyansky P, Sidenko S, Shir V, Peleg E, Binenbaum M, Kaluski E, Krakover R, Vered Z. Two-dimensional strain-a novel software for real-time quantitative echocardiographic assessment of myocardial function. J Am Soc Echocardiogr. 2004;17(10):1021–9. PubMed PMID: 15452466.
4. Mor-Avi V, Lang RM, Badano LP, Belohlavek M, Cardim NM, Derumeaux G, Galderisi M, Marwick T, Nagueh SF, Sengupta PP, Sicari R, Smiseth OA, Smulevitz B, Takeuchi M, Thomas JD, Vannan M, Voigt JU, Zamorano JL. Current and evolving echocardiographic techniques for the quantitative evaluation of cardiac mechanics: ASE/EAE consensus statement on methodology and indications endorsed by the Japanese Society of Echocardiography. J Am Soc Echocardiogr. 2011;24(3):277–313. doi:10.1016/j.echo.2011.01.015. PubMed PMID: 21338865.
5. Helle-Valle T, Crosby J, Edvardsen T, Lyseggen E, Amundsen BH, Smith HJ, et al. New noninvasive method for assessment of left ventricular rotation: speckle tracking echocardiography. Circulation. 2005;112:3149–56.
6. Marwick TH. Measurement of strain and strain rate by echocardiography: ready for prime time? J Am Coll Cardiol. 2006;47:1313–27.
7. Jurcut R, Wildiers H, Ganame J, D'hooge J, De BJ, Denys H, et al. Strain rate imaging detects early cardiac effects of pegylated liposomal Doxorubicin as adjuvant therapy in elderly patients with breast cancer. J Am Soc Echocardiogr. 2008;21:1283–9.
8. Bijnens B, Claus P, Weidemann F, Strotmann J, Sutherland GR. Investigating cardiac function using motion and deformation analysis in the setting of coronary artery disease. Circulation. 2007;116:2453–64.
9. Bjork IC, Rozis E, Slordahl SA, Marwick TH. Incremental value of strain rate imaging to wall motion analysis for prediction of outcome in patients undergoing dobutamine stress echocardiography. Circulation. 2007;115:1252–9.
10. Kukulski T, Jamal F, Herbots L, D'hooge J, Bijnens B, Hatle L, et al. Identification of acutely ischemic myocardium using ultrasonic strain measurements. A clinical study in patients undergoing coronary angioplasty. J Am Coll Cardiol. 2003;41:810–9.

11. Voigt JU, Exner B, Schmiedehausen K, Huchzermeyer C, Reulbach U, Nixdorff U, et al. Strain-rate imaging during dobutamine stress echocardiography provides objective evidence of inducible ischemia. Circulation. 2003;107:2120–6.
12. Weidemann F, Jung P, Hoyer C, Broscheit J, Voelker W, Ertl G, et al. Assessment of the contractile reserve in patients with intermediate coronary lesions: a strain rate imaging study validated by invasive myocardial fractional flow reserve. Eur Heart J. 2007;28:1425–32.
13. Faber L, Prinz C, Welge D, Hering D, Butz T, Oldenburg O, et al. Peak systolic longitudinal strain of the lateral left ventricular wall improves after septal ablation for symptomatic hypertrophic obstructive cardiomyopathy: a follow-up study using speckle tracking echocardiography. Int J Cardiovasc Imaging. 2011;27(3):325–33.
14. Jasaityte R, Dandel M, Lehmkuhl H, Hetzer R. Prediction of short-term outcomes in patients with idiopathic dilated cardiomyopathy referred for transplantation using standard echocardiography and strain imaging. Transplant Proc. 2009;41:277–80.
15. Singh GK, Cupps B, Pasque M, Woodard PK, Holland MR, Ludomirsky A. Accuracy and reproducibility of strain by speckle tracking in pediatric subjects with normal heart and single ventricular physiology: a two-dimensional speckle-tracking echocardiography and magnetic resonance imaging correlative study. J Am Soc Echocardiogr. 2010;23:1143–52.
16. Koopman LP, Slorach C, Hui W, Manlhiot C, McCrindle BW, Friedberg MK, et al. Comparison between different speckle Trucking and color tissue Doppler techniques to measure global and regional myocardial deformation in children. J Am Soc Echocardiogr. 2010;23:919–28.
17. Sengupta PP, Mohan JC, Mehta V, Arora R, Pandian NG, Khandheria BK. Accuracy and pitfalls of early diastolic motion of the mitral annulus for diagnosing constrictive pericarditis by tissue Doppler imaging. Am J Cardiol. 2004;93:886–90.
18. Wang J, Khoury DS, Thohan V, Torre-Amione G, Nagueh SF. Global diastolic strain rate for the assessment of left ventricular relaxation and filling pressures. Circulation. 2007;115:1376–83.
19. Takeuchi M, Nishikage T, Nakai H, Kokumai M, Otani S, Lang RM. The assessment of left ventricular twist in anterior wall myocardial infarction using two-dimensional speckle tracking imaging. J Am Soc Echocardiogr. 2007;20:36–44.
20. Borg AN, Harrison JL, Argyle RA, Ray SG. Left ventricular torsion in primary chronic mitral regurgitation. Heart. 2008;94:597–603.
21. Bertini M, Marsan NA, Delgado V, van Bommel RJ, Nucifora G, Borleffs CJ, et al. Effects of cardiac resynchronization therapy on left ventricular twist. J Am Coll Cardiol. 2009;54:1317–25.
22. Takeuchi M, Borden WB, Nakai H, Nishikage T, Kokumai M, Nagakura T, et al. Reduced and delayed untwisting of the left ventricle in patients with hypertension and left ventricular hypertrophy: a study using twodimensional speckle tracking imaging. Eur Heart J. 2007;28:2756–62.
23. Sengupta PP, Krishnamoorthy VK, Abhayaratna WP, Korinek J, Belohlavek M, Sundt III TM, et al. Disparate patterns of left ventricular mechanics differentiate constrictive pericarditis from restrictive cardiomyopathy. JACC Cardiovasc Imaging. 2008;1:29–38.
24. Rovner A, Smith R, Greenberg NL, Tuzcu EM, Smedira N, Lever HM, et al. Improvement in diastolic intraventricular pressure gradients in patients with HOCM after ethanol septal reduction. Am J Physiol Heart Circ Physiol. 2003;285:H2492–9.
25. Ammar KA, Paterick TE, Khandheria BK, Jan MF, Kramer C, Umland MM, Tercius AJ, Baratta L, Tajik AJ. Myocardial mechanics: understanding and applying three-dimensional speckle tracking echocardiography in clinical practice. Echocardiography. 2012;29(7):861–72. doi:10.1111/j.1540-8175.2012.01712.x. Epub 2012 May 17. PubMed PMID: 22591237.
26. Pérez de Isla L, Balcones DV, Fernández-Golfín C, Marcos-Alberca P, Almería C, Rodrigo JL, Macaya C, Zamorano J. Three-dimensional-wall motion tracking: a new and faster tool for myocardial strain assessment: comparison with two-dimensional-wall motion tracking. J Am Soc Echocardiogr. 2009;22(4):325–30. doi:10.1016/j.echo.2009.01.001. Erratum in: J Am Soc Echocardiogr. 2009 Jun;22(6):745-e1. PubMed PMID: 19345302.
27. Saito K, Okura H, Watanabe N, Hayashida A, Obase K, Imai K, Maehama T, Kawamoto T, Neishi Y, Yoshida K. Comprehensive evaluation of left ventricular strain using speckle tracking

echocardiography in normal adults: comparison of three-dimensional and two-dimensional approaches. J Am Soc Echocardiogr. 2009;22(9):1025–30. doi:10.1016/j.echo.2009.05.021. Epub 2009 Jun 24. PubMed PMID: 19556106.

28. Reant P, Barbot L, Touche C, Dijos M, Arsac F, Pillois X, Landelle M, Roudaut R, Lafitte S. Evaluation of global left ventricular systolic function using three-dimensional echocardiography speckle-tracking strain parameters. J Am Soc Echocardiogr. 2012;25:68–79.

29. Urbano-Moral JA, Patel AR, Maron MS, Arias-Godinez JA, Pandian NG. Three-dimensional speckle-tracking echocardiography: methodological aspects and clinical potential. Echocardiography. 2012;29(8):997–1010. doi:10.1111/j.1540-8175.2012.01773.x. Epub 2012 Jul 12. Review. PubMed PMID: 22783969.

30. Shiota T, editor. 3D Echocardiography. Boca Raton: CRC Press; 2007.

31. Pérez de Isla L, Millán M, Lennie V, Quezada M, Guinea J, Macaya C, Zamorano J. Area strain: normal values for a new parameter in healthy people. Rev Esp Cardiol. 2011;64(12):1194–7. doi:10.1016/j.recesp.2011.03.021. Spanish. PubMed PMID: 21684666.

32. Wen H, Liang Z, Zhao Y, Yang K. Feasibility of detecting early left ventricular systolic dysfunction using global area strain: a novel index derived from three-dimensional speckle-tracking echocardiography. Eur J Echocardiogr. 2011;12(12):910–6. doi:10.1093/ejechocard/jer162. Epub 2011 Sep 6. PubMed PMID: 21900298.

33. Kaku K, Takeuchi M, Tsang W, Takigiku K, Yasukochi S, Patel AR, Mor-Avi V, Lang RM, Otsuji Y. Age-related normal range of left ventricular strain and torsion using three-dimensional speckle-tracking echocardiography. J Am Soc Echocardiogr. 2014;27(1):55–64. doi:10.1016/j.echo.2013.10.002. Epub 2013 Nov 13. PubMed PMID: 24238753.

34. Jasaityte R, Heyde B, D'hooge J. Current state of three-dimensional myocardial strain estimation using echocardiography. J Am Soc Echocardiogr. 2013;26(1):15–28. doi:10.1016/j.echo.2012.10.005. Epub 2012 Nov 11. Review. PubMed PMID: 23149303.

35. Kleijn SA, Aly MF, Terwee CB, van Rossum AC, Kamp O. Reliability of Leith ventricular volumes and function measurements using three-dimensional speckle tracking echocardiography. Eur Heart J Cardiovasc Imaging. 2012;13(2):159–68. doi:10.1093/ejechocard/jer174. Epub 2011 Sep 16. PubMed PMID: 21926118.

36. Muraru D, Cucchini U, Mihăilă S, Miglioranza MH, Aruta P, Cavalli G, Cecchetto A, Padayattil-Josè S, Peluso D, Iliceto S, Badano LP. Left ventricular myocardial strain by three-dimensional speckle-tracking echocardiography in healthy subjects: reference values and analysis of their physiologic and technical determinants. J Am Soc Echocardiogr. 2014;27(8):858–71. e1. doi: 10.1016/j.echo.2014.05.010. Epub 2014 Jun 26. PubMed PMID: 24975996.

37. Kleijn SA, Pandian NG, Thomas JD, Perez de Isla L, Kamp O, Zuber M, Nihoyannopoulos P, Forster T, Nesser HJ, Geibel A, Gorissen W, Zamorano JL. Normal reference values of left ventricular strain using three-dimensional speckle tracking echocardiography: results from a multicentre study. Eur Heart J Cardiovasc Imaging. 2015;16(4):410–6. doi:10.1093/ehjci/jeu213. Epub 2014 Oct 26. PubMed PMID: 25345661.

38. Seo Y, Ishizu T, Enomoto Y, Sugimori H, Yamamoto M, Machino T, Kawamura R, Aonuma K. Validation of 3-dimensional speckle tracking imaging to quantify regional myocardial deformation. Circ Cardiovasc Imaging. 2009;2(6):451–9. doi:10.1161/CIRCIMAGING.109.858480. Epub 2009 Sep 12. PubMed PMID: 19920043.

39. Nesser HJ, Mor-Avi V, Gorissen W, Weinert L, Steringer-Mascherbauer R, Niel J, Sugeng L, Lang RM. Quantification of left ventricular volumes using three-dimensional echocardiographic speckle tracking: comparison with MRI. Eur Heart J. 2009;30(13):1565–73. doi:10.1093/eurheartj/ehp187. Epub 2009 May 29. PubMed PMID: 19482868.

40. Yuda S, Sato Y, Abe K, Kawamukai M, Kouzu H, Muranaka A, Kokubu N, Hashimoto A, Tsuchihashi K, Watanabe N, Miura T. Inter-vendor variability of left ventricular volumes and strains determined by three-dimensional speckle tracking echocardiography. Echocardiography. 2014;31(5):597–604. doi:10.1111/echo.12432. Epub 2013 Nov 6. PubMed PMID: 25070187.

41. Badano LP, Cucchini U, Muraru D, Al Nono O, Sarais C, Iliceto S. Use of three-dimensional speckle tracking to assess left ventricular myocardial mechanics: inter-vendor consistency and reproducibility of strain measurements. Eur Heart J Cardiovasc Imaging. 2013;14(3):285–93. doi:10.1093/ehjci/jes184. Epub 2012 Sep 11. PubMed PMID: 22968525.
42. Gayat E, Ahmad H, Weinert L, Lang RM, Mor-Avi V. Reproducibility and inter-vendor variability of left ventricular deformation measurements by three-dimensional speckle-tracking echocardiography. J Am Soc Echocardiogr. 2011;24(8):878–85. doi:10.1016/j.echo.2011.04.016. Epub 2011 Jun 8. PubMed PMID: 21645991.
43. Yodwut C, Weinert L, Klas B, Lang RM, Mor-Avi V. Effects of frame rate on three-dimensional speckle-tracking-based measurements of myocardial deformation. J Am Soc Echocardiogr. 2012;25(9):978–85. doi:10.1016/j.echo.2012.06.001. Epub 2012 Jul 4. PubMed PMID: 22766029.
44. Thebault C, Donal E, Bernard A, Moreau O, Schnell F, Mabo P, Leclercq C. Real-time three-dimensional speckle tracking echocardiography: a novel technique to quantify global left ventricular mechanical dyssynchrony. Eur J Echocardiogr. 2011;12(1):26–32. doi:10.1093/ejechocard/jeq095. Epub 2010 Aug 24. PubMed PMID: 20736292.
45. Li CH, Carreras F, Leta R, Carballeira L, Pujadas S, Pons-Lladó G. Mechanical left ventricular dyssynchrony detection by endocardium displacement analysis with 3D speckle tracking technology. Int J Cardiovasc Imaging. 2010;26(8):867–70. doi:10.1007/s10554-010-9644-x. Epub 2010 Aug 14. PubMed PMID: 20711677.
46. Tanaka H, Tatsumi K, Matsumoto K, Kawai H, Hirata K. Emerging role of three-dimensional speckle tracking strain for accurate quantification of left ventricular dyssynchrony. Echocardiography. 2013;30(9):E292–5. doi:10.1111/echo.12280. Epub 2013 Jun 6. PubMed PMID: 23741972.
47. Matsumoto K, Tanaka H, Tatsumi K, Miyoshi T, Hiraishi M, Kaneko A, Tsuji T, Ryo K, Fukuda Y, Yoshida A, Kawai H, Hirata K. Left ventricular dyssynchrony using three-dimensional speckle-tracking imaging as a determinant of torsional mechanics in patients with idiopathic dilated cardiomyopathy. Am J Cardiol. 2012;109(8):1197–205. doi:10.1016/j.amjcard.2011.11.059. Epub 2012 Jan 28. PubMed PMID: 22285093.
48. Mochizuki A, Yuda S, Oi Y, Kawamukai M, Nishida J, Kouzu H, Muranaka A, Kokubu N, Shimoshige S, Hashimoto A, Tsuchihashi K, Watanabe N, Miura T. Assessment of left atrial deformation and synchrony by three-dimensional speckle-tracking echocardiography: comparative studies in healthy subjects and patients with atrial fibrillation. J Am Soc Echocardiogr. 2013;26(2):165–74. doi:10.1016/j.echo.2012.10.003. Epub 2012 Nov 8. PubMed PMID: 23140846.
49. Tanaka H, Matsumoto K, Hiraishi M, Miyoshi T, Kaneko A, Tsuji T, Ryo K, Fukuda Y, Tatsumi K, Yoshida A, Kawai H, Hirata K. Multidirectional left ventricular performance detected with three-dimensional speckle-tracking strain in patients with chronic right ventricular pacing and preserved ejection fraction. Eur Heart J Cardiovasc Imaging. 2012;13(10):849–56.
50. Wang Q, Huang D, Zhang L, Shen D, Ouyang Q, Duan Z, An X, Zhang M, Zhang C, Yang F, Zhi G. Assessment of myocardial infarct size by three-dimensional and two-dimensional speckle tracking echocardiography: a comparative study to single photon emission computed tomography. Echocardiography. 2015;32(10):1539–46. doi:10.1111/echo.12901. Epub 2015 Feb 15. PubMed PMID: 25684359.
51. Nagata Y, Takeuchi M, Wu VC, Izumo M, Suzuki K, Sato K, Seo Y, Akashi YJ, Aonuma K, Otsuji Y. Prognostic value of LV deformation parameters using 2D and 3D speckle-tracking echocardiography in asymptomatic patients with severe aortic stenosis and preserved LV ejection fraction. JACC Cardiovasc Imaging. 2015;8(3):235–45. doi:10.1016/j.jcmg.2014.12.009. Epub 2015 Feb 11. PubMed PMID: 25682511.
52. Casas-Rojo E, Fernández-Golfín C, Moya-Mur JL, González-Gómez A, García-Martín A, Morán-Fernández L, Rodríguez-Muñoz D, Jiménez-Nacher JJ, Martí Sánchez D, Zamorano

Gómez JL. Area strain from 3D speckle-tracking echocardiography as an independent predictor of early symptoms or ventricular dysfunction in asymptomatic severe mitral regurgitation with preserved ejection fraction. Int J Cardiovasc Imaging. 2016;9 [Epub ahead of print] PubMed PMID: 27161336.

53. Nemes A, Domsik P, Kalapos A, Lengyel C, Orosz A, Forster T. Comparison of three-dimensional speckle tracking echocardiography and two-dimensional echocardiography for evaluation of left atrial size and function in healthy volunteers (results from the MAGYAR-Healthy study). Echocardiography. 2014;31(7):865–71. doi:10.1111/echo.12485. Epub 2013 Dec 17. PubMed PMID: 24341394.

54. Smith BC, Dobson G, Dawson D, Charalampopoulos A, Grapsa J, Nihoyannopoulos P. Three-dimensional speckle tracking of the right ventricle: toward optimal quantification of right ventricular dysfunction in pulmonary hypertension. J Am Coll Cardiol. 2014;64(1):41–51. doi:10.1016/j.jacc.2014.01.084. PubMed PMID: 24998127.

# Chapter 7
# Guiding Structural Interventions with 3D-Echo

Covadonga Fernández-Golfín Lobán, Alejandra Carbonell San Román, and José Luis Zamorano

## Introduction

Percutaneous catheter-base interventions for the treatment of different valvular and non valvular structural heart disease are increasing. Traditionally, guidance of these procedures has been performed with fluoroscopy and two dimensional transesofageal echocardiography (2D TEE). However, both modalities have limitations. Structural heart diseases procedures requires continuous soft-tissue imaging, which is not possible with fluoroscopy, leading to poor visualization of the target structure and exposing the patients to excessive levels of ionizing radiation. Moreover, being a single plane projection, a comprehensive evaluation of a three dimensional (3D) structure like the heart requires time with multiple X ray projections and expertise. 2D TEE allows a continuous and real time evaluation of cardiac anatomy and function during the procedure. However, being a 2D imaging modality, multiples planes and views are needed to obtain a complete assessment of a certain structure. Catheter detection and visualization is also limited with 2D TEE [1–3].

3D echocardiography and particular 3D TEE allows acquisition of 3D images in real time (1 beat) with good temporal and spatial resolution. This technology allows a better visualization of all relevant cardiac structures at the same time with a better delineation of catheter and wires. 3D TEE provides a better anatomic understanding

**Electronic supplementary material** The online version of this chapter (doi:10.1007/978-3-319-50335-6_7) contains supplementary material, which is available to authorized users.

C.F.-G. Lobán (✉) • A.C.S. Román • J.L. Zamorano
Cardiology Department, University Hospital Ramón y Cajal,
Carretera de Colmenar Km 9.400, 28034 Madrid, Spain
e-mail: covagolfin@yahoo.es

of the different structural abnormalities which is crucial both prior and during the procedure.

As a rule, modalities used for guiding procedures are real time 3D imaging or zoom 3D mode acquisition in one beat. In the first case, a pyramidal set 60° × 30° is displayed in real time with volume rate up to 25 Hz. Increasing or decreasing vertical and lateral width, adjust the volume to the anatomic structure as needed. Lateral and vertical displacement also simplifies the acquisition since the user can move the volume to acquire without moving the probe or changing the plane and all in real time. Zoom 3D acquisition allows acquisition of a truncated pyramidal dataset with variable size and temporal resolution in one beat. Technological advances have simplified acquisition of 3D images. Nowadays, any 3D imaging modality can be used without any restriction in volume sizing on single or multiple beat acquisition. Since high volume rate acquisition is possible in one beat, multiple beat acquisitions needed before to obtain accurate temporal resolution is seldom needed now [1].

In the present chapter, 3D TEE for guiding structural heart disease interventions will be reviewed.

## Atrial Septal Defect

3D TEE has changed the evaluation of the interatrial septum and atrial septal defects. Before the procedure it allows an accurate evaluation of the type and size of the defect as well as its suitability for percutaneous closure. The unique possibility of "en face" visualization the septum either from the left (Fig. 7.1) or right atrium from a 3D volume acquisition is very useful to localize the defect in the septum, evaluate rims and define a single or multiple defects [1, 2, 4]. It is also useful in no secundum atrial septal defects where sometimes interatrial septum anatomy is challenging. Normally acquisition is performed in the bicaval TEE plane with 3D zoom modalities. Lateral and vertical size need to be adjusted to get the whole septum and nearby structures inside the volume. Due to the high volume required for such a large structure, temporal resolution may decrease up to 5 volumes per second. In this case, this is not a limitation since mobility of the interatrial septum is low and high temporal resolution is not needed. Real time 3D acquisition can be used as well after increasing the lateral and vertical width to include the entire atrial septum. In the 3D images a quick and fast evaluation either from the right or left atrium allows a first approach to localize the defect, to rule out multiple defects and to assess size (Fig. 7.2). Both diameters and areas can be easily measured in these images. However for a more accurate assessment of the defect size and rims, multiplanar images obtained from the 3D volume is recommended (Fig. 7.3), especially in complex cases [4, 5].

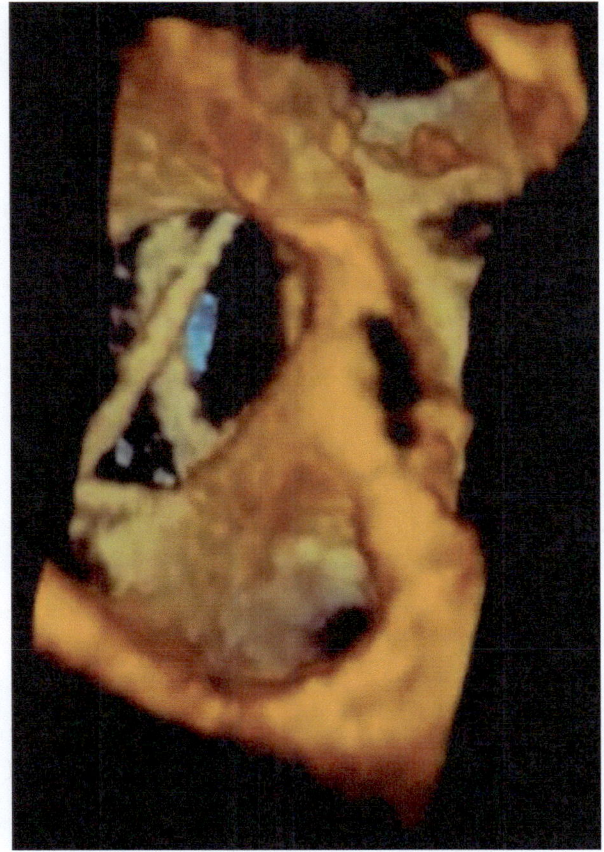

**Fig. 7.1** 3D real time image showing an ostium secundum atrial septal defect from the right atrium with the catheter crossing trough it during percutaneous closure

The closure procedure is very straightforward through a femoral vein access. TEE allows visualization of the sheet trough the defect into de left atrium and the deployment of the device, first the left atrium disc and second the right atrium disc. 3D TEE allows monitoring this procedure by means of real time 3D imaging. 0° four chamber views at the level of the atrial septum is normally an accurate plane to monitor the procedure. By clicking the 3D button, a thin 3D pyramid is obtained. If needed, vertical width can be increase to get a full visualization of the atrial septum form the left atrium by a slight counter clock volume rotation. After implantation and before its release, correct position of the device in the septum needs to be confirmed as well as normal function of the mitral valve and flow in the pulmonary veins. Residual shunt needs to be rules out. With 2D TEE echocardiography different planes need to be performed for a comprehensive evaluation

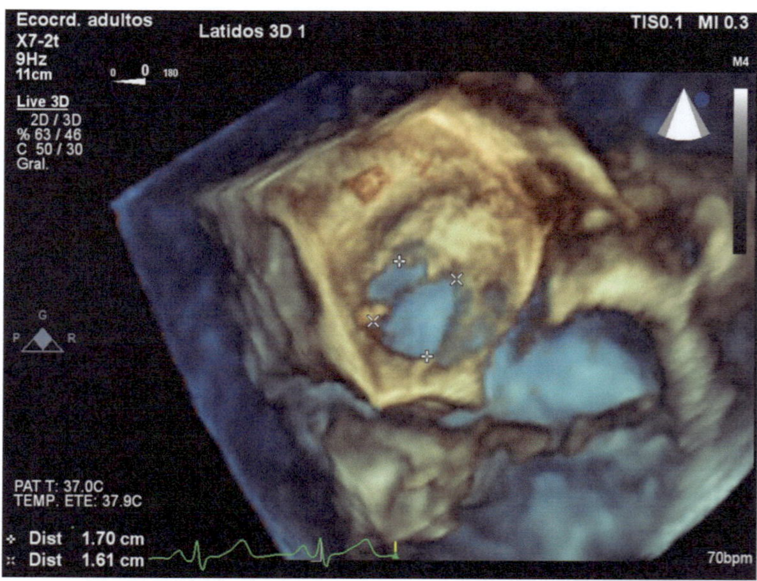

**Fig. 7.2** Live 3D image during percutaneous atrial septal defect closure. En face view of the defect from the left atrial aspect. The location, shape and sixe are clearly seen

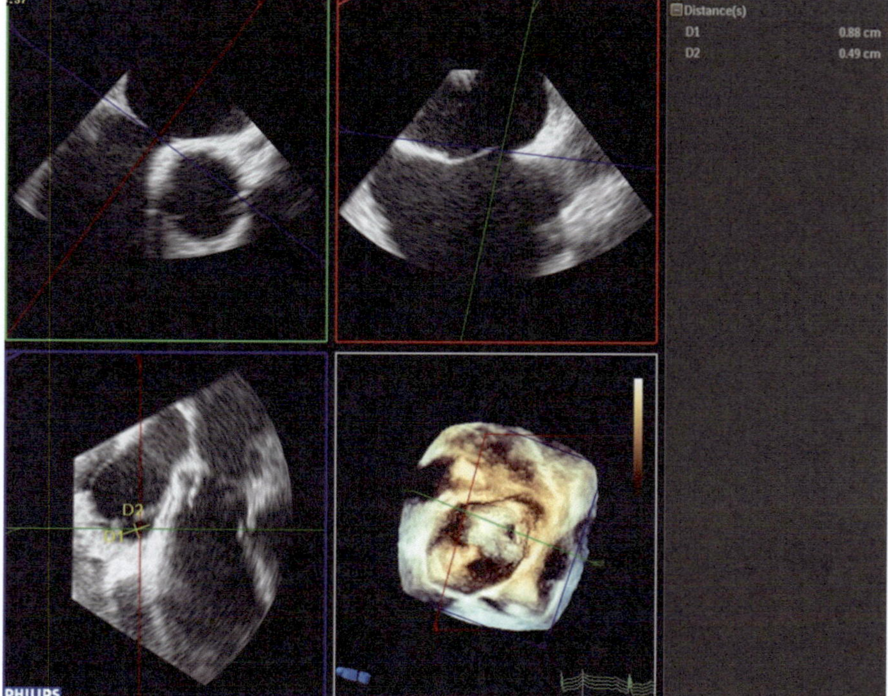

**Fig. 7.3** Multiplanar reconstruction of a small ostium secundum atrial septal defect. Planes are aligned at the level of the defect in the desired moment of the cardiac cycle, perpendicular to each other and final measurement is performed in the "en face" view of the defect, lower left image

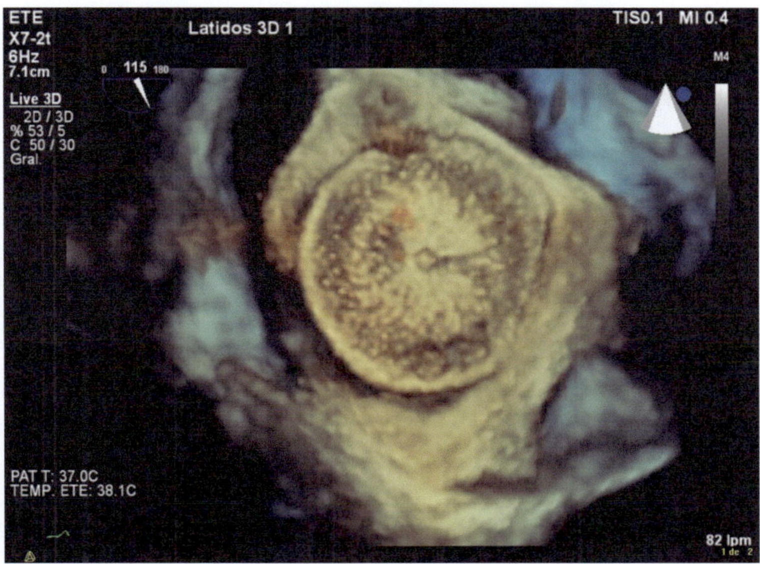


**Fig. 7.4** Live 3D image of the left atrial aspect of the interatrial septum showing the left disc of an Amplatzer devices for atrial septal defect closure

of the results. 3D TEE imaging allows visualization of the septum from different perspectives in the same volume providing a unique "en face" view of the device (Fig. 7.4, Video 7.1).

# Tavi

3D TEE has become a must in the evaluation of patients for TAVI both prior and during the procedure [6, 7].

## *Prior to the Procedure*

Before the procedure to define true severity of the aortic stenosis and to measure the annulus dimensions. This is performed by means of 3D TEE (Table 7.1). Acquisition is performed in the short axis view of the aortic valve (45ª) and in the left ventricular outflow tract view (120°). Normally 3D zoom modality is used with adjustment of the lateral and vertical width to assure that the complete annulus, left ventricular outflow tract and proximal ascending aorta is included. Temporal resolution should be optimized as much as possible with at least 10 volumes/second. This is easily achieved in 1 single beat acquisition mode if the volume is adjusted to the aortic annulus. In some cases however, high volume rate acquisition can be used but

**Table 7.1** 3D imaging prior to TAVI procedure

| | Image plane | 3D modality | Comment |
|---|---|---|---|
| Aortic valve area | TEE 45° and 120ª, aortic valve short axis view and LVOT view | Zoom 3D, adjust volume the aortic valve to optimize temporal resolution | Acquire images with the 3D and 3 2D orthogonal planes visualization to assure relevant structures are inside the acquired volume<br>Analysis is performed in multiplanar reconstructions. Adjust planes perpendicular to the narrowest aortic valve area in systole |
| Aortic annulus diameter | TEE 45° and 120°, aortic valve short axis view and LVOT view | Zoom 3D, adjust volume the aortic valve to optimize temporal resolution | Analysis is performed in multiplanar reconstructions. Adjust planes perpendicular to the aortic annulus in mid-systole when leaflet calcification are no further seen (bellow the calcified aortic annulus plane) |
| Aortic root evaluation | 120° -140° LVOT view | Zoom 3D, adjust volume the aortic valve to optimize temporal resolution | Analysis is performed in multiplanar reconstructions. Adjust planes perpendicular to the aortic wall at different levels in diastole |

spatial resolution and image quality for measurements will decrease. Since the aortic valve in these patients is extensively calcified we recommend acquiring 3D images in both planes so possible limitations due to calcium acoustic shadow are reduced. Multiplane reconstructions from 3D volume acquired are used for both aortic valve area and annulus measurements. Perpendicular adjustment of the reference planes at the level of narrowest valve opening in systole allows aortic valve area tracing (Fig. 7.5). Different papers have shown the superiority of 3D valve area planimetry over 2D in determining aortic stenosis severity. This measurement has also shown a good correlation with both continuity equation valve area and hemodynamic vale area assessment. In the same multiplane images, the image plane can be moved down to the aortic annulus where both diameters, area and perimeter can be easily measured. AV annulus dimensions are measured from the hinge point of the right coronary cusp to the anterior aortic wall, perpendicular to the long axis of the aortic root, in mid-systole where its diameter is at its maximum (Figs. 7.6 and 7.7) Since the aortic annulus is not circular but rather elliptical, 3D sizing of the aortic annulus is superior to the 2D assessment that gives only the sagittal smaller diameter. Different papers have shown the superiority of 3D annulus assessment, both with TEE or computed tomography over 2D [8, 9]. Annulus sizing is more accurate and this translates in better results, reducing the rate of paravalvular regurgitation [10]. Additional information obtained from 3D images are the distance to the right and left main coronary arteries, level of calcification and severity of mitral regurgitation.

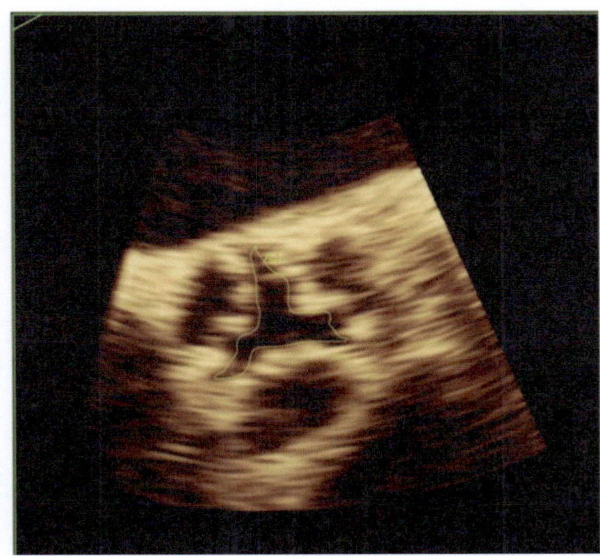

**Fig. 7.5** 3D aortic valve area measurement performed after multiplanar reconstruction selecting the minimum aortic valve area. The plane is place perpendicular to the aortic leaflets in a more distal position where the smaller area is seen

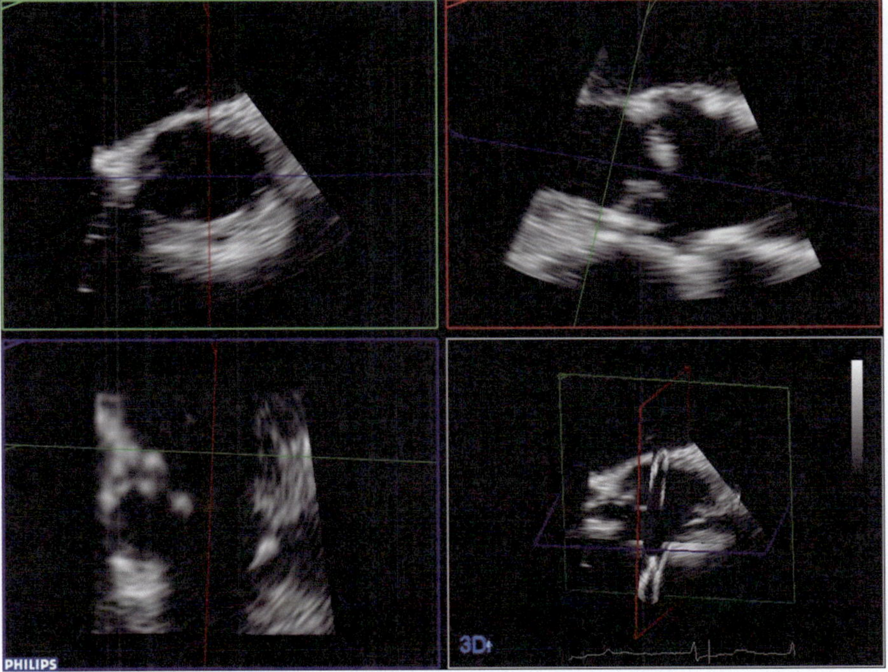


**Fig. 7.6** Multiplanar reconstruction from 3D zoom image acquisition of the aortic annulus. The axes are aligned perpendicular to each other in the 3 orthogonal planes at the level of the aortic annulus

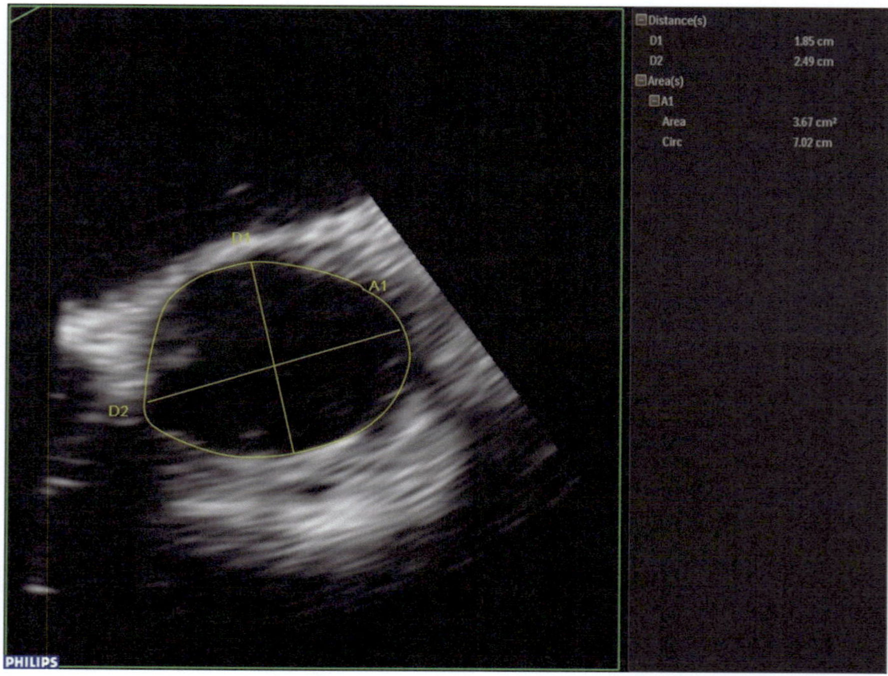


**Fig. 7.7** From multiplanar analysis, the best image of the artic annulus is selected and zoomed for measurements of the diameters area and circumference

## Guiding the Procedure

During the procedure, both 2D and 3D TEE imaging are used. 3D overcomes some of the limitations encountered with 2D; it provides a better visualization of the wires and catheters and both real time orthogonal biplane and 3D imaging helps in different steps of the procedure (Table 7.2). Crossing the stenosed aortic valve may be difficult in some case, real time 3D imaging provides an "en face" view of the valve and may help in this task along with biplane imaging. In the long axis left ventricular outflow tract view, 3D real time imaging allows visualization of wire, valvuloplasty balloon position, inflation and results (Fig. 7.8). In the same way, prostheses advance and positioning is also possible, providing a better delineation of the balloon and prostheses for optimal positioning in the aortic annulus. Edward-Sapiens valve optimal position is 2–4 mm bellow the aortic annulus plane, while Core Valve should be place 5–10 mm bellow [6, 7, 2] After deployment, evaluation of prostheses position, leaflet movement and presence and degree of valvular regurgitation is needed. In this way, assessment of both prostheses position and leaflet movement can be performed with 2D and 3D imaging (Video 7.2). 3D imaging, both real time or zoom 3D allows multiplanar reconstructions in cases where prostheses mal function is suspected or limited evaluation is achieved with 2D echo. Both valvular and paravalvular regurgitation is better evaluated with 3D echo. First biplane

**Table 7.2**  3D imaging during TAVI procedure

|  | Image plane | 3D modality | Comment |
| --- | --- | --- | --- |
| Aortic valve crossing | TEE 45° and 120ᵃ, aortic valve short axis view and LVOT view | Orthogonal biplane imaging, real time 3D short axis view of the aortic valve | Both orthogonal 2D images and real time 3D images with en face view of the aortic valve may be useful in crossing the valve in selected difficult cases |
| Aortic valvuloplasty | TEE 120° LVOT view | Real time 3D image | Evaluation of balloon position during inflation and evaluation of immediate result |
| Aortic prostheses implantation | TEE 120° LVOT view | Real time 3D image | Confirmation of prostheses position in the aortic annulus, evaluation of its deployment and immediate result |
| Evaluation post implantation | TEE 45° and 120ᵃ, aortic valve short axis view and LVOT view | Orthogonal biplane imaging without and with colour Doppler, real time 3D short axis view of the aortic valve, zoom 3D of the aortic valve, zoom 3D with colour | Orthogonal 2D images allow first approach to valve position and leaflet movement. With colour Doppler evaluation of aortic regurgitation, jets, location and extension. Real time 3D imaging complement visualization of leaflet movement and prostheses position. Zoom 3D images with multiplanar reconstruction allows complete assessment of leaflet movement and vena contracta area measurement of the regurgitant jets |

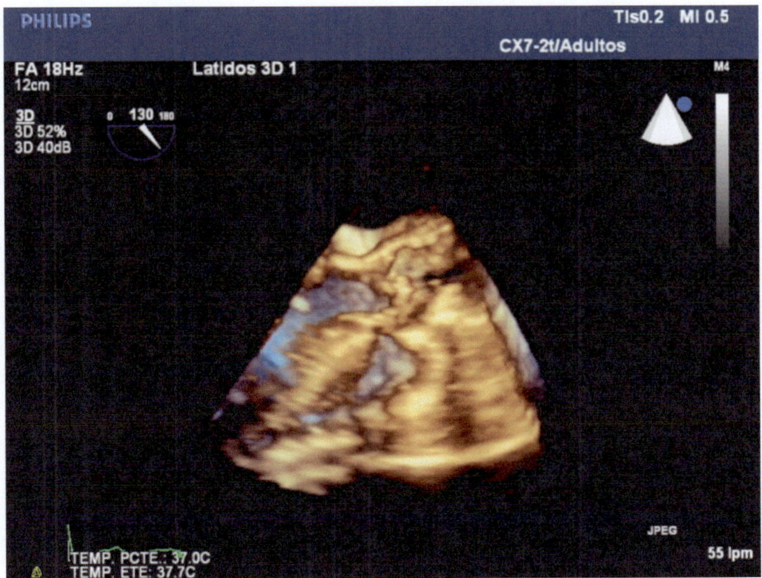

**Fig. 7.8**  Live 3D image, left ventricular outflow tract view, used to monitor percutaneous aortic valve implantation

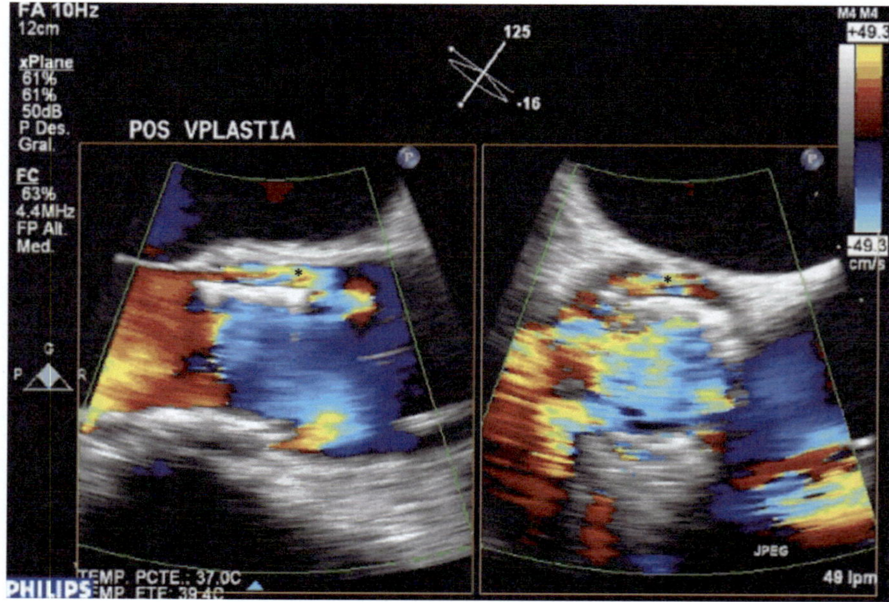

**Fig. 7.9** Biplane 2D color Doppler image showing the aortic prostheses and significant aortic paravalvular regurgitation located posteriorly (*)

simultaneous visualization of the aortic prostheses in the short and long axis view is possible and a first approach to the extension and location of the aortic regurgitation is performed (Fig. 7.9). Color 3D acquisition with 3D zoom modalities allows multiplanar reconstruction to assess origin and size of the regurgitant jet or jets as well as its extension in the annular ring. Vena contracta area can be measured avoiding the limitation of 2D assessment of the regurgitant jets. The VARC recommendations suggest that for paravalvular jets, the proportion of the circumference of the sewing ring occupied by the jet gives a semi-quantitative guide to severity: <10% of the sewing ring suggests mild, 10–29% suggests moderate, and ≥30% suggests severe [11]. This is essential during the procedure because in some cases depending on the degree of valvular regurgitation and prostheses position post-dilatation may be needed. Once prostheses correct position and function is confirmed and before ending the procedure mitral regurgitation severity, left ventricular segmental wall motion, pericardial effusion and aortic wall assessment should be performed to rule out other more rare complications of the procedure.

## MitraClip

Percutaneous mitral valve repair (MVR) using the MitraClip system (MitraClip, Abbott Vascular, Abbott Park, IL, USA) has emerged as an alternative treatment option for patients with severe MR and high surgical risk for MVR. This technique is based on approximating the free edges of the anterior and posterior leaflet with a clip creating a double mitral orifice, increasing valve coaptation and thereby reducing mitral regurgitation. Echocardiography, especially 3D TEE is essential in all the steps of the procedure: patient selection, procedure guiding and evaluation of results. The efficacy and feasibility of MitraClip therapy is dependent on the appropriate patient selection and on the precise evaluation of valve anatomy and function. Implantation requires a correct selection of the patient, guidance of the procedure and evaluation of the result before releasing the device [12, 13].

## *Prior to the Procedure*

Comprehensive assessment of mitral valve is mandatory before MitraClip procedure. 3D TEE overcomes many of the limitations of 2D echocardiography and has proved to be superior in many clinical conditions. Main advantages of 3D TEE in MitraClip patient selection are the evaluation of mitral regurgitation severity and mitral valve morphology [14, 15]. In the first case, direct measurement of the proximal isovelocity surface area and vena contracta without geometric assumptions with 3D TEE, improves accuracy [16, 17]. This is particularly relevant when dealing with functional MR. The asymmetrical deformation of the valve apparatus will generate non-spherical and more funnel-like regurgitant orifices encompassing the coaptation closure line, which can only be completely visualized with 3DTEE. A first color zoom 3D acquisition including the entire mitral valve is normally performed to localize the regurgitant jet; this is very important, since optimal jet origin should be between A2 and P2 segments, being eccentric or more complex jets less suitable. Subsequent, a smaller volume centered in the regurgitant jet (excluding part of the mitral annulus) is acquired with higher temporal resolution for mitral regurgitation vena contracta area analysis (Figs. 7.10 and 7.11). Different papers have shown the higher accuracy of this method compared to 2D TEE evaluation. In the second case, for MV morphologic evaluation, same 3D zoom image offers the advantage of visualization a highly detailed image of the whole MV in a single view (Video 7.3), which can then be rotated and angulated in all image planes; furthermore, additional en face views of the MV from both the LV and LA can be obtained [18]. It has been demonstrated that 3DTEE is more accurate in identifying valve segments compared with 2DTTE as well as clefts, gaps and perforations, frequently missed in 2DTEE. The evaluation of these images allows planning of the procedure, to locate the exact place of maximal mitral regurgitation or even plan a strategy of two clips in cases where mitral regurgitation is very large. Also mitral valve area evaluation by means of planimetry from 3D images (Fig. 7.12) is essential since valve areas bellow 3 cm$^2$ are a contraindication for the procedure (Table 7.3).

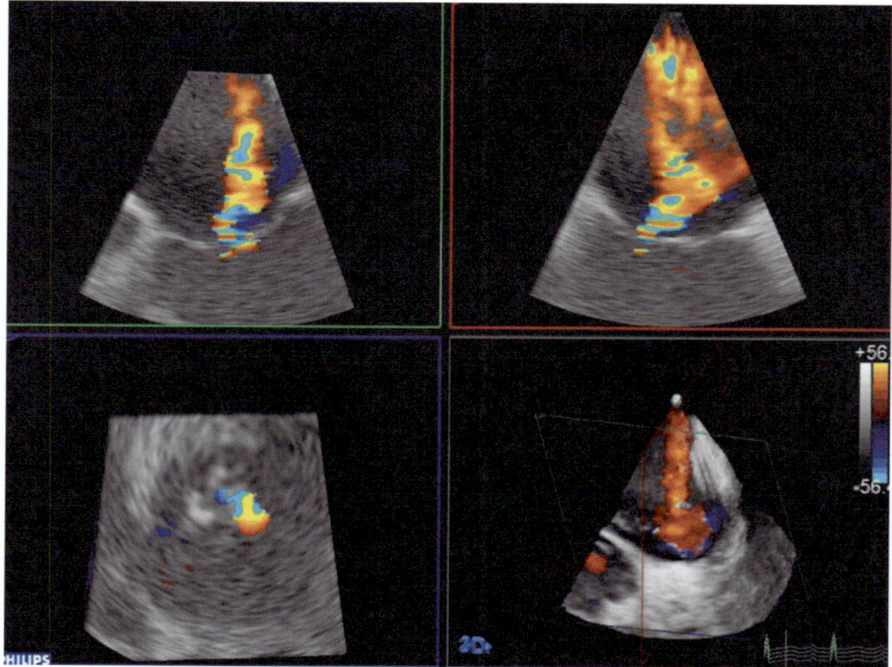

**Fig. 7.10** Color Doppler 3D image, multiplane image showing the jet in the 3 different planes for 3D vena contracta area assessment

## *Guiding the Procedure*

During the procedure there are several steps where 3D imaging is essential (Table 7.4). First, in the transeptal puncture. For MitraClip implantation, a superior and posterior site in the "fossa ovalis" is needed. This position allows manipulation of the catheter in the left atrium and approaching the device towards the mitral valve. A minimum distance of 35–40 mm is required from the puncture site to the mitral valve to assure adequate device manipulation and implantation. 3D TEE probes allow simultaneous visualization of the IAS in a bicaval and short axis views to guide puncture (Fig. 7.13). Also, 3D image acquisition on real time allows en face visualization of the septum to decide optimal site. Once tenting is visualized, assessment of the distance to the mitral valve needs to be assessed in a four-chamber view at 0°. This can be done with 2D TEE, but real time 3D image is very useful since the entire IAS can be visualized and measurement performed (Fig. 7.14) [12, 13, 18].

Once the IAS is crossed, the next step involves the dilation of the orifice to allow the passage of the delivery system into the LA. A superstiff guide wire is then advanced under TEE monitoring to prevent injury of the LA lateral wall or

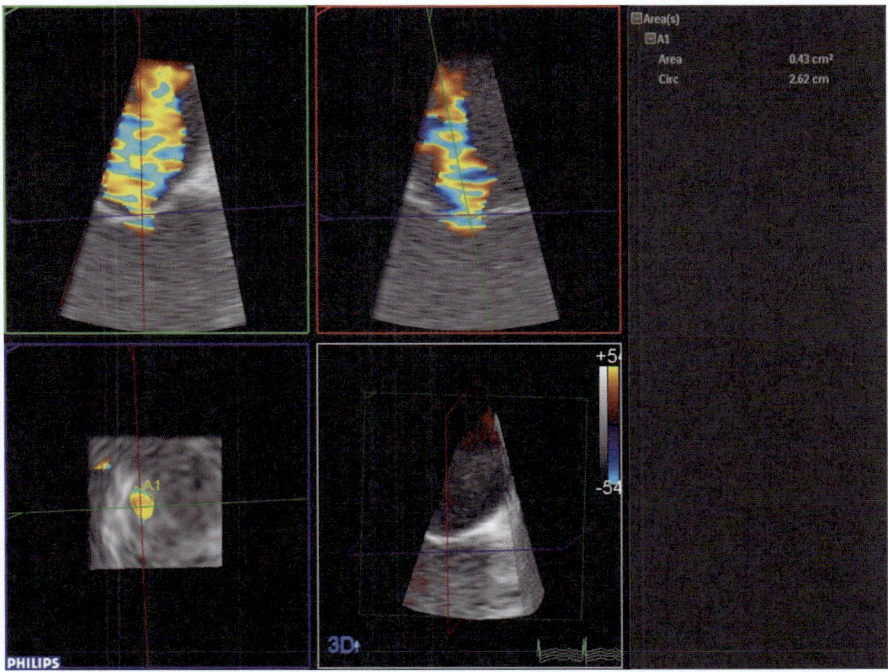


**Fig. 7.11** Measurement of 3D vena contracta. Alignment f the axes is performed perpendicular to the vena contracta. "En face" view of the regurgitant orifice is visible and area can be manually traced (lower let image)

LA appendage; here real time 3D along with biplane images allows visualization of the greater segments of the guide wire. The guide catheter is then advanced in the LA and the guide wire pulled out. Monitoring of the catheter tip with 2DTEE using multiple views should be continuous during manipulations and through the advancement of the clip delivery system, to avoid contact with the surrounding structures. Real-time 3DTEE can obtain in a single perspective visualization of the guide catheter the clip delivery and the anatomical structures. The delivery system is turned inferiorly and angled towards the leaflets, parallel to mitral flow. Correct positioning can be established from the inter-commissural plane at 55–75° and the LV outflow long axis plane at 100–160° using biplane real-time imaging, where the medial-lateral and posterior-anterior alignments can be assessed. The use of 3DTEE in this step can be particularly helpful as the manoeuvre can be tracked in a single perspective with en face anatomical view of the mitral leaflets and the approaching clip (Fig. 7.15) [1, 12, 13].

Optimal Clip position is immediately above the mitral regurgitant orifice. The arms of the clip are positioned orthogonal with the line of coaptation with 3DTEE zoom imaging. Once optimal alignment of the delivery clip system is achieved, it

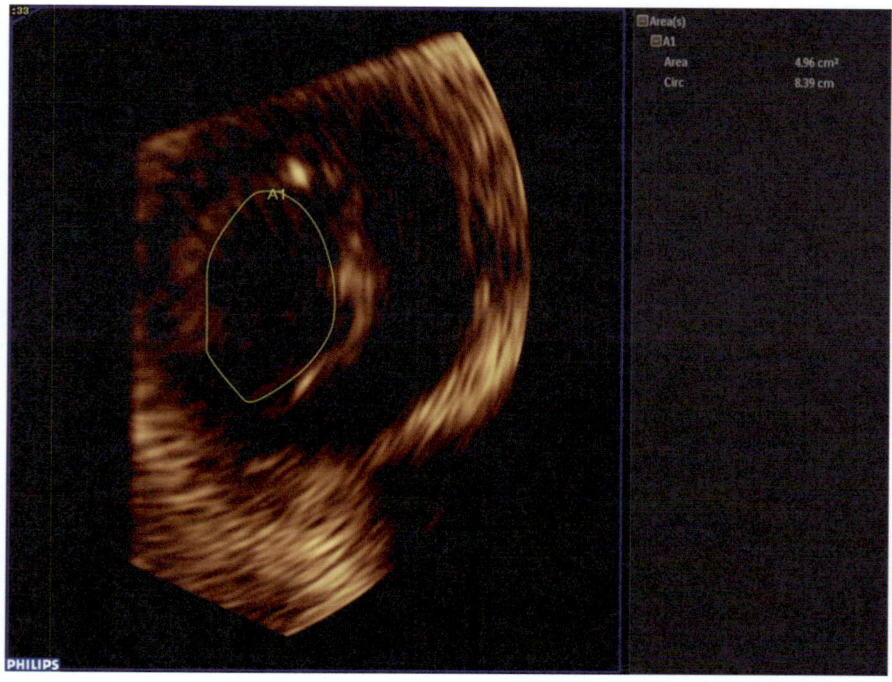


**Fig. 7.12** 3D mitral valve area measurement obtained from multiplane 3D image reconstruction with axes perpendicular to the mitral valve leaflet opening at the level of the narrowest opening point

**Table 7.3** 3D imaging prior to MitraClip procedure

|  | Image plane | 3D modality | Comment |
|---|---|---|---|
| Mitral regurgitation | TEE where best image of the mitral valve and regurgitant jet is seen | Colour zoom 3D, adjust volume to the regurgitant jet to optimize temporal resolution, high volume rate image modality | Acquire images with the 3D and 3 2D orthogonal planes visualization to assure the regurgitant jet origin is inside the acquired volume<br>Analysis is performed in multiplanar reconstructions. Adjust planes perpendicular to the narrowest part of the regurgitant jet. Short axis view in this position is used to trace the effective regurgitant orifice vena contracta area |
| Mitral valve morphology | TEE where best image of the mitral valve is achieved | Zoom 3D, adjust volume the mitral valve to optimize temporal resolution | En face visualization of the mitral valve from the left atrium. Evaluate coaptation defect, clefts and other valve abnormalities |
| Mitral valve area | TEE where best image of the mitral valve is achieved | Zoom 3D, adjust volume the mitral valve to optimize temporal resolution | Analysis is performed in multiplanar reconstructions. Adjust planes perpendicular to mitral leaflets in diastole at the narrowest opening site. Short axis view in this position is used for tracing mitral valve area. |

**Table 7.4**  3D imaging during MitraClip procedure

|  | Image plane | 3D modality | Comment |
|---|---|---|---|
| Transeptal puncture | TEE bicaval plane 90–110° | X-plane or biplane modality | Simultaneous visualization of the bicaval plane (superior and inferior references) and short axis plane (anterior and posterior references) |
| Puncture site confirmation | 0° 4 chambers view | Real time 3D image, increase vertical width to visualize the entire septum and fossa ovalis | Localize tenting site inside the fossa ovalis. Measurement if the distance to the mitral valve can be performed in 3D imaging or using specific software with multiplane reconstructions |
| Catheter advance in the left atrium | TEE 0°–90° | Real time 3D | Follow the catheter's tip in the left atrium and monitor its advance towards the mitral valve |
| Clip alignment | TEE any plane, normally commissural view 55–70° or LVOT view at 120–135° | 3D Zoom | En face view of the mitral valve from the left atrium to confirm alignment of the clip perpendicular to the coaptation line. |
| Evaluation post implantation | TEE any plane with a good image quality of the mitral valve. | 3D Zoom, Colour Doppler 3D zoom | Confirm clip position in the mitral valve, evaluate anterior and posterior leaflet morphology, and assess residual mitral regurgitation, origin and number of jets from an en face view of the mitral valve. Final mitral valve area can be assessed by direct planimetry of the two orifices using multiplane reconstructions. |

*LVOT* left ventricular outflow tract

is advanced into the LV whilst viewed with 2DTEE long-axis left ventricle view from where the opening of the arms can be observed. 3D imaging can quickly reconfirm adequate alignment. The device is pulled back into the LA until the leaflets are firmly captured by the device grippers. Verification of correct leaflet grasping can be performed from the LV outflow and inter-commissural views in x-plane mode, and then the clip gradually closed. Residual MR must be assessed with color Doppler once both leaflets have been successfully clipped. If residual insufficiency is significant, the clip can be repositioned to a more satisfactory position, although implant of a second clip may be necessary. Particularly in this

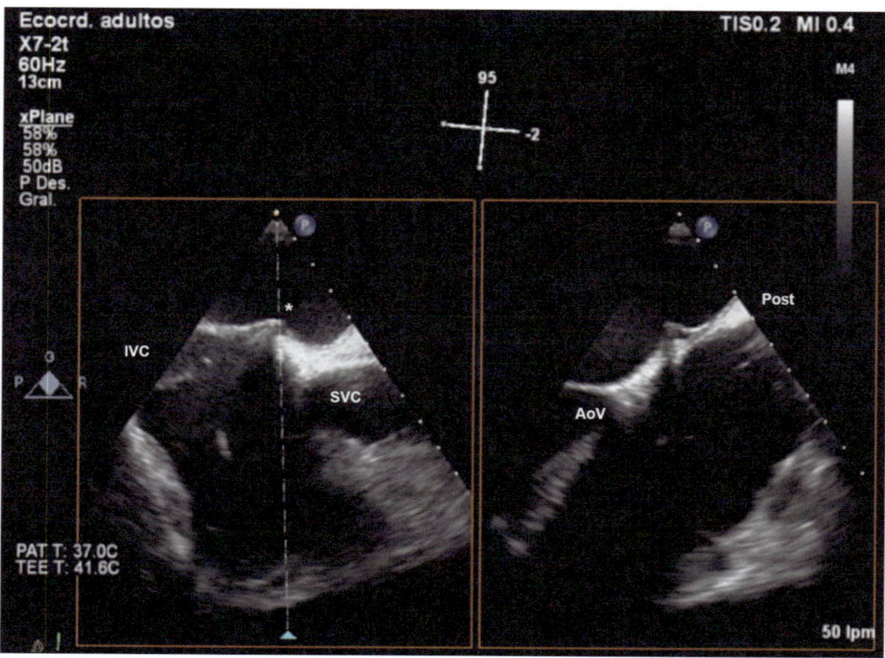

Fig. 7.13 Biplane 2D image during transeptal puncture. Bicaval plane (*left*) and short axis view (*right*) are seen. The tenting (*) in the atrial septum is clearly seen in a superior and central position in the fossa ovalis. SVC: superior vena cava; IVC: inferior vena cava; AoV: aortic valve; Post: posterior

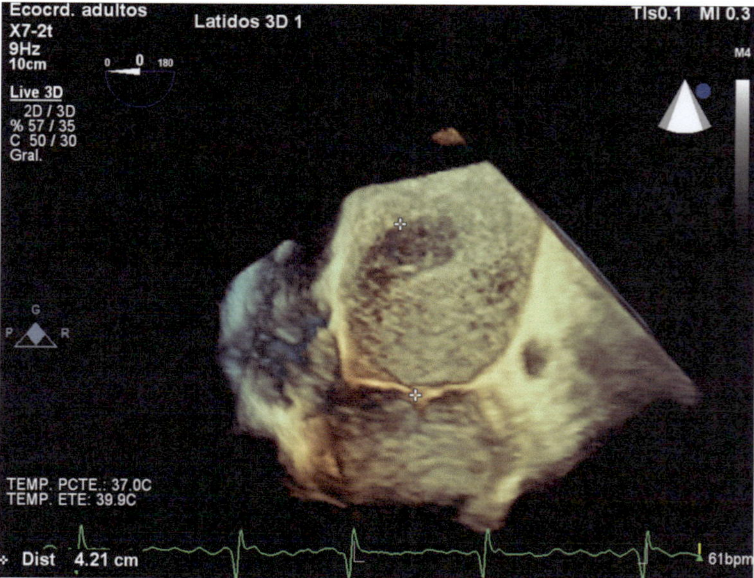

Fig. 7.14 Live 3D image of the atrial septum, view from the left atrium. Measurement of the distance from the tenting site in the septum to the mitral valve is performed confirming an accurate position before real puncture and crossing the septum is done

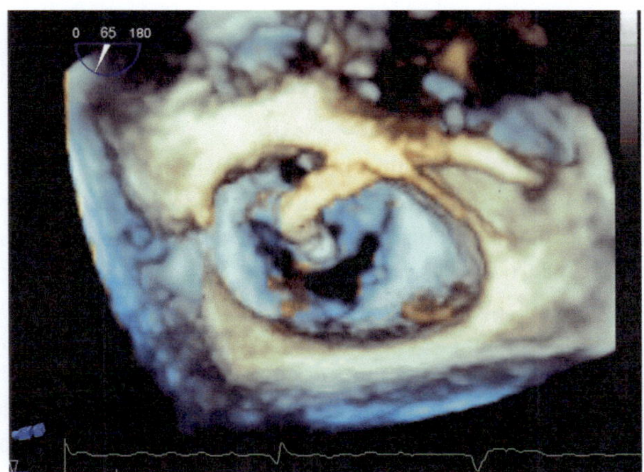


**Fig. 7.15** Zoom 3D image of the mitral valve, en face view (surgical position) from the atrial aspect. The MitraClip delivery catheter is seen crossing the interatrial septum and approaching the mitral valve. The Clip alignment, almost parallel to the coaptation line, can be clearly seen from this perspective

scenario, significant mitral stenosis must be excluded with measurement of trans-valvular gradient using CW Doppler with 2DTEE and planimetry of both orifices with 3DTEE. After final deployment reevaluation of residual MR, degree of mitral stenosis as well as the presence of interatrial shunts using 2D and 3DTEE. Atrial and ventricular views obtained with 3D zoom imaging can be used to determine final clip position (Video 7.4) and identify residual regurgitant jets [12, 13].

## Paravalvular Leak Closure

Paravalvular leaks (PVL) after cardiac valve replacement are rare. They are often incidental findings in routine echocardiographic follow up studies but their clini-cal significance is highly variable: from asymptomatic patients to refractory heart failure and/or severe hemolytic anemia. They can be seen in any cardiac prosthe-ses but frequency is higher in mitral and aortic valves. Diagnosis is based on echo-cardiography. TTE may be able to make the diagnosis in some cases of severe PVL in certain locations, but in most cases, the leak itself is not seen and only indirect Doppler data of high flow across the valve is noted (increased velocity, peak and mean gradients). TEE is always needed to confirm the diagnosis, evalu-ate the shape and size and degree of valvular regurgitation severity. 2D TEE is the first approach but 3D TEE is able to achieve a better assessment of the location, shape, size and degree of regurgitation. All this information is crucial before eval-uating patients for PVL closure. In this setting 3DTEE is clearly superior to 2D TEE [19–21].

## *Prior to the Procedure*

### Mitral Paravalvular Leak

Multiplane 2D TEE allows evaluation of mitral PVL, however a complete assessment of its size and location requires evaluation of the whole annular ring by different 2D and 2D color images acquisition in different exploration angles. (From 0° to 180°). A mental reconstruction is needed afterwards to establish the final diagnosis regarding location, shape and size of the defect. Mitral PVL shape is very variable, being crescent or oblong with tortuous tracks. Evaluation of regurgitation severity is also a challenge. Color Doppler methods are normally used; applying same methods used for native valvular regurgitation specially vena contracta width and PISA effective regurgitant orifice area (EROA). However these methods have important limitations in these patients and the final severity grading should not rely in one parameter but rather in a comprehensive evaluation of the case. 3D TEE overcomes some of these limitations [21]. Regarding anatomic evaluation of the leak, 3D volume acquisition allows a complete visualization of the mitral annular ring with and unique en face view from either the atrial or ventricular aspect. This visualization allows a better assessment of leak location, size and shape (Fig. 7.16 and Video 7.5). In the same way multiple leaks are more easily recognized which is of paramount importance when planning percutaneous PVL closure. Zoom 3D acquisition centered in the mitral prostheses allows this type of images with accurate temporal and spatial resolution in 1 single beat. We recommend to make the acquisition always in the same plane and to visualize the mitral valve in the same orientation to facilitate

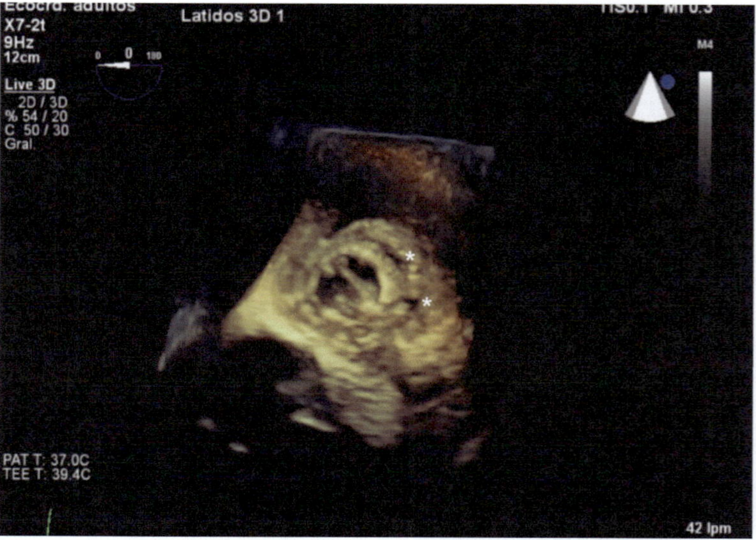


**Fig. 7.16** Live 3D image, "en face" view of a mitral prostheses showing two posterior and posterolateral defects (*), left atrial perspective

a comprehensive evaluation of the prostheses and annular ring. Generally, the clock-face description simulating the surgeon's approach is used for anatomy description in mitral PVL, where the 12-o'clock position of the anterior mitral ring corresponds to the aortic valve, and the 9-o'clock position refers to the left atrial appendage. Possible PVL detected with 3D images need to be confirmed with color 3D images since drop out artifacts are often seen and may mimic an anatomic defect. Color Doppler 3D images can be acquired in any images modality nowadays. Main limitation is temporal resolution and this is the reason high volume rate image acquisition should be used. However, even using high volume rate images temporal resolution may be low. Multiple beat acquisitions will improve temporal resolution but stitching artifacts, especially in patients with atrial fibrillation, will be present. We recommend decreasing the acquisition volume to the region of interest increasing the volume rate and allowing a comprehensive evaluation of the leak. With these images, size, location and shape as well as multiple leaks can be evaluated. Off-line analysis with dedicated software enables the assessment of mitral regurgitation severity by tracing the true area of the vena contracta (EROA) avoiding the limitations described with traditional methods not validated in this scenario. The EROA measured using color Doppler imaging has demonstrated better correlation with the degree or MR than anatomic regurgitant orifice area (AROA) which may overestimate or underestimate the true size due to gain and compression settings [22].

## Aortic Paravalvular Leaks

Aortic PVL are often multiple, eccentric and irregular in shape. Their presence can be masked by reverberation artifacts and acoustic shadowing, making leak identification, visualization and quantification particularly challenging. Although general principles for the assessment of native AR are employed, as in mitral PVL, several of the semi quantitative or quantitative parameters can be inaccurate given the particular nature of the regurgitant jets. As discussed for mitral PVL, multiplane 2D TEE is needed to confirm the diagnosis of aortic PVL. Both mid esofageoual short axis (45°) and left ventricular outflow tract (120°) views are mandatory, however due to the acoustic shadow of the prostheses paravalvular depiction of aortic PVL is difficult, specially those with an anterior location. In some cases, the PVL can be only seen in transgrastric views. Color Doppler is used to assess regurgitant severity, however, vena contracta width or jet width in the LVOT is limited and has not been validated. Extension of the leak in the sewing ring is a better parameters to assess leak severity: <10% being mild regurgitation, 10–30 moderate and >30 severe. Acquisition of 3D zoom images allows a better evaluation of the defect, location and shape. The precise description of the location again remains essential; the surgical view using a clock-face description, would position the tricuspid septal leaflet in the 9-o'clock position. Color 3D image acquisition both with zoom 3D or real time 3D images will help in delineating the true defect, size and shape. As mentioned in mitral PVL, temporal resolution should be optimized. As in mitral PVL, 3D EROA is superior to traditional 2D method prone to errors.

## Guiding the Procedure

PVL closure procedures require TEE guidance. Depending on the location of the leak in the mitral or aortic valve, antegrade trough a transeptal puncture o retrograde access through the aortic valve is decided. In aortic leaks a retrograde approach is used while in mitral leaks either an antegrade or retrograde approach can be used. In mitral leaks a closed loop is sometimes needed to have a close circuit that gives support to the delivery catheter. An initial reassessment to confirm the previous TEE findings is mandatory and can also rule out the presence of thrombi or vegetations [1, 19–21]. Real-time and zoom 3DTEE must identify the anatomic defect to aid the selection of an appropriate closing device, considering its size and position. 2DTTE, but mostly 3DTEE, is essential in guiding the advancement catheters and guide wire and can help manipulation. During the procedure, TEE helps in guiding the transeptal puncture if needed. Afterwards, echo images are essential to confirm that the wire is crossing trough the defect and no trough the prostheses. Once inside, echo images need to confirm the position of the wire in the defect. Even though this can be done with 2D TEE, sometime visualization of the wire is difficult due to acoustic shadows and limitations of wire visualization. 3D TEE overcomes these limitations as it allows a better depiction of the wire and catheter close to the prostheses. Real time 3D images are used with acquired volume size and position adjustment to get best image possible. Delivery sheet is then advanced trough the defect for device deployment. This is normally performed under fluoroscopy and echo guidance, normally 3D. After deployment evaluation of the position is easily performed with 3D images. 3D zoom or real time 3D acquisition allows en face view of the device from the atrial or ventricular aspect to confirm correct position (Fig. 7.17) and absence of complications [21]. Color Doppler is used to evaluate residual regurgitation and location related to the device. 3D color images are superior for evaluation residual regurgitation and location in the sewing ring. If correct position of the device is confirmed with reduction in the severity of regurgitation, it can be safely released and reassessment of the final results can be performed. 3D images are superior to 2D images, especially to better understand the position of the device and its relation to the prostheses ring and other devices.

## Other Applications

### Transeptal Puncture

Transeptal puncture is part of many procedures for the percutaneous treatment of different structural heart disease [1, 2]. Depending on the procedure, a certain location in the fossa ovalis is needed and TEE is mandatory. 3D is superior to 2D since it allows orthogonal simultaneous visualization of the septum with the tenting area, an also because it allows an en face view of the fossa ovalis from the left atria to

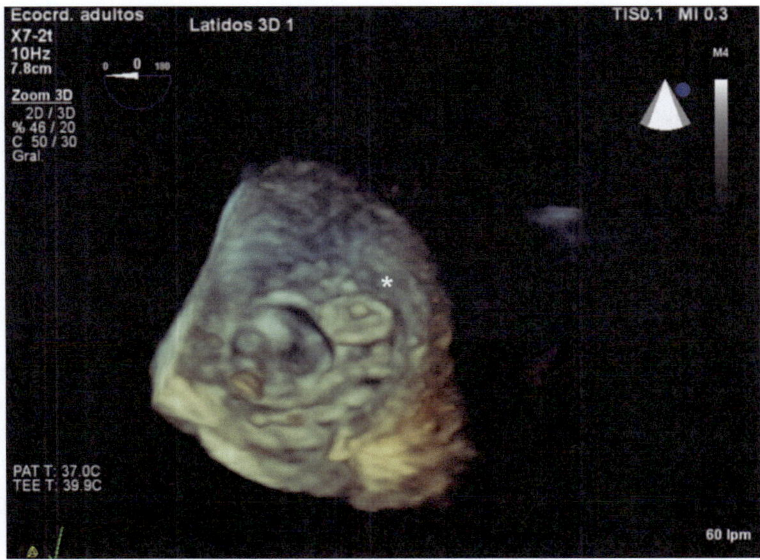

**Fig. 7.17** Live 3D image, "en face" view of a mitral prostheses showing paravalvular leak closure device (*) posterior in the mitral ring (left atrial perspective). Anterior to the device, an smaller defect remains

confirm correct position. X-plane or biplane image modalities are used for the initial tenting evaluation with posterior confirmation through real time 3D images of the septum. Acquisition can be performed in any plane, however, from a 4 chambers view, an excellent evaluation of the septum from the left atrium can be obtained by turning clock-wise the image.

## *Left Atrial Appendage Closure*

Left atrial appendage closure (LAC) has become an alternative to treat patients with high embolic risk atrial fibrillation with contraindications for chronic oral anticoagulation. Based in surgical left atrial appendage ligation, the procedure seals the left atrial appendage with two possible devices (Amplatzer or Watchman) that are deployed inside. Clinical results are promising since the procedure has proved to be safe with and embolic rate in patients treated similar to that of anticoagulated patients. Prior to the procedure LAA thrombus should be ruled out and a comprehensive evaluation of LAA size and shape is mandatory. 2D TEE is able to evaluate LAA dimension and shape but a complete evaluation trough the different 2D planes is needed and images acquires at 0°, 34°, 90°, 120° and 150° evaluated. Size of the ostium and the landing zone (1 cm below the ostium at the level of the left circumflex artery) are measured in the different planes, when the LAA is larger [1, 23]. Maximum diameter obtained in the landing zone is the one used to select the device, which should be 2–4 cm greater in size. Depth of the LAA is also important to assure enough space for the device implantation. Different LAA shapes have been described, chicken wing, cactus, cauliflower and wind stock, which is important to decide procedure strategy in difficult cases. 3D TEE is superior to 2D TEE since it allows a complete evaluation of the LAA from a 3D volume acquisition. Off line analysis and multiplane reconstructions allows evaluation of ostium and landing zone diameter and areas as well as LAA morphology (Fig. 7.18).

Since LAA is a soft tissue structure without calcification or other anatomic landmark visible in fluoroscopy, echo is essential to guide the procedure. First step is transseptal puncture that should be performed inferior and posterior in the fossa oval. The wire is advanced to the LAA and then the delivery catheter is placed in the LAA. TEE both 2D and better 3D allows confirmation of the correct position deep into the LAA for deployment (Fig. 7.19). Deployment is performed under fluoroscopy and echo guidance. Correct position of the device in the LAA, and the outer disc (in the case of Amplatzer device) at the level of the ostium need to be evaluated to confirm complete sealing of the appendage and absence of significant peripheral leak (Fig. 7.20). Normal function of the mitral valve and pulmonary vein flow needs to be assessed as well before de the device can be released [1].

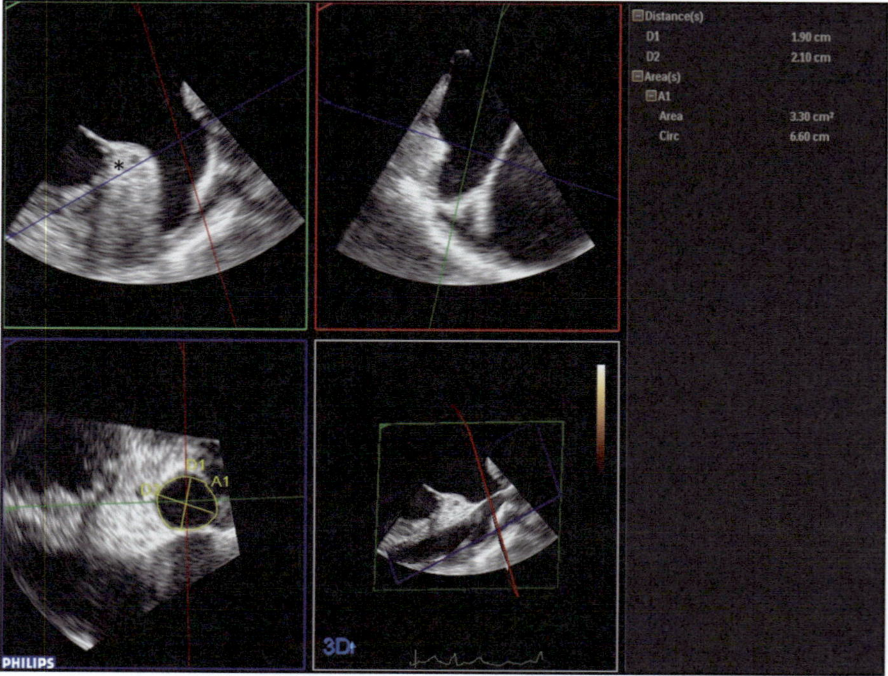


**Fig. 7.18** Multiplanar left atrial appendage reconstruction from a zoom 3D acquisition. Axes area aligned at the level of the landing zone (circumflex artery reference (*), approximately 1 cm below the ostium) where the measurements are performed

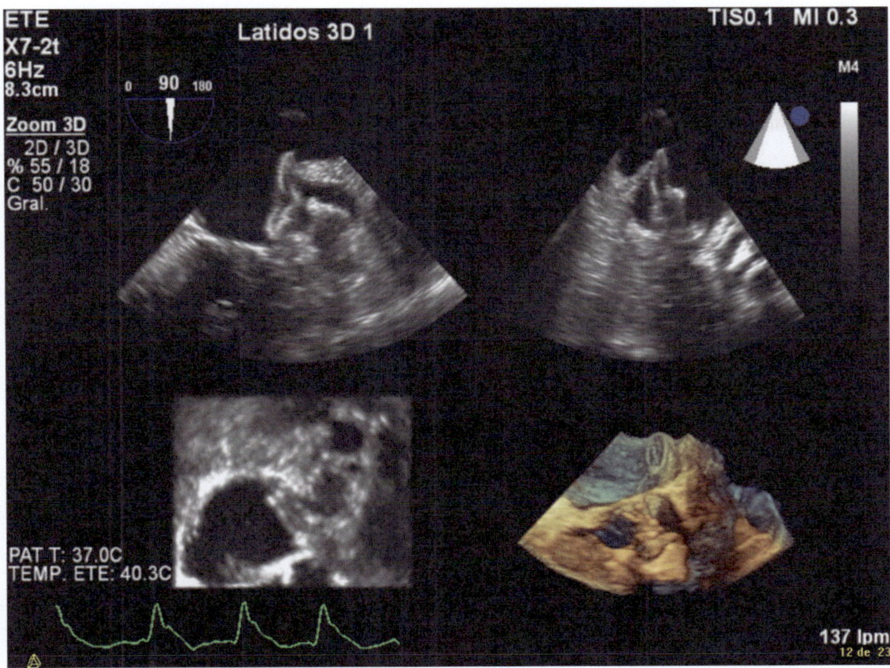

**Fig. 7.19** Zoom 3D image acquisition after left atrial appendage Amplatzer deployment. Evaluation of the position and result can be performed from this images in any plane desired

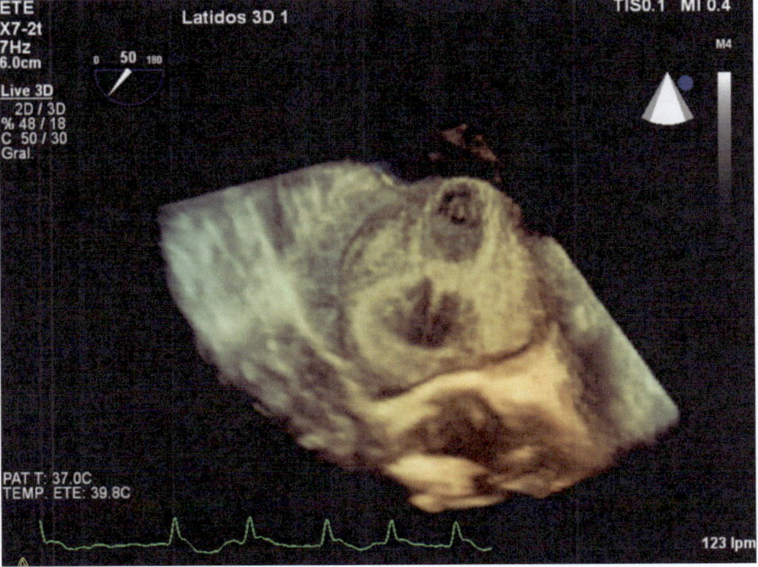

**Fig. 7.20** Live 3D image showing final result after left atrial appendage closure with an Amplatzer device. "En face" view from the left atrial perspective showing the typical "8" image

# References


1. Faletra FF, Pedrazzini G, Pasotti E, et al. 3D TEE during catheter-based interventions. JACC Cardiovasc Imaging. 2014;7:292–308.
2. Balzer J, Kelm M, Kühl HP. Real-time three-dimensional transoesophageal echocardiography for guidance of non-coronary interventions in the catheter laboratory. Eur J Echocardiogr. 2009;10:341–9.
3. Zamorano JL, Badano LP, Bruce C, et al. EAE/ASE recommendations for the use of echocardiography in new transcatheter interventions for valvular heart disease. Eur Heart J. 2011;32:2189–214.
4. Bartel T, Müller S. Device closure of interatrial communications: peri-interventional echocardiographic assessment. Eur Heart J Cardiovasc Imaging. 2013;14:618–24.
5. Kijima Y, Akagi T, Nakagawa K, et al. Three-dimensional echocardiography guided closure of complex multiple atrial septal defects. Echocardiography. 2014;31:E304–6.
6. Zamorano JL, Gonçalves A, Lang R. Imaging to select and guide transcatheter aortic valve implantation. Eur Heart J. 2014;35:1578–87.
7. Smith LA, Monaghan MJ. Monitoring of procedures: peri-interventional echo assessment for transcatheter aortic valve implantation. Eur Heart J Cardiovasc Imaging. 2013;14:840–50.
8. Altiok E, Koos R, Schröder J, et al. Comparison of two-dimensional and three-dimensional imaging techniques for measurement of aortic annulus diameters before transcatheter aortic valve implantation. Heart. 2011;97:1578–84.
9. Smith LA, Dworakowski R, Bhan A, et al. Real-time three-dimensional transesophageal echocardiography adds value to transcatheter aortic valve implantation. J Am Soc Echocardiogr. 2013;4:359–69.
10. Santos N, de Agustin JA, Almeria C, et al. Prosthesis/annulus discongruence assessed by three-dimensional transesophageal echocardiography: a predictor of significant para valvular aortic regurgitation after transcatheter aortic valve implantation. Eur Heart J Cardiovasc Imaging. 2012;13:931–7.
11. Kappetein AP, Head SJ, Généreux P, et al. Updated standardized endpoint definitions for transcatheter aortic valve implantation: the valve academic research consortium-2 consensus document (VARC-2). Eur J Cardiothorac Surg. 2012;42:S45–60.
12. Wunderlich NC, Siegel RJ. Peri-interventional echo assessment for the mitraclip procedure. Eur Heart J Cardiovasc Imaging. 2013;14:935–9.
13. Quaife RA, Salcedo EE, Carroll JD. Procedural guidance using advance imaging techniques for percutaneous edge-to-edge mitral valve repair. Curr Cardiol Rep. 2014;16:452. doi:10.1007/s11886-013-0452-5.
14. Jain S, Malouf JF. Incremental value of 3-D transesophageal echo- cardiographic imaging of the mitral valve. Curr Cardiol Rep. 2014;16:439. doi:10.1007/s11886-013-0439-2.
15. Lancellotti P, Moura L, Pierard LA, et al. European association of echocardiography recommendations for the assessment of valvu- lar regurgitation. Part 2: mitral and tricuspid regurgitation (native valve disease). Eur J Echocardiogr. 2010;11:307–32.
16. Kahlert P, Plicht B, Schenk IM, et al. Direct assessment of size and shape of non-circular vena contracta area in functional versus organic mitral regurgitation using real-time three-dimensional echocardiography. J Am Soc Echocardiogr. 2008;21:912–21.
17. de Agustín JA, Marcos-Alberca P, Fernandez-Golfin C, et al. Direct measurement of proximal isovelocity surface area by single-beat three-dimensional color Doppler echocardiography in mitral regurgitation: a validation study. J Am Soc Echocardiogr. 2012;25:815–23.
18. Faletra FF, Pedrazzini G, Pasotti E, et al. Role of real-time three dimensional transoesophageal echocardiography as guidance imaging modality during catheter based edge-to-edge mitral valve repair. Heart. 2013;99:1204–15.
19. Kliger C, Eiros R, Isasti G, et al. Review of surgical prosthetic paravalvular leaks: diagnosis and catheter-based closure. Eur Heart J. 2013;34:638–49.

20. Kim MS, Casserly IP, Garcia JA, et al. Percutaneous transcatheter closure of prosthetic mitral paravalvular leaks: are we there yet? J Am Coll Cardiol Intv. 2009;2:81–90.
21. Becerra JM, Almeria C, de Isla LP, et al. Usefulness of 3D transoesophageal echocardiography for guiding wires and closure devices in mitral perivalvular leaks. Eur J Echocardiogr. 2009;10:979–81.
22. Franco E, Almería C, de Agustín JA, et al. Three-dimensional color Doppler transesophageal echocardiography for mitral paravalvular leak quantification and evaluation of percutaneous closure success. J Am Soc Echocardiogr. 2014;27:1153–63.
23. Wunderlich NC, Beigel R, Swaans MJ, et al. Percutaneous interventions for left atrial appendage exclusion: options, assessment, and imaging using 2D and 3D echocardiography. JACC Cardiovasc Imaging. 2015;8:472–88.

# Chapter 8
# Fusion of 3D-Echocardiography and Other Imaging Modalities: Hybrid Imaging

Eduardo Casas Rojo and María Valverde Gómez

## History of Fusion Imaging

Since the advent of non-invasive coronary angiography by MDCT there have been numerous works that have validated or proven clinical usefulness of various image fusion systems in order to supplement the anatomical data provided by MDCT with functional information from other imaging modalities. In 2005 Namdar et al. [1] described a system that combined on the same equipment 4 slices MDCT and PET, which obtained hybrid images for visualizing perfusion defects in relation to the corresponding artery or coronary branch, quantifying in 25 patients sensitivity (S), specificity (Sp), positive predictive value (PPV) and negative predictive value (NPV) of 90, 98, 82 and 99%, respectively, taking as the gold standard the combination of PET and invasive coronary angiography. Similar findings have been found in other studies using hybrid equipment with more advanced features.

Gaemperli et al. [2] in 2007 validated a fusion imaging system that did not require hybrid equipment. Instead of that approach this system merged the results of two studies from different machines, in this case 64 slices MDCT and SPECT, which were fused by software. In another publication of the same year [3] the authors showed their clinical experience and demonstrated the incremental value of

When shall we open our minds to the conviction that the ultimate reality of the world is neither matter nor spirit, is no definite thing, but a perspective?

José Ortega y Gasset.

**Electronic supplementary material** The online version of this chapter (doi:10.1007/978-3-319-50335-6_8) contains supplementary material, which is available to authorized users.

E.C. Rojo (✉) • M.V. Gómez
Cardiology Department, Hospital Ramon y Cajal, Madrid, Spain
e-mail: ecasasweb@hotmail.com

© Springer International Publishing AG 2017
E. Casas Rojo et al. (eds.), *Manual of 3D Echocardiography*,
DOI 10.1007/978-3-319-50335-6_8

the merged images vs. interpretation of two separate studies in cases with equivocal or inconsistent findings, allowing to exclude the relevance of 25% of these lesions and showing it in 35% of these cases where the coincidence or "matching" of the anatomical structure with perfusion defect location could not be proven without the help of the combined image. Other studies have increased the documentation of these clinical findings with similar systems [4].

There are also studies that have shown the contribution of fusion of nuclear medicine imaging (SPECT and PET) and MDCT in the therapeutic strategy and revascularization of coronary heart disease due to its ability to accurately locate the artery responsible for the ischemia. The influence of hybrid studies in decision-making and in the number of invasive coronary angiographies required has been proved, and a good reliability of findings in relation to the prognosis of injuries has been assessed [4].

Another approach for obtaining hybrid images with anatomical and functional assessment is to use one technique to acquire two separate studies on the same equipment and then merge them with software. This is the case of the work from White et al. [5] in which 3-Tesla CMR is used to obtain images of the arterial and venous coronary anatomy and to combine them with sequences characterizing the scar in patients with chronic coronary artery disease, suggesting its utility in planning coronary intervention and cardiac resynchronization therapy.

In another work related to image fusion [6], SPECT was combined with pharmacological stress 3D echocardiography in 20 patients with known or suspected coronary artery disease, and in those with available invasive coronary angiography it was found that the hybrid system was superior to individual studies to identify the presence of significant coronary artery disease.

These hybrid systems are promising but have limitations such as high cost (specially when CMR is involved), and radiation dose when using PET or SPECT, because while current MDCT technology has achieved a dramatic reduction in dose, in Nuclear Medicine studies the improvement is not so significant.

## 3D Stress Echocardiography

2D echocardiography at rest may be useful for suspecting coronary disease if abnormal regional contractility is detected. However, in the absence of such anomalies, stress testing, either with exercise or with pharmacological stress (dobutamine, dipyridamole, adenosine), will be necessary for assessing ischaemia. 3D echocardiography (3DE) may add more accurate calculation of volumes and ejection fraction to the rest echocardiography, but the amount of data supporting the advantages of performing 3DE under a stress protocol are limited.

Amhmad et al. [7] tested in 2001 the feasibility of a protocol of dobutamine stress testing with 3DE in addition to 2D. They showed acceptable agreement in the assessing of regional contractility at baseline (84%, Kappa = 0.59) and good agreement at peak (88.9%, Kappa = 0.72); 3DE showed lower interobserver variability, it was acquired in less time and the sensibility for detection of coronary disease was higher compared with 2D.

Matsamura et al. [8] found similar sensitivity, specificity and accuracy of 3D and 2D, taking SPECT as the gold standard, and similar results were obtained in a study with coronary angiography [9]. However in another study with 3D and 3D contrast echocardiography [10], the agreement between both methods was only moderate, probably because of the limitations of a bigger transducer and lower frame rates.

More recently, perfusion by 3D myocardial contrast echocardiography, in addition to contractility assessment, has proven to be feasible [11, 12], but there are not clear advantages over 2D contrast echocardiography at the moment.

In the last years, new approaches like multi-slice mode [13] and high volume-rate scanners [14] with the new small transducers have improved the quality of 3DE during stress, and it has been showed to be superior to 2D specially in the assessment of left anterior descending artery disease, because of a better definition of the apical segments. In another study [15], 2D seems to be better for assessing the base, the mid-inferior and the inferoseptal segments, suggesting that a combined 2D and 3D protocol would be the best.

A new modality for 3DE contractility assessment during stress would be 3DST echocardiography. There are few data available for this approach as a stand-alone protocol, although it is technically feasible (Fig. 8.1), and it may be the key to achieve another way of imaging fusion, as explained on the following section. The protocol for acquiring stress 3DST is the same one which is explained on Chap. 6, with a baseline acquisition before starting exercise or pharmacological stress, followed by a generic 2D stress echocardiography protocol, and an additional acquisition at peak stress, that usually requires to enter the "pause" mode of the stress protocol for changing to 3D probe and acquiring the 3DST images at peak stress.

## Fusion of Coronary Multidetector Tomography and 3D Speckle-Tracking

### *Overview*

In 2008, as explained on Chap. 6, the first 3D echocardiography equipment capable of performing three-dimensional analysis of myocardial deformation in all segments simultaneously from a single apical acquisition (3D-Speckle-tracking, 3DST) was validated. The three-dimensional imaging of the left ventricle with color coding of the degree of myocardial deformation, as volumetric representation or polar map, similar to Gated SPECT, has opened the possibility of performing hybrid imaging systems that combine these images with those obtained by

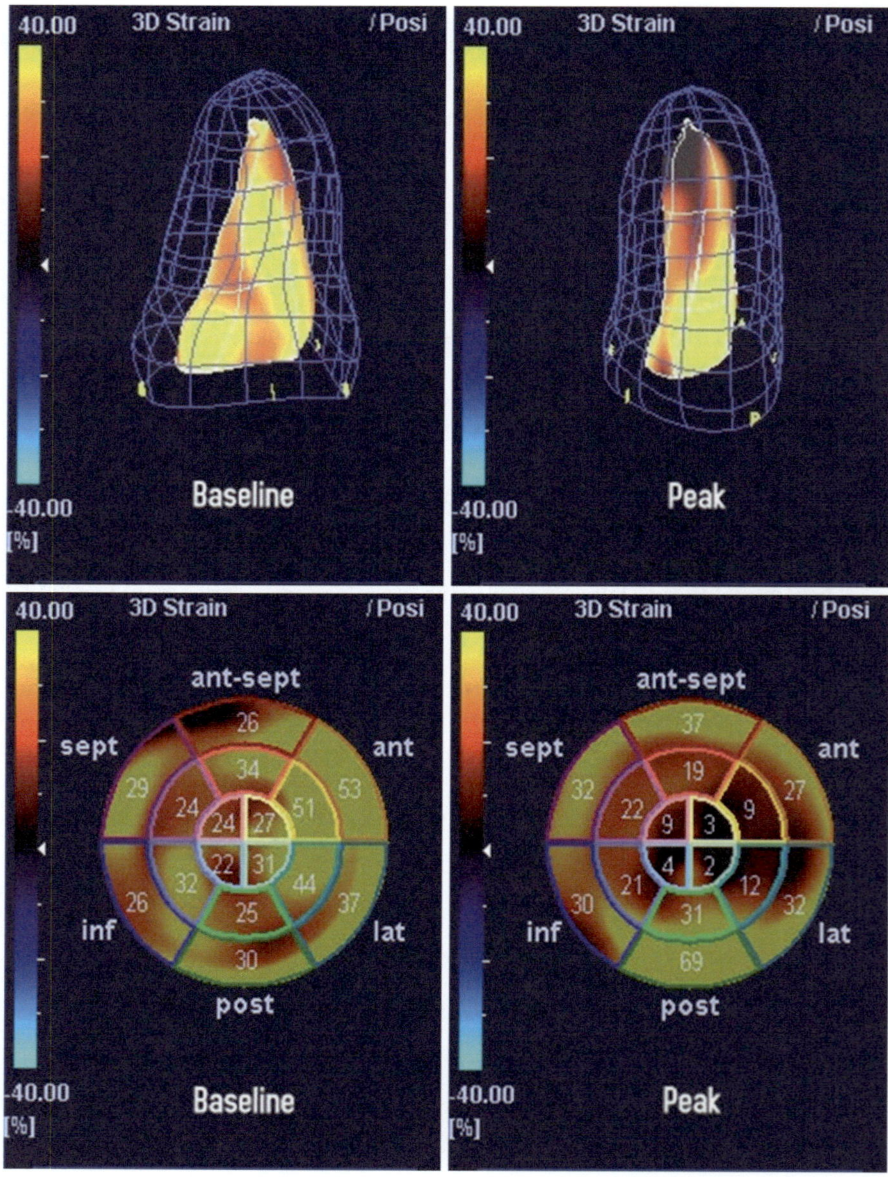


**Fig. 8.1** 3D Speckle-tracking applied to dobutamine stress echocardiography. Plastic bag and polar map views on the left belong to baseline acquisition, with normal LV function and normal regional values of 3D strain. Similar views on the right show acquisition at peak stress, with lower values of strain on apex and anterior/anterolateral wall due to ischaemia, and higher values on the rest of territories, as expected with dobutamine at high dose

MDCT. In 2013 a prototype of hybrid imaging software was introduced. The initial tests explored fusion between MDCT and 3DST rest echocardiography, which may be useful in the presence of regional contractility abnormality at rest (Fig. 8.2);

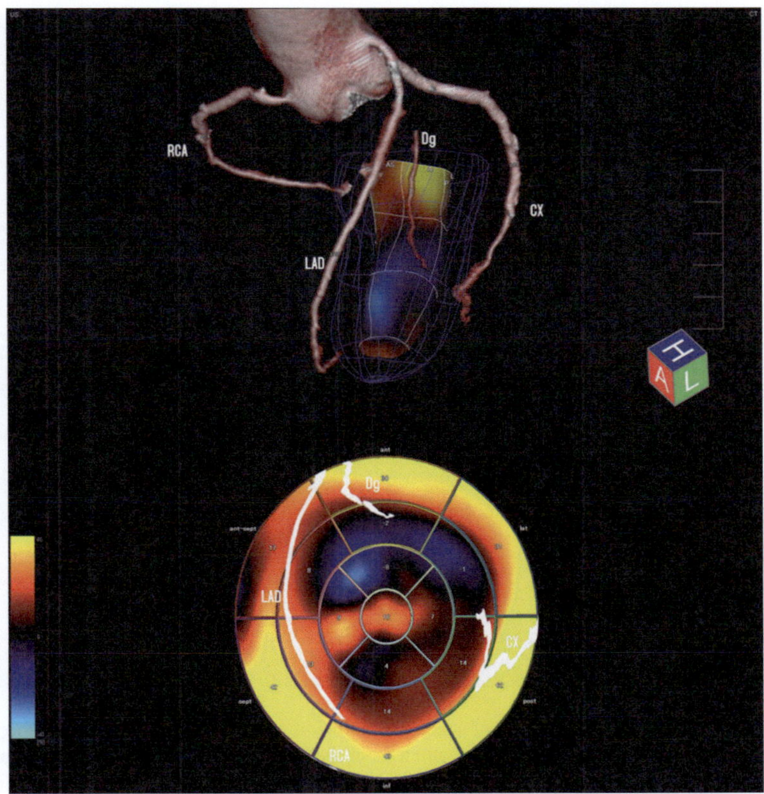


**Fig. 8.2** Fusion of rest 3DST echocardiography and MDCT. The area of low contractility at the apex and anterior wall could easily be interpreted as a sign of LAD disease. The hybrid view made clear that it was related with a sub-occluded Diagonal branch

however our group published the first case in which the hybrid image is used with images of 3D speckle-tracking within a pharmacological stress echocardiography protocol, in order to compare the 3D strain information at rest and at peak stress while assessing the relationship between these changes and the coronary anatomy [16]. See Fig. 8.3 for details. These hybrid images are obtained semi-automatically from the MDCT DICOM files and 3DST echocardiography, through the use of common landmarks that the system easily recognizes. In case of finding inaccuracies the overlapping images can be manipulated for better alignment (Fig. 8.4).

## *Hybrid Imaging Modalities*

- Volumetric 3D reconstruction (Fig. 8.5). It shows the aortic root, the coronary tree and left ventricular volumetric images that can be viewed as still images or moving throughout the cardiac cycle. Different color codes represent the magnitude of the deformation parameter chosen (usually 3D strain, but the representation of the

　　　　　　　　　　　　　　　　　　　　　　　　　　　　　　　E.C. Rojo and M.V. Gómez

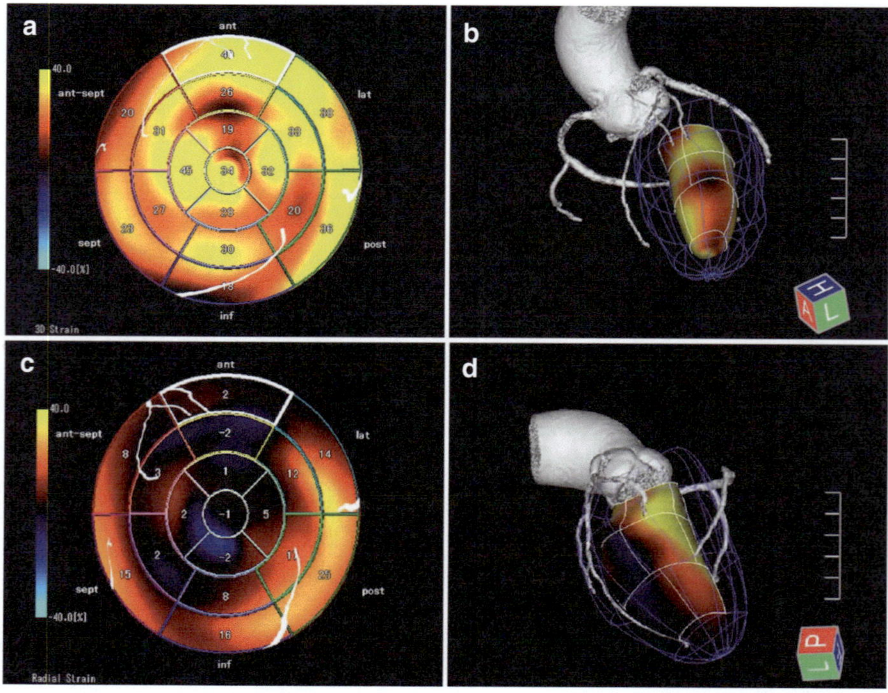

**Fig. 8.3** First case ever documented of stress 3DST fusion with MDCT. A patient with three vessels disease underwent dobutamine stress and a large area of septal, apical and anterior ischaemia was assessed. The hybrid view showed the relationship of this area with the LAD artery. Images A/B belong to the baseline study and C/D belong to the peak stress

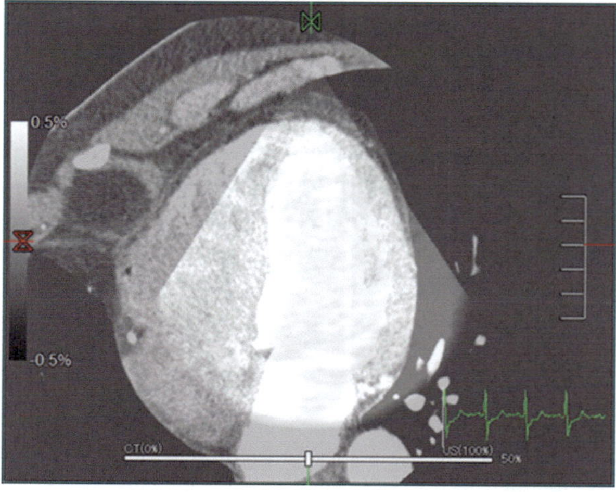

**Fig. 8.4** Overlapping of MDCT and ultrasound images of the left ventricle for fusion

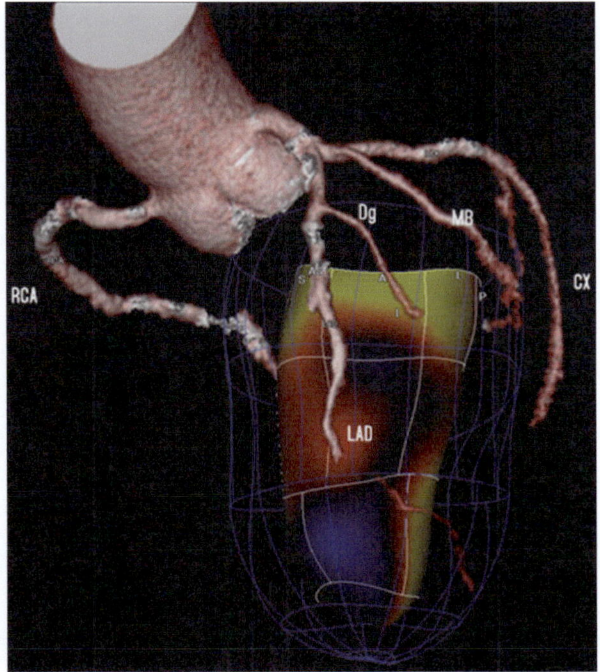


**Fig. 8.5** Volumetric 3D reconstruction of the aortic root, coronary arteries and left ventricle. A critical stenosis of the distal LAD matches with an area of low 3D strain at the apex

radial, longitudinal strain, area-strain, etc. can be chosen). In the most common encoding, the dark blue areas correspond to regions with hypokinesia, and areas of yellow color mark segments with greater contractility. The visualization of the coronary arteries and the LV strain at the same time allows to visually check the "matching" between the coronary stenosis and hypokinetic regions.

- Polar map or bullseye view (Fig. 8.6). It shows 16 or 17 myocardial segments (depending on the selected model) with the average strain in each segment, and the middle-distal segments of the coronary arteries superimposed on them. The color code of the polar map is the same as for encoding the LV volumetric reconstruction. There is also an *anatomic coronary territories map* (Fig. 8.7) that depending on the size and shape of the arteries of each particular patient, sets three areas that would belong to Left Anterior Descending, Circumflex and Right Coronary artery. This approach may be more useful that the usual assignation of certain myocardial segments to certain coronary arteries. Moreover, the average strain for each area can be shown, and the increase or decrease of strain during stress testing can be quantified. If this system is validated in the near future, quantitative stress echocardiography may be a reality.

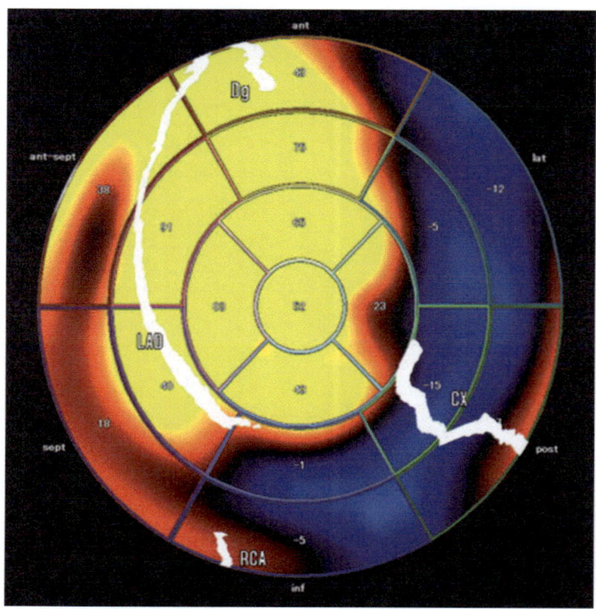


**Fig. 8.6** Polar map with myocardial segments, coronary arteries and radial strain color coding in a patient with prior myocardial infarction involving occlusion of the CX. Fusion was performed after stenting. The dark area on the anterolateral and inferolateral wall matches with the CX territory

## Advantages of the Hybrid TC + 3D-ST System

The advantages of the combination of coronary anatomy and functional assessment have been already tested with SPECT/PET and MDCT fusion, as explained in the first section of this chapter. The simultaneous assessment of both aspects of the disease on the same image provides an incremental value over the separate interpretation of both tests. This information may influence the decisions of physicians, and the matching of anatomic and functional findings correlates with prognosis. The new strategy of using echocardiography has an obvious advantage over SPECT or PET and is the absence of harmful radiation. With the same coronary tree as reference, several studies may be compared in the follow-up of a patient without additional radiation.

## Limitations of the Technique

The inclusion of echocardiography as a functional component of these hybrid systems instead of perfusion techniques such as PET or SPECT has the limitation on not assessing perfusion directly, but the impact of such perfusion on cardiac mechanics. Also, 3DST technology allows for spectacular images thanks to automated endocardial and epicardial border detection, but the accuracy of these systems is highly dependent on the quality of the ultrasonic window. When this is not optimal, manual corrections are often needed, and the reproducibility of the studies may be not as good.

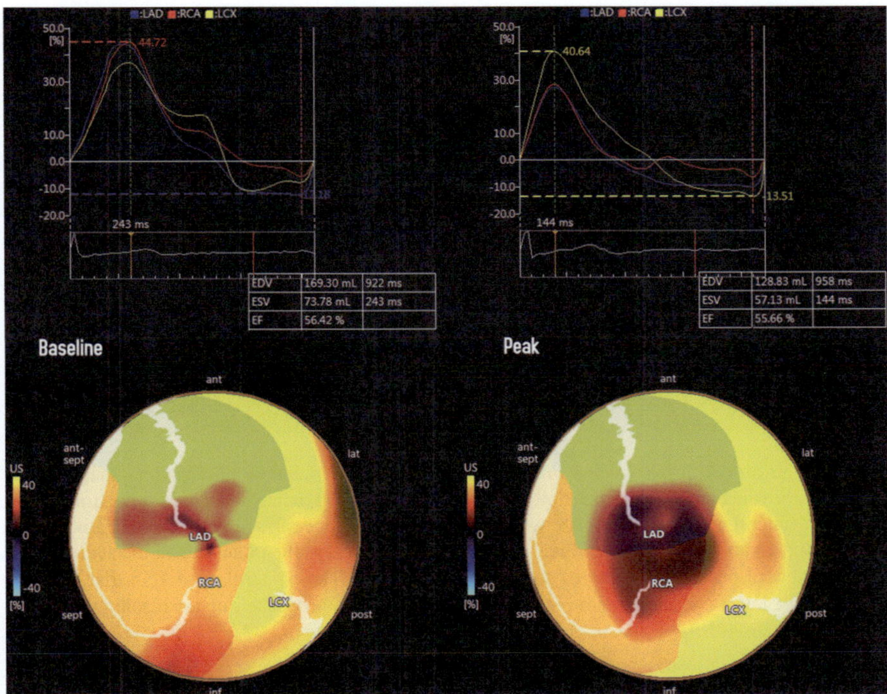

**Fig. 8.7** Anatomic coronary territories in a patient with three vessels disease and ischaemic response on dobutamine stress. This modality of polar map shows the distribution of myocardium in relation with each coronary vessel, and graphics show curves of 3D strain for each territory. At baseline (left figures) strain is normal all over the surface of the polar map, and curves show high proportions of strain for the three territories; at peak (right figures) an area of low strain appears at the apex with extension to both LAD and RCA territories. The graphics show a decrease of strain in LAD and RCA related territory and an increase in CX territory

In addition, the frame rate of these studies (usually around 20–25 vps), is a major limitation, especially when used in patients with elevated heart rates, as it occurs during exercise or pharmacological stress, which is precisely the moment when the hybrid image has more clinical utility. However clinical validation studies of the system that are ongoing will provide the real clinical utility of the technique.

## *Future Directions*

One line of research is the emerging application of the hybrid system for visualizing coronary veins in combination with image speckle-tracking, in this case fusion is aimed at locating the segments with the latest activation of contraction and their relationship with a particular coronary vein (Fig. 8.8). A clinical case applying this approach has been already published [17]. The hybrid image in this context might be helpful for locating the most appropriate vein for left ventricular pacing in cardiac resynchronization therapy.

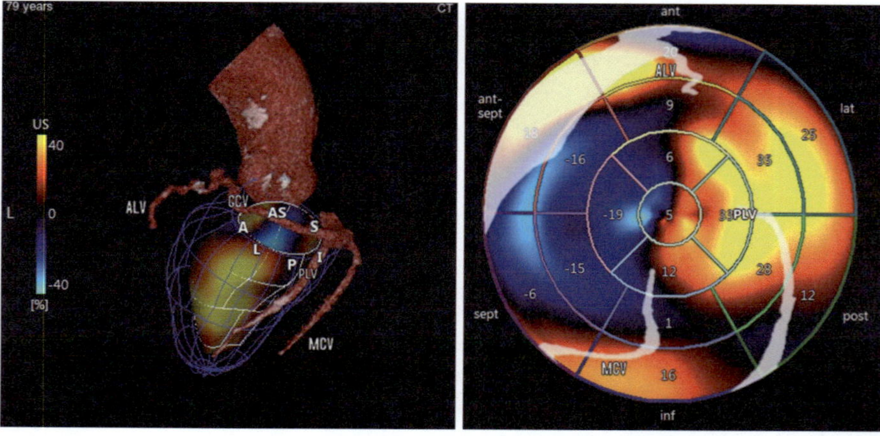


**Fig. 8.8** Fusion of coronary veins MDCT and 3DST-derived radial strain. The left image shows the coronary veins and the left ventricle at late systole, showing the area of latest activation in yellow color (lateral wall). The opposite wall (septal), with earlier contraction, shows negative strain at that moment and it is colored in blue. The right image displays the polar map at the same frame. The differences between both areas suggest dyssynchrony. The posterolateral vein that emerges just from the latest contraction area, would probably be the appropriate one for placing the lead if resynchronization therapy was applied

It is also expected further development of 3DST technology for increasing image quality, reliability of the automatic detection and tracking of endocardial and epicardial borders, and the frame rate. Additionally, a system with vendor independence allowing to use data from different 3DST systems would increase the clinical applicability on daily practice.

# 3D Echocardiography and Fluoroscopy: Echo Navigator

Minimally-invasive cardiovascular interventions are becoming wider and wider spread because of their demonstrated effectiveness and safety. Two-dimensional (2D) X-ray imaging used to be the dominant imaging modality for guiding this kind of cardiac procedures. It offers some advantages, such as its high definition of catheters, valves and metallic and calcified structures, as well as its good temporal resolution. However, fluoroscopy has also some pitfalls. It is inadequate to visualize soft tissues, only provides 2D imaging and implies contrast and radiation.

That is why echocardiography has turned into an essential tool inside the Cath Lab. It has all the attributes that fluoroscopy lacks: it is a non-radiation, non-contrast technique, that allows continuous soft tissue imaging. Moreover, if implemented, transesophageal echocardiography (TEE) and 3D echocardiography provide better understanding of morphology and spatial relation of intracardiac structures than transthoracic and 2D echocardiography (TTE) [18].

During interventional procedures, fluoroscopy for catheter and device visualization and echocardiography for anatomy and soft tissue imaging are most frequently used. But up to now, none of them offered a simultaneous evaluation of both types of structures, thus requiring several screens and extensive effort of coordination and communication between imagers and operators.

Recently, a new navigation system (EchoNavigator, Philips Healthcare, Best, the Netherlands) has been introduced which synchronizes echocardiography and fluoroscopy in real-time. This new imaging technology seeks to improve the communication between the echocardiographer and the interventionalist, to increase the confidence and anatomical awareness, to assist in guidance, and to increase procedural efficiency [19, 20].

The EchoNavigator places the two imaging modalities in the same coordinate system and is based on the localization and tracking of the TEE probe. After synchronization of TEE and fluoroscopy images, the system automatically tracks and follows the movements of the c-arm gantry. This way, if the c-arm is moved, echocardiography images are updated and reconstructed with the same angulation, allowing rapid understanding of the anatomy and the relation between cardiac structures and devices during complex interventions.

Furthermore, Markers (dots or crosses) can be set to highlight important structures on the echocardiography image, and they are automatically displayed and updated in real time on the fluoroscopy image. It appears particularly useful for guiding complex catheter or device manipulations with the target of the displayed marker, potentially reaching an important reduction of time and radiation.

In a more practical focus, we are going to describe how the usual performance of this technology is, how the images are presented and what its main clinical applications are.

At the beginning of a procedure the TEE probe is co-registered by the acquisition of two angulated fluoroscopy projections [21]. Once the algorithm recognizes the TEE probe and its orientation, the TEE and x-ray images are combined and can be manipulated.

The system offers a four image display (Fig. 8.9) usually displaying the following views: (1) the fluoroscopy view; (2) the c-arm gantry view, in which the echocardiographic view is oriented in the same plane as the x-ray view (and automatically updated by each movement of the c-arm); (3) the echocardiographic view which is the standard TEE projection showing up on the echocardiographer's screen; and (4) a free image that can be rotated or cropped.

Therefore, EchoNavigator allows the physician (usually very experienced in the use of fluoroscopic images but less so in using ultrasonic images) to use the more intuitive perspective of fluoroscopic images but with the additional information, specifically 3-D soft-tissue visualization, provided by echocardiography. Major spatial transformations such as the mental rotation of ultrasound images displayed in an unfamiliar perspective, no longer have to be performed by the physician after the automatic registration of ultrasound with x-ray and the display of the modalities in a familiar perspective [22].

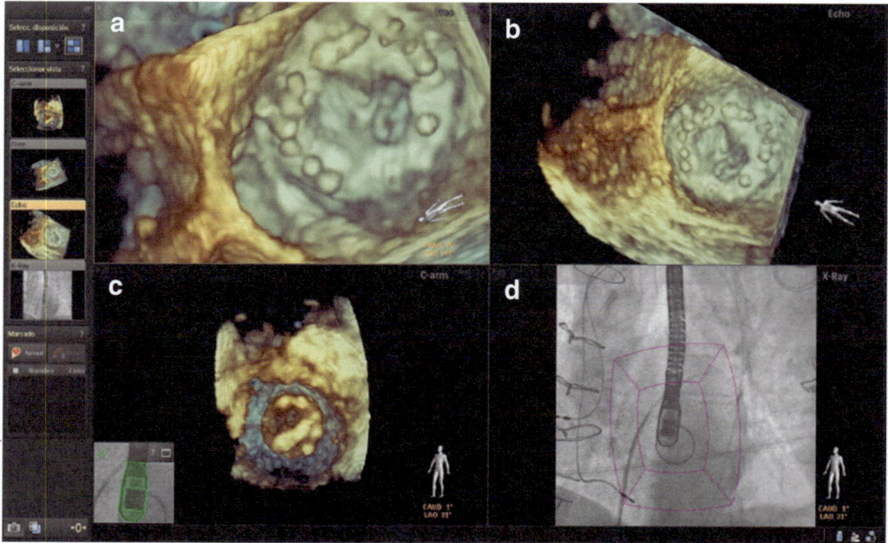

**Fig. 8.9** Echo-Navigator. Whole screen with four simultaneous real-time imaging modalities during mitral prosthesis leak closure. Two upper images from 3D TEE show different points of view for showing the interventional cardiologist the situation of the leak and its relationship with the surrounding structures. On the right inferior image, the fluoroscopy view matches with the pyramidal 3D echo display on the left inferior display, and both images are synchronized for moving together when the X-ray arm is being moved

In Chap. 7, guiding of interventional procedures is explained in detail. However in the following sections we will summarize the specific role of Echonavigator in the most common procedures.

## *Transcatheter Aortic Valve Replacement (TAVR)*

With all the features described above, it seems easy to recognize the utility of a coordinated system of fluoroscopy and echocardiography in TAVR. There are certain steps in the whole procedure (as balloon valvuloplasty, prosthesis implantation) where the possibilities of EchoNavigator improve the communication of the heart team, getting a safer and more effective intervention. For the Sapien valve, roughly half of the device should be above and below the aortic annulus. For the CoreValve, TEE should confirm that the nitinol stent is well within the borders of the calcified native annulus. Visualizing the valve during the time of rapid pacing and balloon inflation (for the Sapien valve) or deployment of the CoreValve provides an immediate verification of correct valve placement [23].

Probably the most recognizable application of EchoNavigator in TAVR is in patients with less calcified valves, where visualizing the aortic annulus in fluoroscopy may be more challenging. The level of the annulus can be marked in an echocardiography image and these markers will be automatically transposed and set in the fluoroscopy image (Figs. 8.10 and 8.11), allowing the use of this reference for catheter guidance and evaluation of prosthesis implantation depth [24].

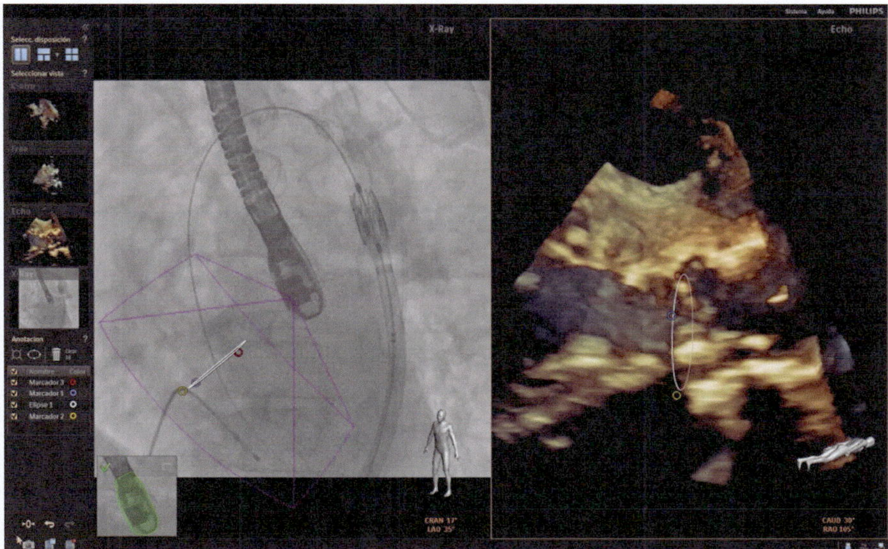

**Fig. 8.10** Echo-Navigator. On the right, 3D TEE of the left ventricle outflow tract. 3 color markers and a ellipse have been drawn for locating the aortic annulus. On the left, fluoroscopy guided by a synchronized display of the color markers and the ellipse

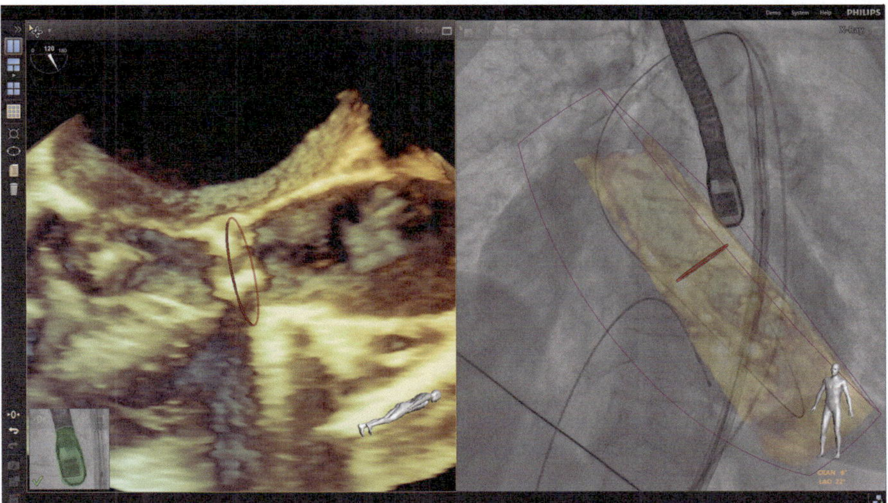

**Fig. 8.11** Echo-Navigator. Fusion image combining fluoroscopy and 3D TEE on the same display, with the aortic annulus previously marked with a red ellipse

## *Percutaneous Mitral Valve Repair*

The complexity of structural heart disease interventions such as edge-to edge mitral valve repair requires integration of multiple highly technical imaging modalities. This integration usually occurs in the brain of experienced interventionalist viewing at least two different image display monitors and mentally fusing the individual datasets. EchoNavigator has significantly impacted the display of critical image targets. This combined display technology allows rotation and orientation of both dataset at the discretion of the interventionalist in perspectives necessary to define targets and guidance of device manipulation [22].

The use of the EchoNavigator during MitraClip interventions is of particular interest during two procedural steps: puncture of the interatrial septum, and catheter steering for optimal clip placement. The former must be performed in a specific site (posterior and superior location, in the interatrial septum, and 4 cm above the mitral annulus) that allows manipulation of the system inside the left atrium (LA) and grasping of leaflets. The optimal puncture site is identified in the TEE four-chamber view (or roughly 0°) where the required distance can easily be measured [imagen, si no nuestra de 5, 5a]. For the perforation however, the TEE angle is increased to roughly 45° and the simultaneous biplane or multiple plane function activated. The bicaval view is then used as an overlay on top of the fluoroscopy. This ensures a fast but nevertheless safe and very precise puncture of the interatrial septum [25].

Once the interatrial septum is perforated and the sheet in place, steering the MC delivery system down to the mitral valve can be challenging on two- dimensional fluoroscopy. Erroneous steering may lead to long radiation and procedure time and potentially damage the left atrium free wall. Fusing live 2D and 3D echocardiography with fluoroscopy is safe and feasible in most patients and shows a trend towards reduction of fluoroscopy and procedure time [26].

It is worth mentioning that this kind of hybrid imaging has also a potencial impact in the possible new future of Transcatheter Mitral Valve Replacement, especially in valve-in-native-valve procedures [27].

## *Atrial Septal Defect (ASD) Closure*

The EchoNavigator system is particularly appreciated in the presence of multi-fenestrated ASD. In this case the precise placement of the device is at least as important as the choice of the appropriate device size, and the simultaneous visualization of the echocardiographic and x-ray images facilitates passage of the largest defect [19].

So, without echocardiographic imaging, there is a high likelihood that the wire will pass the septum in a non-targeted manner. Overlay image and/or the use of a marker ensure passage of the correct perforation and lead to complete ASD/PFO closure. Overlay imaging supports fast and safe deployment of the device since there is constant control of the correct position of the sheet orifice within the left atrium. Using overlay imaging, this procedure can be performed without the use of contrast agents [28].

## *Left Atrial Appendage (LAA) Closure*

In this context, where EchoNavigator has its best application is in the guidance of transseptal puncture. Most operators prefer an inferoposterior, others a mid to superior and posterior puncture. Anyway, the use of markers is helpful to localize the otherwise invisible LAA structures on fluoroscopy and prevent catastrophic complications (as perforation of the LAA wall and laceration of the pulmonary artery). Such markers can be placed at the LAA orifice (at the level of the circumflex artery), the orifice of the left upper pulmonary vein (warfarin ridge), or the tip or bottom of the LAA. That done, the overlay imaging facilitate and ensure correct device position [29].

## *Paravalvular Leaks (PVL) Closure*

Three-dimensional TEE is currently one of the preferred techniques, both for pre-procedural assessment and for intra-intervention guidance, due to its capacity to provide a better identification of multiple defects and accurate measurement of irregularly shaped orifices [29, 30]. But it is not enough in the case of mechanical prosthesis, because of the possible shadowing. In such scenarios, the challenge is overtaken thanks to its combination with fluoroscopy: that is, EchoNavigator.

In mitral leaks, the closure can be performed using either a retrograde or anterograde approach [31]. EchoNavigator results really helpful defining together both soft tissues (in the echocardiographic images) and wires and metal structures (in the X-ray ones). It is almost mandatory, as previously mentioned, in the transseptal puncture (if the anterograde approach is chosen) and really clarifying in detecting the leaks and positioning the devices. Also, Real-time 3DE provides an en face view of the mitral prosthesis, allowing accurate assessment of the number, localization, size, and shape of the paravalvular dehiscence [32].

In para-Aortic leaks (where retrograde transaortic approach is usually preferred), also, 3D-TEE and fluoroscopy are used as guidance to ensure the correct wire placement. Using markers and real-time overlay imaging facilitates localizing the perforation site and enables wire passage with- out the use of contrast.

Chapter 8 – Videos

VIDEO 1 – 3DST/CT fusion. Suboclussion of diagonal branch matches with 3D strain anterolateral area.

VIDEO 2 – 3DST/CT fusion. Anterior, anterolateral and apical hypokynesia during dobutamine stress in a patient with 3 vessel disease. Hybrid images can be rotated and tilted.

VIDEO 3 – 3DST/CT fusion. Comparison between rest and stress study displaying coronary areas. for the particular anatomy of the patient. Ischaemia on LAD and RCA territories is best assessed when stopping the loop at peak systole.

VIDEO 4 – Echo Navigator. Fusion between 2D echocardiography and fluoroscopy during transseptal puncture.

VIDEO 5 – Echo Navigator. Fusion between 3D TEE and fluoroscopy during left atrial appendage closure.

# References


1. Namdar M, Hany TF, Koepfli P, Siegrist PT, Burger C, Wyss CA, Luscher TF, von Schulthess GK, Kaufmann PA. Integrated PET/CT for the assessment of coronary artery disease: a feasibility study. J Nucl Med. 2005;46(6):930–5. PubMed PMID: 15937302
2. Gaemperli O, Schepis T, Kalff V, Namdar M, Valenta I, Stefani L, Desbiolles L, Leschka S, Husmann L, Alkadhi H, Kaufmann PA. Validation of a new cardiac image fusion software for three-dimensional integration of myocardial perfusion SPECT and stand-alone 64-slice CT angiography. Eur J Nucl Med Mol Imaging. 2007;34(7):1097–106. Epub 2007 Jan 24. PubMed PMID: 17245532
3. Gaemperli O, Schepis T, Valenta I, Husmann L, Scheffel H, Duerst V, Eberli FR, Luscher TF, Alkadhi H, Kaufmann PA. Cardiac image fusion from stand-alone SPECT and CT: clinical experience. J Nucl Med. 2007;48(5):696–703. Erratum in: J Nucl Med. 2007;48(7):1095. PubMed PMID: 17475956
4. Gaemperli O, Saraste A, Knuuti J. Cardiac hybrid imaging. Eur Heart J Cardiovasc Imaging. 2012;13(1):51–60. doi:10.1093/ejechocard/jer240. Epub 2011 Nov 17. Review. PubMed PMID: 22094239
5. White JA, Fine N, Gula LJ, Yee R, Al-Admawi M, Zhang Q, Krahn A, Skanes A, MacDonald A, Peters T, Drangova M. Fused whole-heart coronary and myocardial scar imaging using 3-T CMR. Implications for planning of cardiac resynchronization therapy and coronary revascularization. JACC Cardiovasc Imaging. 2010;3(9):921–30. doi:10.1016/j.jcmg.2010.05.014. PubMed PMID: 20846626
6. Walimbe V, Jaber WA, Garcia MJ, Shekhar R. Multimodality cardiac stress testing: combining real-time 3-dimensional echocardiography and myocardial perfusion SPECT. J Nucl Med. 2009;50(2):226–30. doi:10.2967/jnumed.108.053025. Epub 2009 Jan 21. PubMed PMID: 1916423
7. Ahmad M, Xie T, McCulloch M, Abreo G, Runge M. Real-time three-dimensional dobutamine stress echocardiography in assessment stress echocardiography in assessment of ischemia: comparison with two-dimensional dobutamine stress echocardiography. J Am Coll Cardiol. 2001;37(5):1303–9. PubMed PMID: 11300439
8. Matsumura Y, Hozumi T, Arai K, Sugioka K, Ujino K, Takemoto Y, Yamagishi H, Yoshiyama M, Yoshikawa J. Non-invasive assessment of myocardial ischaemia using new real-time three-

dimensional dobutamine stress echocardiography: comparison with conventional two-dimensional methods. Eur Heart J. 2005;26(16):1625–32. Epub 2005 Apr 7. PubMed PMID: 15817607

9. Aggeli C, Giannopoulos G, Misovoulos P, Roussakis G, Christoforatou E, Kokkinakis C, Brili S, Stefanadis C. Real-time three-dimensional dobutamine stress echocardiography for coronary artery disease diagnosis: validation with coronary angiography. Heart. 2007;93(6):672–5. Epub 2006 Nov 3. PubMed PMID: 17085530; PubMed Central PMCID: PMC1955206

10. Takeuchi M, Otani S, Weinert L, Spencer KT, Lang RM. Comparison of contrast-enhanced real-time live 3-dimensional dobutamine stress echocardiography with contrast 2-dimensional echocardiography for detecting stress-induced wall-motion abnormalities. J Am Soc Echocardiogr. 2006;19(3):294–9. PubMed PMID: 16500492

11. Bhan A, Kapetanakis S, Rana BS, Ho E, Wilson K, Pearson P, Mushemi S, Deguzman J, Reiken J, Harden MD, Walker N, Rafter PG, Monaghan MJ. Real-time three-dimensional myocardial contrast echocardiography: is it clinically feasible? Eur J Echocardiogr. 2008;9(6):761–5. doi:10.1093/ejechocard/jen143. Epub 2008 May 1. PubMed PMID: 18490290

12. Aggeli C, Felekos I, Roussakis G, Kazazaki C, Lagoudakou S, Pietri P, Tousoulis D, Pitsavos C, Stefanadis C. Value of real-time three-dimensional adenosine stress contrast echocardiography in patients with known or suspected coronary artery disease. Eur J Echocardiogr. 2011;12(9):648–55. doi:10.1093/ejechocard/jer103. Epub 2011 Jul 19. PubMed PMID: 21771801

13. Yoshitani H, Takeuchi M, Mor-Avi V, Otsuji Y, Hozumi T, Yoshiyama M. Comparative diagnostic accuracy of multiplane and multislice three-dimensional dobutamine stress echocardiography in the diagnosis of coronary artery disease. J Am Soc Echocardiogr. 2009;22(5):437–42. doi:10.1016/j.echo.2009.02.005. PubMed PMID: 19307099

14. Badano LP, Muraru D, Rigo F, Del Mestre L, Ermacora D, Gianfagna P. Proclemer High volume-rate three-dimensional stress echocardiography to assess inducible myocardial ischemia: a feasibility study. J Am Soc Echocardiogr. 2010;23(6):628–35. doi:10.1016/j.echo.2010.03.020. PubMed PMID: 20434877

15. Johri AM, Chitty DW, Hua L, Marincheva G, Picard MH. Assessment of image quality in real time three-dimensional dobutamine stress echocardiography: an integrated 2D/3D approach. Echocardiography. 2015;32(3):496–507. doi:10.1111/echo.12692. Epub 2014 Jul 24. PubMed PMID: 25059625

16. Casas-Rojo E, Fernández-Golfín C, Zamorano J. Hybrid imaging with coronary tomography and 3D speckle-tracking stress echocardiography fusion. Eur Heart J Cardiovasc Imaging. 2014;15(5):555. doi:10.1093/ehjci/jet236. Epub 2013 Nov 7. PubMed PMID: 24204034

17. Casas-Rojo E, Fernández-Golfín C, Ana G-M, Gorissen W, Zamorano J. Fusion between cardiac venous coronary computed tomography and three-dimensional speckle-tracking for selecting the appropriate vein for resynchronization therapy. Eur Heart J Cardiovasc Imaging. 2016; doi:10.1093/ehjci/jew091.

18. Perk G, Kronzon I. Interventional echocardiography in structural heart disease. Curr Cardiol Rep. 2013;15(3):338. doi:10.1007/s11886-012-0338-y.

19. Corti R, Biaggi P, Gaemperli O, et al. Integrated x-ray and echocardiography imaging for structural heart interventions. EuroIntervention. 2013;9(7):863–9. doi:10.4244/EIJV9I7A140.

20. Gao G, Penney G, Ma Y, et al. Registration of 3D trans-esophageal echocardiography to X-ray fluoroscopy using image-based probe tracking. Med Image Anal. 2012;16(1):38–49. doi:10.1016/j.media.2011.05.003.

21. Clegg SD, Chen SJ, Nijhof N, et al. Integrated 3D echo-X ray to optimize image guidance for structural heart intervention. JACC Cardiovasc Imaging. 2015;8(3):371–4. doi:10.1016/j.jcmg.2014.06.024.

22. Quaife RA, Salcedo EE, Carroll JD. Procedural guidance using advance imaging techniques for percutaneous edge-to-edge mitral valve repair. Curr Cardiol Rep. 2014;16(2):452. doi:10.1007/s11886-013-0452-5.

23. Holmes DR, Mack MJ, Kaul S, et al. 2012 ACCF/AATS/SCAI/STS expert consensus document on transcatheter aortic valve replacement. J Am Coll Cardiol. 2012;59(13):1200–54. doi:10.1016/j.jacc.2012.01.001.
24. Smith LA, Dworakowski R, Bhan A, et al. Real-time three-dimensional transesophageal echocardiography adds value to transcatheter aortic valve implantation. J Am Soc Echocardiogr. 2013;26(4):359–69. doi:10.1016/j.echo.2013.01.014.
25. Philip F, Athappan G, Tuzcu EM, Svensson LG, Kapadia SR. MitraClip for severe symptomatic mitral regurgitation in patients at high surgical risk: a comprehensive systematic review. Catheter Cardiovasc Interv. 2014;84(4):581–90. doi:10.1002/ccd.25564.
26. Sündermann SH, Biaggi P, Grünenfelder J, et al. Safety and feasibility of novel technology fusing echocardiography and fluoroscopy images during MitraClip interventions. EuroIntervention. 2014;9(10):1210–6. doi:10.4244/EIJV9I10A203.
27. Cheung A, Stub D, Moss R, et al. Transcatheter mitral valve implantation with Tiara bioprosthesis. EuroIntervention. 2014;10(Suppl. U):115–9. doi:10.4244/EIJV10SUA17.
28. Biaggi P, Fernandez-Golfín C, Hahn R, Corti R. Hybrid imaging during transcatheter structural heart interventions. Curr Cardiovasc Imaging Rep. 2015;8:33. doi:10.1007/s12410-015-9349-6.
29. Rodríguez Muñoz D, Lázaro Rivera C, Zamorano Gómez JL. Guidance of treatment of perivalvular prosthetic leaks. Curr Cardiol Rep. 2014;16(1):430. doi:10.1007/s11886-013-0430-y.
30. Gonzalves A, Almeria C, Marcos-Alberca P, et al. Three-dimensional echocardiography in paravalvular aortic regurgitation assessment after transcatheter aortic valve implantation. J Am Soc Echocardiogr. 2012;25(1):47–55. doi:10.1016/j.echo.2011.08.019.
31. Lázaro C, Hinojar R, Zamorano JL. Cardiac imaging in prosthetic paravalvular leaks. Cardiovasc Diagn Ther. 2014;4(4):307–13. doi:10.3978/j.issn.2223-3652.2014.07.01.
32. González A, Zamorano JL. Review of ESC 2014 Barcelona. Spain Eur Med J. 2014;2(October):54–60.

# Chapter 9
# Cardiac Congenital Disease and 3D-Echocardiography

Michael Grattan and Luc Mertens

## Introduction

Three-dimensional (3D) echocardiography (3DE) has been used in pediatric and adult patients with congenital heart disease (CHD) for over 20 years [1–3]. Early 3DE was limited by long acquisition and post-processing times. It was not until the advent of real time 3D echocardiography (RT3DE) using matrix array probes that the technology became feasible as a clinical tool [4].

CHD encompasses a broad spectrum of lesions, ranging from simple septal defects and minor valve abnormalities to complex lesions involving abnormal atrio-ventricular and ventriculo-arterial connections, and significant alterations in the spatial orientation of the heart structures. Patients with CHD often require intricate surgeries and interventional procedures to correct or palliate their lesions. 3D echocardiography can improve the understanding of CHD, aid in the surgical planning for these patients, and provide additive information in their pre- and post-operative follow-up.

## Assessing Morphology in Congenital Diseases with 3D

RT3DE has been shown to aid in the diagnosis and understanding of both simple and complex CHD. It allows structures of the heart to be visualized anatomically instead of using arbitrary 2-dimensional (2D) cut planes, and may be more intuitive for surgeons and other non-echocardiographers. Importantly, it allows cardiac structures to be simultaneously viewed anatomically *and* physiologically (in a beating

M. Grattan • L. Mertens (✉)
The Hospital for Sick Children, University of Toronto, Toronto, ON, Canada
e-mail: luc.mertens@sickkids.ca

© Springer International Publishing AG 2017

211

E. Casas Rojo et al. (eds.), *Manual of 3D Echocardiography*,
DOI 10.1007/978-3-319-50335-6_9

heart), something surgical views in the operating room cannot provide. 3D imaging allows visualization of cardiac structures in the entire context of the heart and aids in the comprehension of the spatial relations of different structures. It can provide an in depth visualization of valves and their support apparatus without the need for multiple images and sweeps.

Guidelines have been published for 3DE image acquisition and display in adults with structurally normal hearts [5]. These and additional pediatric/congenital-specific guidelines [6] can be applied to patients with CHD. RT3DE is limited by relatively low spatial and temporal resolution. High quality image acquisition is fundamental to maximize the spatial resolution when acquiring 3D datasets. RT3DE can distinguish between cardiac structures in the axial, lateral and elevation planes, with the optimal spatial resolution obtained in the axial plane (Fig. 9.1). To maximize spatial resolution for 3D datasets, all cardiac structures of interest should ideally be imaged orthogonally, in the axial plane, with appropriate focal length and position (Table 9.1). Temporal resolution also must be maximized, especially in small patients with fast heart rates. Multiple-beat acquisition can improve frame rates but can introduce stitch artifact. Cooperative patients can be guided through appropriate breath-holding techniques, but unco-operative patients may require sedation or anesthesia. Careful adjustment of the lateral and elevation sector width to only include areas of interest can often improve the temporal resolution such that high quality data sets can be obtained from a single beat.

An advantage of 3D datasets is that structures can be displayed in many unique orientations. Guidelines have been published for RT3DE image display in adults with structurally normal hearts to reduce variability and confusion [5] and additional guidelines are available for patients with CHD [6]. Echocardiographic images can be displayed using typical 2D cuts (with added depth), anatomically (similar views to cross-sectional imaging), and surgically [6]. 3D echocardiography provides the most added value through its ability to display cardiac structures from the

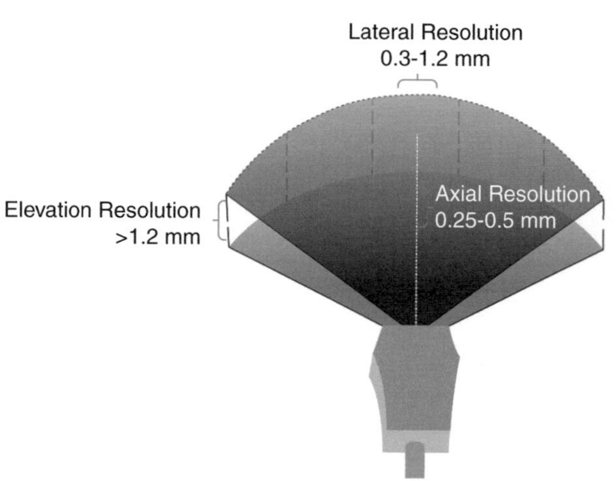


**Fig. 9.1** Relative spatial resolution in axial, lateral and elevation planes

**Table 9.1**   Optimal approach for RT3DE of CHD

| Structure | TTE | TEE | Additional information |
|---|---|---|---|
| MV/LAVV | A4C<br>PLAX<br>PSAX en face (live 3D) | ME 4C (0°)<br>TG SAX<br>(0–45°) | PLAX useful for valve support apparatus |
| TV/RAVV | A4C – RV centric PLAX | ME 4C (0°) | RV centric A4C – probe shifted rightward |
| AoV/truncal valve | High PLAX<br>High right PLAX<br>PSAX en face (live 3D) | ME SAX<br>(30–45°) | Full volume/3D zoom preferred<br>High/right PLAX allows axial approach |
| PV | PLAX, PSAX<br>Subcostal RAO | (Limited use )<br>ME SAX<br>(60–75°) | Subcostal RAO limited as decreased resolution in far field |
| Atrial septum | Subcostal short/long<br>Right PLAX A4C | ME 4C (0°)<br>ME sagittal<br>(80–90°) | A4C → decreased resolution, alternative if no subcostal window |
| Ventricular septum | Subcostal short<br>PLAX, PSAX<br>A4C | TG SAX<br>(0–45°)<br>ME 4C (0°) | A4C → decreased resolution, alternative if no subcostal window<br>Parasternal views for PMVSD |
| LV/RV | A4C<br>Subcostal | ME 4C (0°) | RV centric view for RV<br>May require subcostal views to include entire ventricle |

Full volume datasets and 3D zoom generally provide optimal spatial and temporal resolution
*TTE* transthoracic echocardiography, *TEE* transesophageal echocardiography, *MV* mitral valve, *LAVV* left atrioventricular valve, *A4C* apical 4 chamber view, *PLAX* parasternal long axis view, *PSAX* parasternal short axis view, *3D* 3 dimension, *ME* mid-esophageal, *4C* 4 chamber, *TG* transgastric, *SAX* short axis, *TV* tricuspid valve, *RAVV* right atrioventricular valve, *AoV* aortic valve, *PV* pulmonary valve, *RAO* right anterior oblique view

surgeon's view but in a beating heart. We recommend including surgical views if possible when presenting 3DE images.

Early on, the addition of RT3DE was shown to improve diagnostic accuracy compared to 2D echocardiography alone [7]. 2D Echocardiography of complex CHD can be especially challenging, even for experienced cardiologists. Multiple imaging planes and the use of 2D sweeps can improve diagnostic accuracy, but often the cardiac anatomy is not fully understood until the cardiac anatomy has been exposed in the operating room. Information about the spatial relationship of different cardiac structures may dictate what type of surgical repair is performed and whether patients will be able to undergo complete repair versus single ventricle palliation. RT3DE has been shown to improve the understanding and diagnostic accuracy of CHD compared to traditional 2D echocardiography, especially for complex defects [8]. Use of the multiplanar reformatting (MPR) setting provides unique 2D views and allows imagers to optimize images offline and perform virtual sweeps. It has aided in the determination surgical strategy (1 versus 2 ventricle repair) as well as the assessment of valve morphology and vascular anatomy in complex CHD [9]. RT3DE is especially helpful in the evaluation of extracardiac structures, VSDs with complex anatomy, the assessment of atrioventricular valve abnormalities and very complex CHD [10].

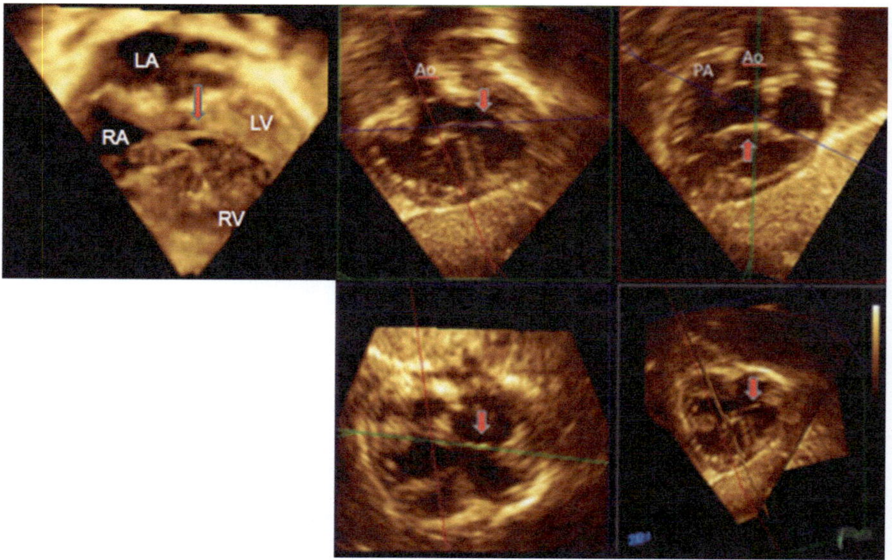



**Fig. 9.2** Double outlet right ventricular with straddling of the tricuspid valve. The MPR shows straddling of the tricuspid valve with attachments of the tricuspid valve leaflet in the LV. This precludes closure of the interventricular communication and connecting the LV to the aorta as this would damage the tricuspid valve subvalvar apparatus

One of the most difficult cardiac lesions to understand can be double outlet right ventricle. In this lesion both outflow tracts arise from the right ventricle; however their orientation to each other can be quite variable. A VSD is almost always present, but its location and orientation fluctuates with variable commitments either to the aorta, pulmonary artery, both arteries or neither. Even experienced pediatric echocardiographers using high quality 2D echocardiography struggle to determine the commitment of these structures to each other. 3D imaging using MRI [11] and RT3DE [12] can significantly improve the understanding of these complex spatial arrangements. Specifically, RT3DE can provide important information regarding the ability to baffle the VSD to the aorta without obstructing the tricuspid valve (TV), the need for an RV to pulmonary artery conduit, and the need for VSD enlargement [12]. Figure 9.2 shows and example how straddling of the tricuspid valve can interfere with potential biventricular repair of a double outlet right ventricle. Using MPR reconstruction the 3D dataset substantial attachments were demonstrated to attach in the LV precluding closure of the interventricular communication and connecting the LV to the aorta.

## Congenital Heart Disease Involving the Atrioventricular Valves

3DE is widely recognized as a valuable tool for assessing mitral valve (MV) and TV morphology and function in the adult population. Assessing congenital abnormalities of these valves can be particularly challenging due to their abnormal and variable morphology, presence of previous interventions, and asymmetric and variable flow dynamics. 3DE has improved our understanding of valve function and dysfunction in this population by allowing visualization of the entire valve apparatus at once, including valve, chords, and papillary muscles. It has been shown to improve diagnostic accuracy in certain mitral valve abnormalities, and importantly, can provide the surgeon with surgical views in a physiologic beating state.

The optimal echocardiographic views for 3D assessment of the atrioventricular valves are the apical four chamber (standard and RV-centric) and the parasternal long axis views (Table 9.1). The apical four-chamber view provides the highest spatial resolution of the left and right AV valve tissue and the parasternal long axis view provides the highest spatial resolution of the left AV valve support apparatus as well as good views of the right AV valve. Full volume and 3D zoom datasets provide the highest spatial and temporal resolution, although live 3D views can be beneficial to augment 2D 'en face' views. The use of 3D colour Doppler is very important to differentiate defects in coaptation from image dropout. It is recommended that colour Doppler always accompanies RT3DE assessment of any valve [13].

## *Congenital Mitral Valve Disease*

With the exception of MV prolapse, congenital diseases of the MV are rare [14]. They include abnormalities predominantly of the valve tissue (isolated MV clefts and MV dysplasia) and abnormalities of the valve and support apparatus (double orifice MV, parachute MV and arcade MV). These abnormalities can lead to stenosis, regurgitation or both, and can be challenging to surgically repair.

RT3DE allows visualization of the entire valve and support apparatus in one image. Early 3DE improved our understanding of the normal MV structure and function, including its saddle shape, influences on leaflet stress and dynamic changes throughout systole and diastole [15]. Early studies on the normal MV paved the way for its assessment in CHD. There have been many reports of RT3DE aiding in the diagnosis of congenital MV disease including MV prolapse, double orifice MV [16, 17] (Fig. 9.3), arcade MV [18], isolated MV dysplasia, cleft MV (Fig. 9.4) and parachute MV [19]. In addition RT3DE has contributed to the diagnosis of abnormalities of the supravalvar area including cor triatriatum [20] and supramitral ring [21]. In a larger cohort, Takahashi et al. [22] showed that RT3DE had improved accuracy compared to 2D echocardiography in detecting leaflet and commissural abnormalities and correlated well with surgical findings.

RT3DE can improve the assessment and quantification of mitral regurgitation. 2D echocardiography provides adequate assessment of central, symmetric jets of mitral regurgitation. However, mitral regurgitation jets in congenital MV disease are often eccentric, irregularly shaped and displaced towards a specific anatomic abnormality (i.e. cleft). The assessment of mitral regurgitation with RT3DE does not

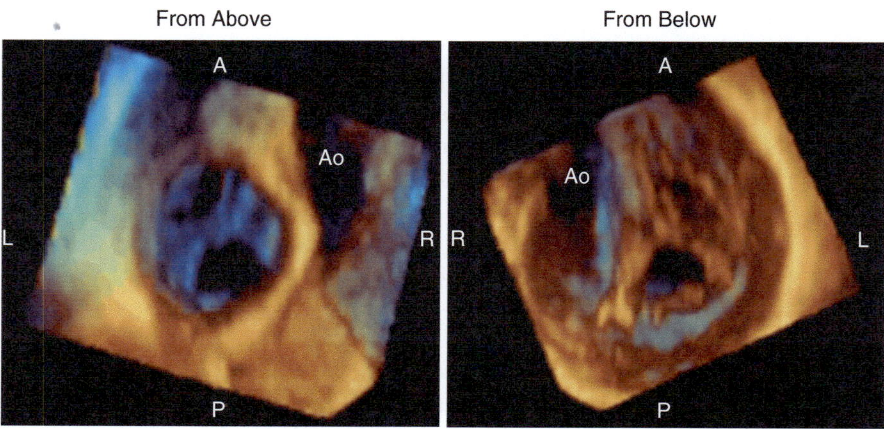



**Fig. 9.3** Double orifice mitral valve as seen from the left atrium (*left panel*) and left ventricle (*right panel*)

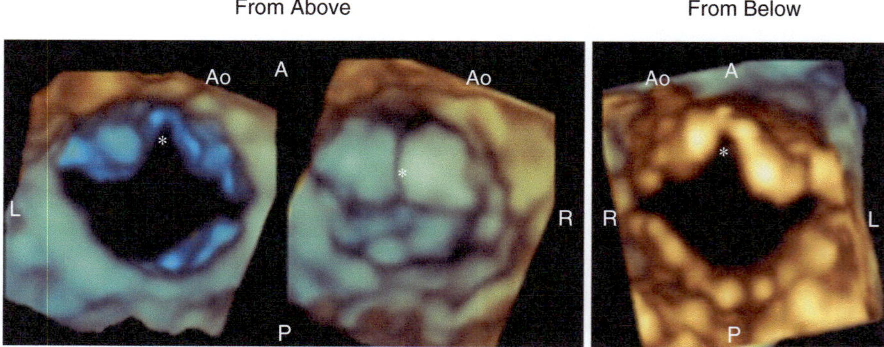



**Fig. 9.4** Isolated MV cleft. As visualized by 3-D echo. A cleft directed anteriorly is noted in the anterior mitral leaflet. Left and middle panels show the mitral valve from the LA with the leaflets opened and closed. The right panel visualizes the valve from the left ventricle with the leaflets opening in diastole

require assumptions about the jet shape, and has been shown to be superior to 2D echocardiography in the detection and assessment of commissural regurgitation [22]. Importantly, the assessment of regurgitation using RT3DE occurs in a physiologic state, which makes it superior to surgical saline testing, especially for commissural regurgitation and clefts [22]. Many studies have been performed in adults with structurally normal MV comparing 3D derived vena contracta area (Fig. 9.5) to traditional measures of mitral regurgitation [23–25], with excellent correlation between RT3DE and MRI. In patients with atrioventricular septal defects (AVSD), vena contracta area correlates well with 2D-derived measures of regurgitation [26]. However, no studies have compared RT3DE-derived vena contracta area with MRI-derived regurgitant fraction in patients with CHD, and no normal values have been established in the pediatric population.

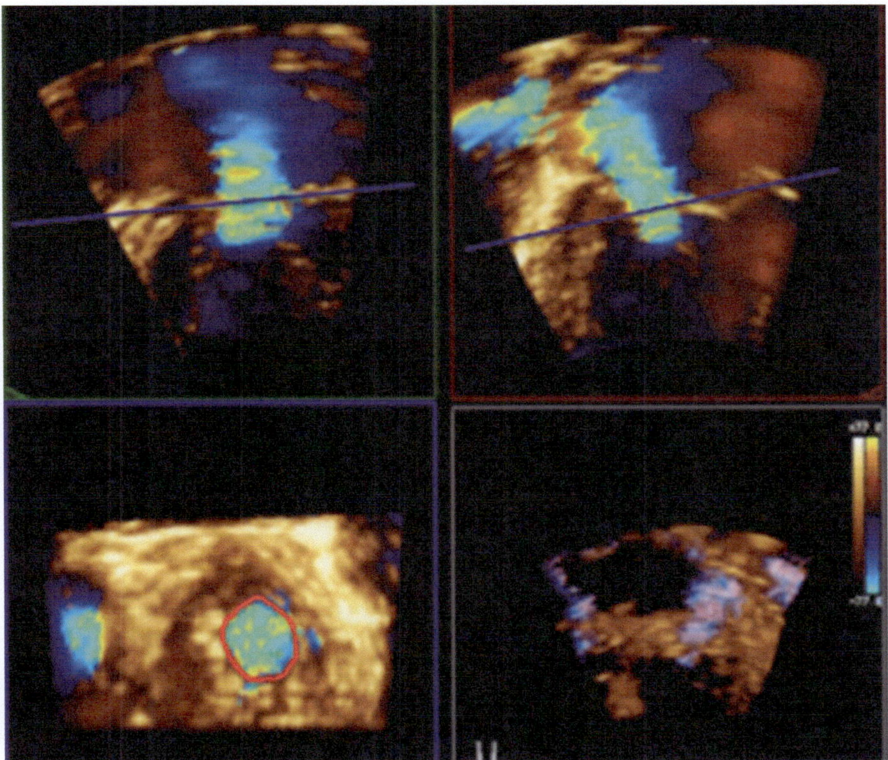

**Fig. 9.5** MPR mode to assess vena contracta area in MR. Using the upper two cut planes, a short axis section of the MV is obtained at the exact vena contract. The vena contracta 'en face' is displayed in the lower left frame and can be traced to determine the vena contracta area. 2D echocardiography can produce similar views, but cannot guarantee that the image displayed is at the true vena contracta

## *Left Atrioventricular Valve in Atrioventricular Septal Defects*

The defining feature of an atrioventricular septal defect is a common atrioventricular junction with a trileaflet left atrioventricular valve and an unwedged aortic valve (Fig. 9.6). The presence and severity of inter-atrial and inter-ventricular shunting is variable. Although sometimes called a MV, the left atrioventricular valve is unique, as it is composed of three leaflets. The so-called cleft is actually the zone of apposition between the superior and inferior bridging leaflets and is often a source of significant regurgitation (Figs. 9.6 and 9.7). Even in the current surgical era, regurgitation and stenosis of the left atrioventricular valve cause significant long-term morbidity.

RT3DE has been shown to provide additional anatomic and functional information both prior to AVSD repair [27] and afterwards [28, 29]. RT3DE correlates better with surgical findings compared to 2D echocardiography [30], specifically in the detection of commissural abnormalities and related regurgitation and in assessing for a residual cleft post repair [27].

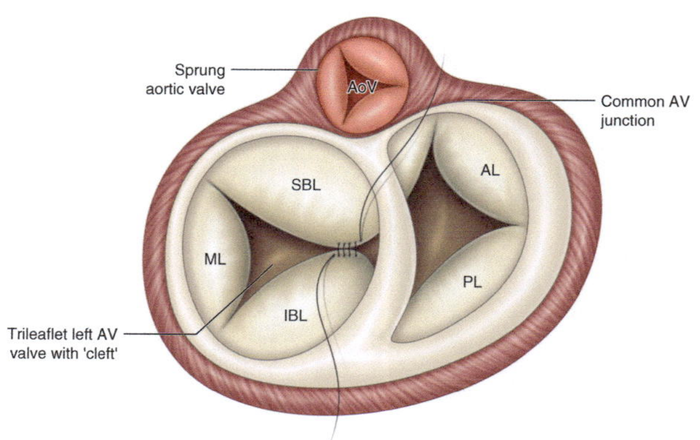


**Fig. 9.6** Anatomy of the atrioventricular junction in an atrioventricular septal defect. *AL* anterior leaflet, *AoV* aortic valve, *IBL* inferior bridging leaflet, *ML* mural leaflet, *PL* posterior leaflet, *SBL* superior bridging leaflet

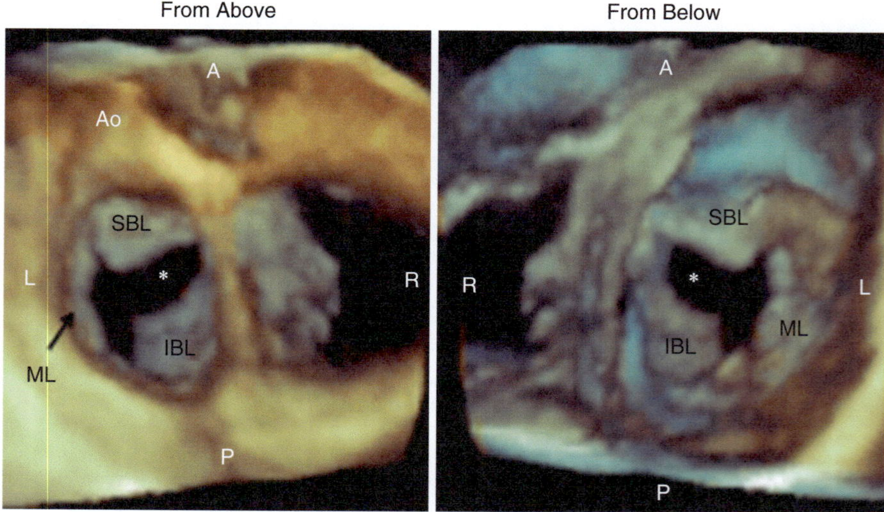


**Fig. 9.7** RT3DE of an atrioventricular septal defect with no ventricular shunt (primum defect). Left panel shows the surgical view from the left atrium. Right panel shows the view from the left ventricle. * so-called cleft (zone of apposition between the superior and inferior bridging leaflets). *A* anterior, *P* posterior, *Ao* aorta, *L* left, *R* right, *ML* mural leaflet, *IBL* inferior bridging leaflet, *SBL* superior bridging leaflet

It is still poorly understood why some AV valves are at increased risk of dysfunction after AVSD repair compared to others. RT3DE has provided important information regarding valve function and physiology in patients with AVSD and aided in the determination of risk factors for regurgitation and optimal surgical strategies. Unlike 2D echocardiography RT3DE is able to quantify valve prolapse area, and it is now clear that increased prolapse is associated with increased AV valve regurgitation pre- and post-operatively

[26]. RT3DE also allows the quantification of valve tethering, through the measurement of valve and support apparatus angles. Increased tethering, often associated with asymmetric commissures, is associated with increased valve regurgitation post-operatively, even in patients with minimal pre-operative valve dysfunction [28, 31]. This has led some institutions to perform routine RT3DE assessments of the left atrioventricular valve in patients with AVSD and alter their surgical approach in high-risk patients [31].

## Congenital Tricuspid Valve Disease

Congenital tricuspid valve (TV) disease usually includes TV dysplasia and Ebstein's anomaly of the TV. The TV is more difficult to visualize compared to the mitral valve and there is no standard 'en face' view available using 2D echocardiography. It is often even more difficult to visualize the TV in patients with Ebstein's anomaly due to the displacement and rotation of the functional valve orifice. The regurgitant jet is often very eccentric and difficult to evaluate.

RT3DE allows the TV to be visualized 'en face' and has been shown to be more accurate for detecting abnormalities in the TV anatomy and sources of regurgitation compared to 2D echocardiography alone [22] (Fig. 9.8). In Ebstein's anomaly RT3DE has been helpful in visualizing the TV anatomy and assessing tricuspid regurgitation using the vena contracta area [32, 33]. It has proven valuable in evaluating the RV size and function in this lesion [32, 33]. More recently, the MPR mode has allowed a more accurate determination of dysplastic versus Ebsteinoid TV, and has correlated well with surgical findings [34].

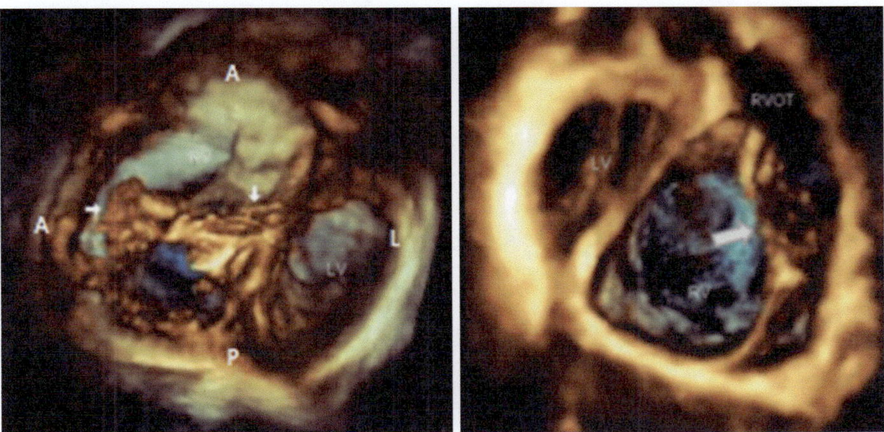


**Fig. 9.8** Ebstein's anomaly of the tricuspid valve. Left panel show a view from the RV,. Notice the attachments on the septal leaflet to the interventricular septum. Also note the abnormal attachments of the anterior leaflet of the tricuspid valve to the RV free wall resulting in tethering of the anterior leaflet. Finally there is significant displacement and tethering of the deficient posteroinferior leaflets. On the right panel the opening of the tricuspid valve in the direction of the right ventricular outflow tract can be appreciated (*arrow*)

## *Atrioventricular Valve Disease in Single Ventricles*

Despite advances in pre-operative, surgical and post-operative care, the morbidity and mortality in patients with single ventricle physiology remains high. These patients are at risk of significant AV valve regurgitation, which puts them at even higher risk. These valves can be challenging to image as they are often structurally different from mitral or tricuspid valves and commonly additional abnormalities including clefts, prolapse and tethering (Fig. 9.9).

RT3DE has significantly improved our ability to visualize the atrioventricular valve anatomy in single ventricles, as well as our understanding of the mechanisms of regurgitation. In patients with normal cardiac anatomy, it is well known that there are ventricular-ventricular interactions that can affect atrioventricular valve function. These interactions are altered in patients with single ventricle physiology and may lead to ventricular dysfunction and valvar regurgitation. In patients with hypoplastic left heart syndrome, RT3DE has shown that the tricuspid valve annulus shape is flatter, more circular, more dilated and less dynamic throughout the cardiac cycle [34, 35]. These changes and chordal abnormalities may lead to tethering and prolapse and are associated with increased regurgitation [34, 35]. Not only does this information improve our understanding of valve function in these lesions. It may help predict high-risk patients. Kutty et al. has shown that patients with increased tethering and a flatter annulus prior to stage 1 palliation are at increased risk of tricuspid regurgitation post operatively [35]. Interestingly, they did not find significant

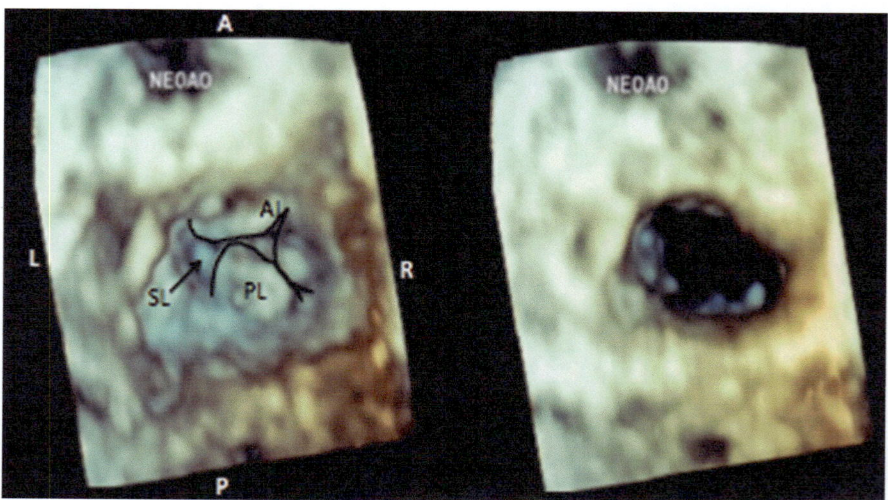


**Fig. 9.9** TV in hypoplastic left heart syndrome. The septal leaflet is tethered while the anterior valve has prominent small 'cleft' between scallops. Often with progressive dilatation of the tricuspid annulus, this can be region where regurgitation is common. Finally there is some anterior and posterior leaflet prolapse contributing to the regurgitation in this patient

prolapse at this stage, and propose that prolapse may develop over a longer time period in these patients.

Quantification of valve regurgitation in these patients is often difficult and qualitative. RT3DE has been used to quantify tricuspid regurgitation (vena contracta area) in structurally normal hearts, with excellent correlation with 2D echocardiography [36]. This method has a superior correlation with MRI quantification in the evaluation of other cardiac valves compared to 2D echocardiography, and is often used as the gold standard for assessment of regurgitation. Although definitive studies have not been performed to evaluate quantification of AV valve regurgitation in the single ventricle population using RT3DE, this method is promising in improving the ability to quantify regurgitation in this population.

## Atrial and Ventricular Septal Defects

### *Atrial Defects*

Atrial septal defects (ASDs) are one of the most common CHD, occurring in 19% of CHD [14]. Traditionally ASDs were closed surgically; however more defects are now amenable to interventional device closure in the cardiac catheterization laboratory. The appropriate selection of patients for device ASD closure is critical and requires specific information on the number, size and shape of defects, as well as their relation to other cardiac structures. In some patients, these factors can be difficult to determine using 2D echocardiography alone.

In children, the atrial septum is a thin structure that is prone to dropout artifact, and maximizing the spatial resolution during image acquisition is important. Subcostal and right parasternal transthoracic views, and mid-esophageal TEE (0 and 90 degrees) views maximize spatial resolution by imaging in the axial plane. In older children and adults with limited subcostal views, apical 4 chamber views can be cropped to visualize the atrial septum 'en face'. Although the spatial resolution is decreased, it is often sufficient in older patients with a thicker atrial septum [37]. The addition of colour Doppler to 3D images can help to distinguish defect from dropout. Anatomic and surgical views from the right and left atria [38], as well as standard 2D views with added depth can be used to display the anatomy (Fig. 9.10).

RT3DE has aided in the diagnosis of all types of inter-atrial communications [39], but its true value has been aiding the characterization and management of secundum ASDs. Early on, RT3DE was shown to provide additive information on the size and shape of ASDs as well as the size of their rims that correlated well with catheter and surgical findings [40–42]. In larger studies, RT3DE has been shown to be similar to 2D echocardiography in determining rim size, but superior in evaluating the number and shape of defects [43, 44]. RT3DE is especially advantageous for characterizing patients with multiple defects, as determining the relative size and shape of multiple defects is difficult using 2D echocardiography [45].

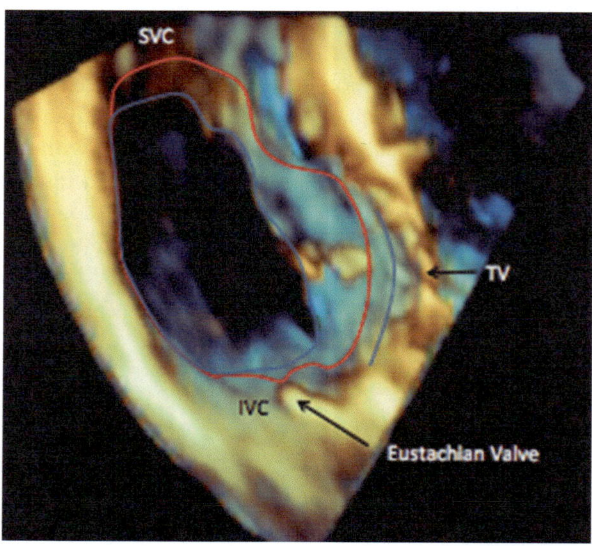


**Fig. 9.10** Visualization of atrial communications. A large ASD as viewed from the right atrium. *Red circle* outlines the anatomic atrial septum. *Blue circle* outlines the atrial septal defect. There is insufficient rim separating the atrial septal defect from the IVC and the posterior atrial wall.

The faster acquisition and post-processing times, and the improving resolution of 'live-3D' has made RT3DE TEE feasible in guiding ASD closure and evaluating the position of ASD devices in the cardiac catheterization laboratory [46]. The added depth that RT3DE provides has made it easier to identify and follow catheters and wires [37] and we postulate that in the future this technology may lead to decreased fluoroscopy time. RT3DE has also been used in the catheter laboratory to aid in device sizing, and has been shown to correlate better than 2D echocardiography for balloon sizing. RT3DE still underestimates the defect size compared to balloon sizing methods, but may ultimately provide more accurate measurements [47].

## Ventricular Septal Defects

Ventricular septal defects (VSDs) are the most common CHD. Similar to ASDs, their closure traditionally occurred surgically. Increasingly VSDs, especially muscular defects are being closed interventionally. Although 2D echocardiography can determine the general type and size of VSD, it is difficult to define the exact location and shape of defect.

The optimal imaging plane for evaluating VSDs depends on their location. Subcostal and transgastric views generally provide the most orthogonal imaging planes and the highest spatial resolution. Parasternal long axis views provide high quality imaging of the mid-muscular and perimembranous septum. Modified apical 4 chamber views can also achieve high quality images of the muscular septum. RT3DE allows viewers to visualize the ventricular septum anatomically in three dimensions rather than necessitating the construction of a virtual 3D image from multiple cut planes. Viewing defects from the RV aspect provides a more typical surgical view, but may be problematic by prominent trabeculations. Viewing defects from the LV aspect and the addition of colour Doppler can distinguish true defects from dropout artifact and prominent trabeculations (Fig. 9.11) [48].

The advantages of RT3DE over 2D echocardiography for assessment of VSDs are the ability to more accurately and intuitively visualize the defect size (see Fig. 9.11), shape and position, as well as the relationship of the defects to other cardiac structures, including the tricuspid and aortic valves [49–52]. RT3DE can be especially beneficial when multiple defects are present. It may improve the ability to surgeons to accurately and efficiently locate and close defects, and may provide important information to guide the specific operative approach [51]. It can also be used to provide additional information about associated lesions including aortic valve prolapse, AV valve straddle and RV outflow tract obstruction [48].

Muscular VSDs are increasingly being closed in the catheterization laboratory. Similar to ASDs, RT3DE can be used to guide catheter and wire course as well as confirm appropriate device deployment. RT3DE may increase efficiency and decrease fluoroscopy time by allowing visualization of all rims in one image that does not need to be altered throughout the case [53].

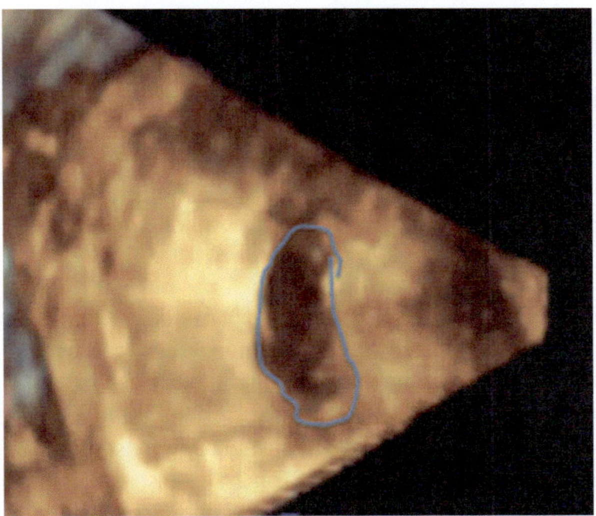

**Fig. 9.11** En face view of the interventricular septum from the LV side. A large muscular ventricular septal defect can be identified (*blue line* defines the borders of the defect). The real size of the VSD was underestimated by 2D imaging

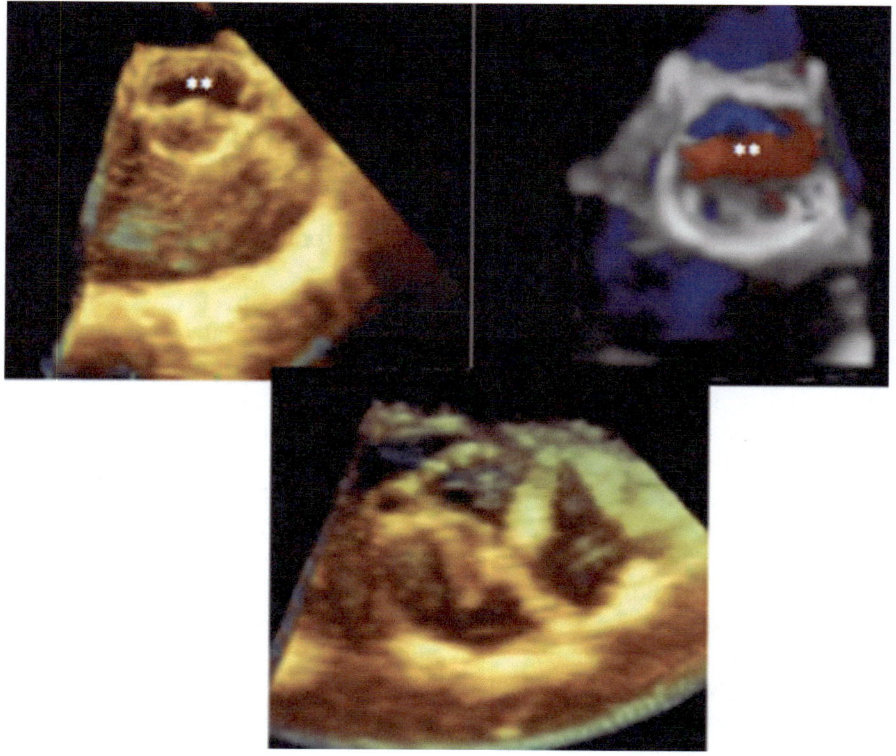

**Fig. 9.12** Transesophageal 3DTEE in an adolescent undergoing aortic valve repair for severe aortic insufficiency. This patient underwent balloon aortic valvuloplasty because severe aortic stenosis. There is a large hole in the anterior leaflet of the bicuspid aortic valve (**). Through this deficiency there is severe aortic regurgitation. The TEE contribute to describing the exact mechanism of regurgitation. The patient underwent a successful leaflet repair using a pericardial patch technique with excellent result. The lower panel shows the valve after repair. There was only mild residual regurgitation

## Aortic and Pulmonary Valve Disease

The utility of RT3DE in the assessment of aortic valve disease is identical in pediatric and congenital patients compared to the adult population with acquired aortic valve disease [54]. RT3DE has been proven useful in the assessment of LV outflow tract dimensions and in the assessment of the aortic valve annulus. Also for the evaluation of LV mass and volume, RT3DE has plays a role although most of the guideline recommendations for valve intervention, are based on 2-D measurements. During transcatheter valve implantation, 3-D TEE guidance adds important spatial information which can be helpful during the procedure [55]. In perioperative cases, especially of aortic leaflet repair 3D TEE is particularly useful for defining the valve anatomy, the mechanism of valve disease and for describing the immediate surgical result Fig. 9.12). 3D imaging allows an intuitive surgical view, which helps surgeons in tailoring their surgical approach. As no pediatric 3-D TEE probe is currently available, application of this technology for children with congenital heart disease remains problematic for children below 20 kg. Epicardial 3-D is possible but technically not easy for the aortic valve.

For the pulmonary valve, there is much less experience in us of RT3DE. The difficulty for transthoracic representation is that the pulmonary valve is in the near field of the volumes and can be hard to visualize well. For TEE imaging the valve is positioned far from the probe, which can limit the use of 3D TEE. In a recent study it was demonstrated that RT3DE can provide better images of the pulmonary valve in patients before tetralogy of Fallot correction with more accurate measurements of the pulmonary valve annulus when compared to the surgical annulus sizing [56]. 3DRTE could play additional role in describing the 3-D complexity of right ventricular outflow tract obstruction.

## 3-D Echocardiography After Surgery for Congenital Heart Disease

For the post-operative assessment of patients with congenital heart disease, 3DRTE can be used for different defects. A detailed description of the potential use of 3DRTE for all indications after congenital heart surgery goes beyond the scope of the current chapter. We will focus on two different relatively common applications. The first one is the use of 3DRTE for the assessment of RV volumes in patients after tetralogy of Fallot repair. The second example is the 3-D assessment of atrioventricular valve structure and function in patients post repair of atrioventricular septal defect.

Assessment of RV size and function is important in post-operative tetralogy of Fallot patients [57]. Post surgical repair severe pulmonary regurgitation is a common problem, particularly in patients who underwent transannular patch repair. Severe pulmonary regurgitation results in progressive right ventricular dilation and can result be associated with RV dysfunction. Cardiac MRI is generally considered to be the reference technique for assessment of RV volumes and ejection fraction [58]. 3DRTE is a good alternative that has been applied to this patient population. Different studies have looked at the feasibility and accuracy of RV volumetric measurements in patients after surgical repair for congenital heart disease. The technical feasibility of including the entire RV volume in the image acquisition may be difficult especially in dilated RVs [59]. 3DRTE has been demonstrated to underestimate RV volumes when compared to those measured by cMRI, especially for the more dilated RVs [60] although this systematic error was not confirmed in all studies [61]. Further improvements in automated border detection algorithms or knowledge-based reconstruction methods based on databases of tetralogy patients, will further result in more accurate and user-friendly 3-D methods [62].

A second illustration of the utility of 3DRTE is the postoperative assessment of patients after atrioventricular septal defect repair for the assessment of the mechanism of residual valve regurgitation. Visualising the atrioventricular valve 'en face' together with color-Doppler imaging allows to identify the anatomical substrate for the residual leakage and better understand the mechansims involved [27, 31, 63]. This allows better planning of surgical reinterventions.

## (Other Applications and) Future Directions

The main limitations of RT3DE are its limited spatial and temporal resolution, the lack of pediatric-specific TEE probes, and our limited ability to display images in three dimensions.

New ultrasound technologies are becoming available that will hopefully solve the issue of temporal resolution, as they can provide frame rates for 2D images of over 1000 fps [64]. This technology will revolutionize the entire field of echocardiography including the use of RT3DE. We are hopeful that in the near future, there will be a pediatric-specific 3D TEE probe that will facilitate high quality 3D imaging for smaller patients with poor transthoracic acoustic windows and for intraoperative assessment.

Images obtained from RT3DE are usually displayed in two dimensions, with different 'imaging tricks' to allow viewers to comprehend the images in 3D. Software for viewing and cropping these images can still be quite finicky and challenging, especially for inexperienced users. Some images can be displayed on 3D screens using stereo 3D viewing glasses. Many additional avenues for 3D image display have been described including 3D printed hearts [65], holographic images that can be manipulated in real time and virtual reality [66]. 3D cardiac printing has become well-established using MRI, and additional techniques have investigated hybrid printing using both technologies [67].

Additional potential uses for 3D echocardiography include the assessment of fetuses with CHD. In animal models, RT3DE combined with videocardioscopy has also facilitated the intracardiac, patch surgical closure of ASDs (any size) in beating hearts [68, 69].

## References


1. Bates JR, Tantengco MV, Ryan T, Feigenbaum H, Ensing GJ. A systematic approach to echocardiographic image acquisition and three-dimensional reconstruction with a subxiphoid rotational scan. J Am Soc Echocardiogr. 1996;9:257–65.
2. Ludomirsky A, Vermilion R, Nesser J, et al. Transthoracic real-time three-dimensional echocardiography using the rotational scanning approach for data acquisition. Echocardiography. 1994;11:599–606.
3. Salustri A, Spitaels S, McGhie J, Vletter W, Roelandt JR. Transthoracic three-dimensional echocardiography in adult patients with congenital heart disease. J Am Coll Cardiol. 1995;26:759–67.

4. Balestrini L, Fleishman C, Lanzoni L, et al. Real-time 3-dimensional echocardiography evaluation of congenital heart disease. J Am Soc Echocardiogr. 2000;13:171–6.
5. Lang RM, Badano LP, Tsang W, et al. EAE/ASE recommendations for image acquisition and display using three-dimensional echocardiography. J Am Soc Echocardiogr. 2012;25:3–46.
6. Simpson J, Miller O, Bell A, Bellsham-Revell H, McGhie J, Meijboom F. Image orientation for three-dimensional echocardiography of congenital heart disease. Int J Cardiovasc Imaging. 2012;28:743–53.
7. Seliem MA, Fedec A, Cohen MS, et al. Real-time 3-dimensional echocardiographic imaging of congenital heart disease using matrix-array technology: freehand real-time scanning adds instant morphologic details not well delineated by conventional 2-dimensional imaging. J Am Soc Echocardiogr. 2006;19:121–9.
8. Chen GZ, Huang GY, Tao ZY, Liu XQ, Lin QS. Value of real-time 3-dimensional echocardiography sectional diagnosis in complex congenital heart disease evaluated by receiver operating characteristic analysis. J Am Soc Echocardiogr. 2008;21:458–63.
9. Bharucha T, Roman KS, Anderson RH, Vettukattil JJ. Impact of multiplanar review of three-dimensional echocardiographic data on management of congenital heart disease. Ann Thorac Surg. 2008;86:875–81.
10. Del Pasqua A, Sanders SP, de Zorzi A, et al. Impact of three-dimensional echocardiography in complex congenital heart defect cases: the surgical view. Pediatr Cardiol. 2009;30:293–300.
11. Farooqi KM, Uppu SC, Nguyen K, et al. Application of virtual three-dimensional models for simultaneous visualization of intracardiac anatomic relationships in double outlet right ventricle. Pediatr Cardiol. 2016;37:90–8.
12. Pushparajah K, Barlow A, Tran VH, et al. A systematic three-dimensional echocardiographic approach to assist surgical planning in double outlet right ventricle. Echocardiography. 2013;30:234–8.
13. Kutty S, Colen TM, Smallhorn JF. Three-dimensional echocardiography in the assessment of congenital mitral valve disease. J Am Soc Echocardiogr. 2014;27:142–54.
14. Mozaffarian D, Benjamin EJ, Go AS, et al. Heart disease and stroke statistics-2016 update: a report from the American Heart Association. Circulation. 2016;133:e38–e360.
15. Salgo IS, Gorman 3rd JH, Gorman RC, et al. Effect of annular shape on leaflet curvature in reducing mitral leaflet stress. Circulation. 2002;106:711–7.
16. Anwar AM, McGhie JS, Meijboom FJ, Ten Cate FJ. Double orifice mitral valve by real-time three-dimensional echocardiography. Eur J Echocardiogr. 2008;9:731–2.
17. Pizzino F, Piccione MC, Trio O, Zito C, Monaco M, Carerj S. Isolated double orifice mitral valve in a young asymptomatic woman. J Cardiovasc Med. 2015.
18. Espinola-Zavaleta N, Vargas-Barron J, Keirns C, et al. Three-dimensional echocardiography in congenital malformations of the mitral valve. J Am Soc Echocardiogr. 2002;15:468–72.
19. Valverde I, Rawlins D, Austin C, Simpson JM. Three-dimensional echocardiography in the management of parachute mitral valve. Eur Heart J Cardiovasc Imaging. 2012;13:446.
20. Sew D, Kostolny M, Carr M, Cook AC, Marek J. Complex left atrial cor triatriatum associated with supravalvar mitral membrane, coronary sinus defect and persistent left superior caval vein. 3D echocardiography navigates surgeon to successful repair. Int J Cardiol. 2014;173:e58–62.
21. Jone PN, Bremen C, DiMaria M, et al. Three-dimensional echocardiography enhances diagnostic accuracy of supramitral ring. Echocardiography. 2015;32:1048–50.
22. Takahashi K, Mackie AS, Rebeyka IM, et al. Two-dimensional versus transthoracic real-time three-dimensional echocardiography in the evaluation of the mechanisms and sites of atrioventricular valve regurgitation in a congenital heart disease population. J Am Soc Echocardiogr. 2010;23:726–34.
23. Little SH, Pirat B, Kumar R, et al. Three-dimensional color Doppler echocardiography for direct measurement of vena contracta area in mitral regurgitation: in vitro validation and clinical experience. JACC Cardiovasc Imaging. 2008;1:695–704.

24. Marsan NA, Westenberg JJ, Ypenburg C, et al. Quantification of functional mitral regurgitation by real-time 3D echocardiography: comparison with 3D velocity-encoded cardiac magnetic resonance. JACC Cardiovasc Imaging. 2009;2:1245–52.
25. Zeng X, Levine RA, Hua L, et al. Diagnostic value of vena contracta area in the quantification of mitral regurgitation severity by color Doppler 3D echocardiography. Circ Cardiovasc Imaging. 2011;4:506–13.
26. Takahashi K, Mackie AS, Thompson R, et al. Quantitative real-time three-dimensional echocardiography provides new insight into the mechanisms of mitral valve regurgitation post-repair of atrioventricular septal defect. J Am Soc Echocardiogr. 2012;25:1231–44.
27. Takahashi K, Guerra V, Roman KS, Nii M, Redington A, Smallhorn JF. Three-dimensional echocardiography improves the understanding of the mechanisms and site of left atrioventricular valve regurgitation in atrioventricular septal defect. J Am Soc Echocardiogr. 2006;19:1502–10.
28. Bharucha T, Sivaprakasam MC, Haw MP, Anderson RH, Vettukattil JJ. The angle of the components of the common atrioventricular valve predicts the outcome of surgical correction in patients with atrioventricular septal defect and common atrioventricular junction. J Am Soc Echocardiogr. 2008;21:1099–104.
29. Hlavacek AM, Crawford Jr FA, Chessa KS, Shirali GS. Real-time three-dimensional echocardiography is useful in the evaluation of patients with atrioventricular septal defects. Echocardiography. 2006;23:225–31.
30. Barrea C, Levasseur S, Roman K, et al. Three-dimensional echocardiography improves the understanding of left atrioventricular valve morphology and function in atrioventricular septal defects undergoing patch augmentation. J Thorac Cardiovasc Surg. 2005;129:746–53.
31. Colen TM, Khoo NS, Ross DB, Smallhorn JF. Partial zone of apposition closure in atrioventricular septal defect: are papillary muscles the clue. Ann Thorac Surg. 2013;96:637–43.
32. Patel V, Nanda NC, Rajdev S, et al. Live/real time three-dimensional transthoracic echocardiographic assessment of Ebstein's anomaly. Echocardiography. 2005;22:847–54.
33. Vettukattil JJ, Bharucha T, Anderson RH. Defining Ebstein's malformation using three-dimensional echocardiography. Interact Cardiovasc Thorac Surg. 2007;6:685–90.
34. Bharucha T, Anderson RH, Lim ZS, Vettukattil JJ. Multiplanar review of three-dimensional echocardiography gives new insights into the morphology of Ebstein's malformation. Cardiol Young. 2010;20:49–53.
35. Kutty S, Colen T, Thompson RB, et al. Tricuspid regurgitation in hypoplastic left heart syndrome: mechanistic insights from 3-dimensional echocardiography and relationship with outcomes. Circ Cardiovasc Imaging. 2014;7:765–72.
36. Velayudhan DE, Brown TM, Nanda NC, et al. Quantification of tricuspid regurgitation by live three-dimensional transthoracic echocardiographic measurements of vena contracta area. Echocardiography. 2006;23:793–800.
37. Silvestry FE, Cohen MS, Armsby LB, et al. Guidelines for the echocardiographic assessment of atrial septal defect and patent foramen ovale: from the American Society of Echocardiography and Society for Cardiac Angiography and Interventions. J Am Soc Echocardiogr. 2015;28:910–58.
38. Pushparajah K, Miller OI, Simpson JM. 3D echocardiography of the atrial septum: anatomical features and landmarks for the echocardiographer. JACC Cardiovasc Imaging. 2010;3:981–4.
39. Roberson DA, Cui W, Patel D, et al. Three-dimensional transesophageal echocardiography of atrial septal defect: a qualitative and quantitative anatomic study. J Am Soc Echocardiogr. 2011;24:600–10.
40. Mehmood F, Vengala S, Nanda NC, et al. Usefulness of live three-dimensional transthoracic echocardiography in the characterization of atrial septal defects in adults. Echocardiography. 2004;21:707–13.
41. Acar P, Dulac Y, Aggoun Y. Images in congenital heart disease. Atrial septal defect within the oval fossa with enlarged coronary sinus: three-dimensional echocardiography. Cardiol Young. 2002;12:560.

42. van den Bosch AE, Ten Harkel DJ, McGhie JS, et al. Characterization of atrial septal defect assessed by real-time 3-dimensional echocardiography. J Am Soc Echocardiogr. 2006;19:815–21.
43. Taniguchi M, Akagi T, Watanabe N, et al. Application of real-time three-dimensional transesophageal echocardiography using a matrix array probe for transcatheter closure of atrial septal defect. J Am Soc Echocardiogr. 2009;22:1114–20.
44. Seo JS, Song JM, Kim YH, et al. Effect of atrial septal defect shape evaluated using three-dimensional transesophageal echocardiography on size measurements for percutaneous closure. J Am Soc Echocardiogr. 2012;25:1031–40.
45. Taniguchi M, Akagi T, Kijima Y, Sano S. Clinical advantage of real-time three-dimensional transesophageal echocardiography for transcatheter closure of multiple atrial septal defects. Int J Cardiovasc Imaging. 2013;29:1273–80.
46. Lodato JA, Cao QL, Weinert L, et al. Feasibility of real-time three-dimensional transoesophageal echocardiography for guidance of percutaneous atrial septal defect closure. Eur J Echocardiogr. 2009;10:543–8.
47. Hascoet S, Hadeed K, Marchal P, et al. The relation between atrial septal defect shape, diameter, and area using three-dimensional transoesophageal echocardiography and balloon sizing during percutaneous closure in children. Eur Heart J Cardiovasc Imaging. 2015;16:747–55.
48. Charakida M, Pushparajah K, Anderson D, Simpson JM. Insights gained from three-dimensional imaging modalities for closure of ventricular septal defects. Circ Cardiovasc Imaging. 2014;7:954–61.
49. Chen FL, Hsiung MC, Nanda N, Hsieh KS, Chou MC. Real time three-dimensional echocardiography in assessing ventricular septal defects: an echocardiographic-surgical correlative study. Echocardiography. 2006;23:562–8.
50. Cheng TO, Xie MX, Wang XF, Wang Y, Lu Q. Real-time 3-dimensional echocardiography in assessing atrial and ventricular septal defects: an echocardiographic-surgical correlative study. Am Heart J. 2004;148:1091–5.
51. Mercer-Rosa L, Seliem MA, Fedec A, Rome J, Rychik J, Gaynor JW. Illustration of the additional value of real-time 3-dimensional echocardiography to conventional transthoracic and transesophageal 2-dimensional echocardiography in imaging muscular ventricular septal defects: does this have any impact on individual patient treatment? J Am Soc Echocardiogr. 2006;19:1511–9.
52. Mehmood F, Miller AP, Nanda NC, et al. Usefulness of live/real time three-dimensional transthoracic echocardiography in the characterization of ventricular septal defects in adults. Echocardiography. 2006;23:421–7.
53. Charakida M, Qureshi S, Simpson JM. 3D echocardiography for planning and guidance of interventional closure of VSD. JACC Cardiovasc Imaging. 2013;6:120–3.
54. Capoulade R, Pibarot P. Assessment of aortic valve disease: role of imaging modalities. Curr Treat Options Cardiovasc Med. 2015;17:49.
55. Hahn RT. Guidance of transcatheter aortic valve replacement by echocardiography. Curr Cardiol Rep. 2014;16:442.
56. Hadeed K, Hascoet S, Amadieu R, et al. 3D transthoracic echocardiography to assess pulmonary valve morphology and annulus size in patients with Tetralogy of Fallot. Arch Cardiovasc Dis. 2016;109:87–95.
57. Villafane J, Feinstein JA, Jenkins KJ, et al. Hot topics in tetralogy of Fallot. J Am Coll Cardiol. 2013;62:2155–66.
58. Valente AM, Cook S, Festa P, et al. Multimodality imaging guidelines for patients with repaired tetralogy of fallot: a report from the AmericanSsociety of Echocardiography: developed in collaboration with the Society for Cardiovascular Magnetic Resonance and the Society for Pediatric Radiology. J Am Soc Echocardiogr. 2014;27:111–41.
59. Khoo NS, Young A, Occleshaw C, Cowan B, Zeng IS, Gentles TL. Assessments of right ventricular volume and function using three-dimensional echocardiography in older children and

adults with congenital heart disease: comparison with cardiac magnetic resonance imaging. J Am Soc Echocardiogr. 2009;22:1279–88.

60. Grewal J, Majdalany D, Syed I, Pellikka P, Warnes CA. Three-dimensional echocardiographic assessment of right ventricular volume and function in adult patients with congenital heart disease: comparison with magnetic resonance imaging. J Am Soc Echocardiogr. 2010;23:127–33.

61. Dragulescu A, Grosse-Wortmann L, Fackoury C, Mertens L. Echocardiographic assessment of right ventricular volumes: a comparison of different techniques in children after surgical repair of tetralogy of Fallot. Eur Heart J Cardiovasc Imaging. 2012;13:596–604.

62. Dragulescu A, Grosse-Wortmann L, Fackoury C, et al. Echocardiographic assessment of right ventricular volumes after surgical repair of tetralogy of Fallot: clinical validation of a new echocardiographic method. J Am Soc Echocardiogr. 2011;24:1191–8.

63. Colen T, Smallhorn JF. Three-dimensional echocardiography for the assessment of atrioventricular valves in congenital heart disease: past, present and future. Semin Thorac Cardiovasc Surg Pediatr Card Surg Annu. 2015;18:62–71.

64. Cikes M, Tong L, Sutherland GR, D'Hooge J. Ultrafast cardiac ultrasound imaging: technical principles, applications, and clinical benefits. JACC Cardiovasc Imaging. 2014;7:812–23.

65. Samuel BP, Pinto C, Pietila T, Vettukattil JJ. Ultrasound-derived three-dimensional printing in congenital heart disease. J Digit Imaging. 2015;28:459–61.

66. Xue H, Sun K, Yu J, et al. Three-dimensional echocardiographic virtual endoscopy for the diagnosis of congenital heart disease in children. Int J Cardiovasc Imaging. 2010;26:851–9.

67. Kurup HK, Samuel BP, Vettukattil JJ. Hybrid 3D printing: a game-changer in personalized cardiac medicine? Expert Rev Cardiovasc Ther. 2015;13:1281–4.

68. Suematsu Y, Martinez JF, Wolf BK, et al. Three-dimensional echo-guided beating heart surgery without cardiopulmonary bypass: atrial septal defect closure in a swine model. J Thorac Cardiovasc Surg. 2005;130:1348–57.

69. Vasilyev NV, Martinez JF, Freudenthal FP, Suematsu Y, Marx GR, del Nido PJ. Three-dimensional echo and videocardioscopy-guided atrial septal defect closure. Ann Thorac Surg. 2006;82:1322–6. discussion 1326

# Index




© Springer International Publishing AG 2017
E. Casas Rojo et al. (eds.), *Manual of 3D Echocardiography*,
DOI 10.1007/978-3-319-50335-6